Child Maltreatment

Contemporary Issues in Research and Policy

Volume 5

Series editors
Jill E. Korbin, Ph.D., Professor of Anthropology, Associate Dean, College of
Arts and Sciences, Director, Schubert Center for Child Studies, Crawford Hall,
7th Floor, 10900 Euclid Avenue, Cleveland, OH 44106-7068, USA
jill.korbin@case.edu

Richard D. Krugman, MD, Distinguished Professor of Pediatrics and Dean,
University of Colorado School of Medicine, Room C-1003 Bldg 500,
Anschutz Medical Campus, 13001 E. 17th Place, Aurora, CO 80045, USA
richard.krugman@ucdenver.edu

This series provides a high-quality, cutting edge, and comprehensive source offering the current best knowledge on child maltreatment from multidisciplinary and multicultural perspectives. It consists of a core handbook that is followed by two or three edited volumes of original contributions per year. The core handbook will present a comprehensive view of the field. Each chapter will summarize current knowledge and suggest future directions in a specific area. It will also highlight controversial and contested issues in that area, thus moving the field forward. The handbook will be updated every five years. The edited volumes will focus on critical issues in the field from basic biology and neuroscience to practice and policy. Both the handbook and edited volumes will involve creative thinking about moving the field forward and will not be a recitation of past research. Both will also take multidisciplinary, multicultural and mixed methods approaches.

More information about this series at http://www.springer.com/series/8863

Deborah Daro • Anne Cohn Donnelly
Lee Ann Huang • Byron J. Powell
Editors

Advances in Child Abuse Prevention Knowledge

The Perspective of New Leadership

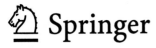
Springer

Editors
Deborah Daro
Chapin Hall
University of Chicago
Chicago, IL, USA

Lee Ann Huang
Chapin Hall
University of Chicago
Chicago, IL, USA

Anne Cohn Donnelly
Northwestern University
Evanston, IL, USA

Byron J. Powell
Center for Mental Health Policy
   and Services Research
Department of Psychiatry
Perelman School of Medicine
University of Pennsylvania
Philadelphia, PA, USA

ISSN 2211-9701   ISSN 2211-971X (electronic)
Child Maltreatment
ISBN 978-3-319-16326-0   ISBN 978-3-319-16327-7 (eBook)
DOI 10.1007/978-3-319-16327-7

Library of Congress Control Number: 2015938162

Springer Cham Heidelberg New York Dordrecht London

Printed on acid-free paper

Springer International Publishing AG Switzerland is part of Springer Science+Business Media (www.springer.com)

Preface

This outstanding volume, *Advances in Child Abuse Prevention Knowledge: The Perspective of New Leadership*, is important in several key ways to the future of the related fields of child maltreatment research and practice. Most importantly, it is primarily authored by the participants in the *Doris Duke Fellowships for the Promotion of Child Well-Being* initiative, who are poised to lead the joint fields in the future. The Doris Duke fellows have together tackled core challenges to the joint fields in thoughtful and knowledgeable ways. The chosen format, with teams of Doris Duke fellows coauthoring chapters, represents the future of child maltreatment research and practice: engaging the team approach to enhance learning and effectiveness, an approach most likely to produce the best outcomes for this multi-disciplinary, systemic field. Embracing both research and practice is a noteworthy focus of the Doris Duke Fellowship program, increasing the likelihood that both will be more rigorous, relevant, and impactful as a result. The structure of the fellows program and the volume are most impressive!

While I have not been a researcher in this specific field, I chaired both the initial National Research Council study more than 20 years ago, *Understanding Child Abuse and Neglect* (National Research Council 1993) and the recent one, *New Directions in Child Abuse and Neglect Research* (Institute of Medicine/National Research Council 2014). Apparently the primary criterion for chairing the study was to be in a related field of research—in my case, developmental science—but not centrally involved in studying child maltreatment. (I did add measures on the experience of child maltreatment to my longitudinal study in the field following the first National Research Council report, but I could not report on them because of state laws regarding mandatory reporting of any evidence on child maltreatment.) With the first study, I agreed to participate because of the importance of the problem for children, their families, and society; while the field of child maltreatment research was at a much earlier stage in terms of the knowledge base, I believe that the initial report was able to identify ways for a field to come together around key questions. With the second study, I was motivated by exciting advances in knowledge over the intervening 20 years, emerging from the 20-fold increase in publications on the topic, creating a new science of child abuse and neglect. The Institute of Medicine study was again importantly sponsored by the Federal Administration on Children and Families (and specifically the Children's Bureau).

The key findings of this most recent report include centrally that child abuse and neglect produces problems not only in childhood but throughout the life course, with cascading effects on all areas of individual functioning as well as affecting families and communities, with an estimated annual cost to a society of $80.3 billion. The effects of child maltreatment have now been documented not only in behavior but also in underlying genetic changes as well as brain consequences, making clear how the effects become pervasive and perhaps explaining intergenerational transmission processes. Significant research progress has also been made with preventive and treatment efforts, something the Institute of Medicine volume explores in several chapters. Given the documentation of dire, lifelong, and systemic consequences, the studies documenting positive results of treatment and, especially, prevention give us hope for a better future for reducing child maltreatment and its effects, especially when a more systemic approach is taken. At the same time, there remains much to be learned from future research, increasing the importance of leaders such as the Doris Duke fellows.

The Doris Duke fellows volume builds upon the recent Institute of Medicine report in important ways. In addition, it implements one of the key recommendations: to develop new leadership for the field. With only a single smaller research agency and similarly smaller scientific/professional societies guiding the field, it is even more important that there be key leadership groups working with them and others to form a collective vision for the field. The volume makes clear that the Doris Duke fellows are prepared to take leadership roles, something that they have already begun on many fronts.

Advances in Child Abuse Prevention Knowledge tackles several key problems in the field and generally takes highly innovative approaches. For example, the volume places understanding of the field in the context of related fields of work: developmental science, trauma and other forms of risk and challenge to growing individuals, prevention and treatment more generally, and sociocultural underpinnings of all work with human groups. Indeed, the fact that the systemic approach—indeed, the multisystem approach—is required for effective understanding of any change efforts underlies all of the thinking in the volume. Such complex conceptualization is only possible, in my view, when teams have diverse experience and knowledge. At the same time, the fellows realize the importance of creating opportunities for innovation and identifying opportunities for learning and implementation. Advancing the fields of research and practice will require this thoughtful combination of systematic work together with capitalizing on opportunities such as natural experiments and policy changes.

The volume includes some surprises, such as the chapter on adolescence. My research has focused largely on that age period and yet I had never reflected on the underreporting in official records of child maltreatment among this group relative to the voluminous body of work identifying the pervasive experience of maltreatment reported by adolescents themselves. The linkage between child maltreatment and adolescent pregnancy alone is an important contribution that I hope will receive further attention. The chapters identifying improvements to current practice also represented fresh new ideas to me that I hope will lead to much follow-up work.

Some of the chapters discuss biobehavioral maltreatment research that I believe will clarify many current questions and provide greater specificity needed for effective practice. Recent human evidence amplifies animal research from the past decade demonstrating that behavior affects biology and that understanding the biological consequences of trauma such as child maltreatment will help us target key processes for intervention. For example, recent human research from several laboratories shows the effects of trauma (such as child abuse) on genes (through epigenetic processes) and on brain structure and function.

This recent generation of research also involves some novel and important research collaborations of key biological researchers partnering with leading child abuse prevention researchers as well as child maltreatment researchers with important longitudinal samples. Biological researchers have identified child maltreatment not only as an important societal problem to be addressed but also as a key target for testing hypotheses about underlying mechanisms. For example, this newer research begins to explain "resilience," or why not all children experiencing similar exposure durations and forms of child maltreatment show the same behavioral outcomes. Indeed, a large body of research on differential sensitivity has demonstrated that various kinds of behavioral experiences have better or worse outcomes depending on genetic status.

Further, intergenerational transmission of child maltreatment is now being studied in multigenerational epigenetic studies of sexual abuse. All this recent activity demonstrates that researchers of diverse backgrounds see the importance of child maltreatment as a social and health problem. And despite the complexity and challenges of the field, significant advances in definition, research, and treatment of child maltreatment make it a better example for studying basic processes of stress, violence, and trauma.

This volume and the Doris Duke fellows' role as leaders in child maltreatment research and practice give me great hope for the future of these joint fields. The strategic framing of the fellowship program is reflected in the volume and demonstrates the knowledge, creativity, and effectiveness of these emerging scholars. The field is enriched and advanced by their contributions in the volume and may be transformed by them. The novel collaborations demonstrated through the writing of chapters in the volume are also effective as research collaborations—both basic and intervention research collaborations. I have full confidence that these Doris Duke fellows will seek out and be pursued for many novel collaborations in their careers and will thereby lead the field to important new discoveries in research and practice. Thanks to the Doris Duke Charitable Foundation and the leaders of this important program for creating an effective and strategic training opportunity. This program is a gift to knowledge development as well as an effective approach to improve humanity.

University of Michigan   Anne Peterson
Ann Arbor, MI, USA

Acknowledgments

An underlying premise of this edited volume is the power of collective discourse in improving our ability to understand complex issues and to generate new, innovative solutions. Just as the Doris Duke fellows have collaborated in crafting their respective chapters, we, as editors, have benefited from each other's perspectives and the support of our colleagues. We are deeply appreciative of the Doris Duke Charitable Foundation for their initial and continued support of the fellowship. The vision and commitment of our initial Project Officer, Mary Bassett, and our current Project Officer, Lola Adedokun, have created a dynamic program where individual fellows are encouraged to both learn from and teach each other. Chapin Hall is honored to be part of this effort and for the opportunity it provides us to contribute to building a new generation of scholars committed to using research to promote more effective policy and practice.

As noted in several chapters, the research reported on in these pages also reflects the investments of multiple funders. Building a truly generative and innovative field requires not only new leadership but also continuous investment by an array of funders from both the public and private sectors.

This project has benefited directly from the efforts of many individuals including Jill Korbin who, as a member of the fellowship advisory board, initially suggested this project as a unique learning opportunity for the fellows. We are very grateful to Jill and Richard Krugman, the coeditors of the Springer Child Maltreatment series, for allowing this project to be part of their ongoing efforts to summarize and promote new learning around the difficult issues facing the child maltreatment field. We are also grateful to the eight "veterans" in the field who shared their insights on how the field has changed over time. The reflections provided by Todd Herrenkohl, James Garbarino, Cathy Spatz Widom, Ellen Penderhughes, Lisabth Schorr, Larry Palinkas, Lucy Berliner and Bryan Samuels remind us all that moving forward requires careful attention to what has been tried and learned in the past.

Finally, we would like to extend a special thanks to Matthew Brenner, member of Chapin Hall's public affairs staff, for his yeoman effort in copy editing all the chapters and insuring consistency in style and structure. We would not have been able to complete this project without his assistance.

Contents

Introduction

Improving efforts to prevent child abuse and neglect requires continuous and critical assessment of what we believe we know and how best to create and use new learning. From the onset, efforts to prevent child maltreatment have been defined by a dual emphasis on practice and research. This reflects work of early pioneers such as Henry Kempe, Vincent DeFrancis, Brandt Steele, and Elizabeth Elmer, who drew on their dual roles as skilled practitioners and researchers. Reflecting this foundational base, investments in basic and applied research on child abuse and neglect for the past 50 years have been informed by a continuous interplay between research and practice (Daro 2009; Daro and Cohn Donnelly 2002). Initial questions regarding the underlying causes and incidence of child maltreatment and its impacts on child health and development have given way to more nuanced questions regarding these issues as well as rigorous research on the impacts of various treatment and preventive interventions. Our understanding of the problem has deepened and our capacity to respond is encouraging, a conclusion reflected in a recent report on the state of the field issued by the Institute of Medicine/National Research Council, *New Directions in Child Abuse and Neglect Research* (IOM/NRC 2014). New scientific methods, particularly in the area of neurobiological science, have underscored the complexity of the problem, its differential impacts across populations and contexts, and the challenge in replicating and sustaining effective interventions. While progress has been impressive, significant gaps remain in our understanding of child maltreatment and how best to respond.

As the field moves into its next 50 years, new research methods and standards of evidence are emerging. The traditional scientific process of small clinical research efforts is being expanded to include more diverse ways of learning. Increasingly, rigorous research designs incorporate statistical methods that model randomized conditions, draw on administrative data systems to track population-level changes, and conduct detailed implementation studies which provide practitioners and participants with immediate feedback on a program's efficacy.

In addition to utilizing advanced methodologies, this next wave of research will be conducted by a new generation of diverse scholars, many of whom are just now entering the field. These emerging scholars, while informed by what has gone on in the past, will bring their own perspectives to the issue, apply different statistical methods in addressing their core research questions, and access a range of innovative technologies. They are able to obtain and share critical information on program performance in a more time sensitive and accurate manner. Social networking systems and Internet access also make it easier for scholars to review information from both the peer review and policy domains and to communicate with their colleagues from different institutions and disciplines. Such linkages create a rich context for generating policy- and practice-relevant research questions that will guide the field in potentially new directions.

The purpose of this book is to examine current research gaps and new learning opportunities through the eyes of these emerging scholars. Specifically, the book examines how these researchers are using new frameworks to shape their work, apply their findings, and define their learning communities. The primary chapter authors are individuals who are enrolled in or have recently completed their doctoral studies in a variety of disciplines. They have worked together as part of the *Doris Duke Fellowships for the Promotion of Child Well-Being—seeking innovations to prevent child abuse*. The fellowship is funded by the Doris Duke Charitable Foundation and administered by Chapin Hall at the University of Chicago. Established in 2010, the fellowship identifies promising doctoral students from diverse disciplines and works with them over a 2-year period to deepen their understanding of the child maltreatment problem, foster an interdisciplinary learning community that creates synergies across their individual work, and improve their capacity to apply research and empirical methods to the field's policy and practice decisions. The fellowship's ultimate goal is to contribute to a new generation of leaders capable of and interested in guiding the field's response to the inevitable changes that occur in families and the contexts in which they live. Through a robust self-generating learning network and the continued support of both academic and policy mentors, fellows mirror the dual commitment to research rigor and policy and practice relevance that reflect the field's foundational base. Collectively, these conditions create a unique and important opportunity to model the type of learning environment needed to successfully address the opportunities and challenges facing those working in the social sciences today. This book creates an important vehicle to showcase the individual contributions of these emerging scholars as well as the power of collective effort.

Chapter Content

The fellows address two broad sets of issues in their chapters—issues involving the nature of the problem and issues involving the nature of the response. Under the first topic, fellows examine the current context and continued research challenges for addressing how we define the problem, understand its etiology and differential developmental impacts, and understand its interface with the issue of culture. In considering how best to respond, the fellows address growing concern within the practice and policy communities regarding how best to identify, replicate, and sustain high quality interventions as well as the relative merits of adopting a protective factors framework for guiding our overall response. Each chapter also includes a short essay authored by an established scholar in the field commenting on how knowledge (or lack of knowledge) in a specific area has influenced their own research or practice over the years and shaped their current thinking.

Prior to the content chapters, book editors Deborah Daro and Anne Cohn Donnelly provide an historical overview of the child maltreatment field and outline the role a new generation of scholars might play in balancing this historical evolution with their own conceptualizations of the problem and research priorities. After briefly reviewing this historical context, they present some of the salient challenges that continue to plague the field and the barriers that exist in supporting sustained progress. The chapter also examines strategies for identifying and training a new generation of scholars to address this issue, drawing on the experiences of the fellows participating in the *Doris Duke Fellowships for the Promotion of Child-Well Being*.

In Chap. 2, Duke Fellows Amanda Van Scoyoc, Jessica S. Wilen, Kate Daderko, and Sheridan Miyamoto challenge the perception of maltreatment subpopulations, noting that 33–94 % of children involved in the child welfare system experience multiple types of abuse and neglect. In addition, abuse and neglect often co-occur with other early stressful experiences such as chronic poverty, maternal substance abuse, and domestic violence, making it difficult to discern the unique effects of maltreatment on a child's developmental trajectory. The chapter highlights the programmatic and policy implications of addressing child maltreatment as a set of unique subpopulations versus viewing the problem as part of a broader and highly complex social dilemma. The authors outline a research agenda that adopts a person-centered approach to understanding maltreatment's impact and discuss how administrative data systems can be altered to document the problem at a level commensurate with its complexity. Todd Herrenkohl, professor at the University of Washington School of Social Work, authored the essay on this topic.

In Chap. 3, Carly B. Dierkhising, Jennifer Mullins Geiger, Tamara E. Hurst, Carlomagno Panlilio, and Lisa Schelbe address the unique issues surrounding the identification and response to maltreated adolescents. Although population-based studies suggest adolescents experience similar or higher rates of maltreatment as young children, they are less likely to be formally reported for maltreatment. Lower reporting rates may reflect a prevailing notion that adolescents are better able to protect themselves from abusive caretakers and, if necessary, leave abusive homes. Challenging this perception, the chapter explores the incidence rates among adolescents and the underlying causal connections between maltreatment and subsequent involvement in the juvenile justice system and, in some cases, commercial sexual exploitation. The authors call for more consistent documentation and public recognition of adolescent maltreatment and its consequences on adolescent development. Equally important is developing common protocols for identifying and addressing the needs of abused adolescents involved in the child welfare and juvenile justice systems as well as those youth being sexually exploited. James Garbarino, professor and Maude C. Clarke Chair in humanistic psychology at Loyola University Chicago, authored the essay on this topic.

Jennifer Mullins Geiger, Lisa Schelbe, Megan J. Hayes, Elisa Kawam, Colleen Cary Katz, and J. Bart Klika address the intergenerational transmission of maltreatment in Chap. 4. While it is commonly assumed that individuals with a history of child maltreatment may be at an increased risk of maltreating their own children, this process is poorly understood and far from self-evident. The authors' review of current research suggests that intergenerational transmission of child abuse is most likely among those individuals maltreated as children who also experience other adversities such as intimate partner violence, child welfare involvement, aging out of foster care, families with limited social support, or psychological distress due to traumatic experiences. Further, research suggests that safe, stable, and nurturing relationships and environments can reduce the occurrence of child maltreatment and may be a useful framework in understanding those who break this cycle of violence. In response to the problem, the authors suggest expanded use of innovative evidence-based, trauma-informed methods of practice with specific high-risk groups, such as foster care youth and those experiencing interpersonal violence and poverty. The authors explain how employing these methods and improving the use of more sophisticated administrative data systems to track the immediate and distal outcomes of children in the child welfare system will provided a more comprehensive and holistic examination of risk and resiliency. Cathy Spatz Widom, distinguished professor of psychology at John Jay College, authored the essay on this topic.

In Chap. 5, Megan Finno-Velasquez, Elizabeth A. Shuey, Chie Kotake, and J. Jay Miller tackle cultural considerations in refining intervention designs. Culture is often defined monolithically, using physically evident characteristics like race and ethnicity. However, the authors view culture as a fluid construct that is formulated by the assimilation of cultural tools across successive generations and a family's individual needs, experiences with, and interpretations of these tools. As such, the role of culture in parenting and child maltreatment may be best understood when examined through an interdisciplinary, multidimensional lens and through its intersection with race and ethnicity, social stratification, ecological context, and individual family experiences. The authors discuss approaches for applying this expanded framework in determining appropriate interventions and professional development strategies. The authors also call for greater integration between those examining family characteristics and ecological contexts and those exploring cultural values and beliefs. Ellen Pinderhughes, associate professor of child development at Tufts University, authored the essay on this topic.

Chapter 6 authors Paul Lanier, Kathryn Maguire-Jack, Joseph Mienko, and Carlomagno Panlilio address what we know about determining if, how, and when prevention can work. To be successful in practice with families and to gain support for further dissemination, the authors suggest maltreatment prevention interventions must accomplish two goals: develop and implement a logic model informed by theory that targets known causes of child maltreatment and demonstrate evidence of program effectiveness with rigorous methodological designs that isolate program effects. To that end, the chapter begins with a discussion of how theories on mal-treatment etiology inform logic models for existing prevention programs ("causes of known effects") and then outlines a range of statistical methods for inferring causality in observational studies ("effects of known causes"). While the authors agree on the importance of program evaluations using random assignment to fully understand program impacts, they also suggest program evaluators should not limit their designs to regression-based analyses. Strong alternative designs, including propensity score analysis, instrumental variables, regression discontinuity, and directed acyclic graphs, should be explored. Lisbeth Schorr, senior fellow at the Center for the Study of Social Policy and founding cochair of the Aspen Institute's Roundtable on Community Change, authored the essay on this topic.

In Chap. 7, authors Byron J. Powell, Emily A. Bosk, Jessica S. Wilen, Christina M. Danko, Amanda Van Scoyoc, and Aaron Banman address the challenge of successfully integrating evidence-based programs into standard agency practice. Evidence-based programs and practices pertinent to the prevention and treatment of child abuse and neglect remain underutilized in community settings. Drawing on the emerging field of implementation science, the authors review the extant research and offer innovative examples that demonstrate how implementation science and practice can contribute to the promotion of child well-being. Specifically, they discuss research that can inform both early (exploration, adoption decision/preparation) and later stages (active implementation and sustainment) of implementation. After highlighting a number of contextual factors that influence the implementation processes, the authors present eight areas critical to advancing the science and practice of implementation, and ultimately, the well-being of children and families. Lawrence Palinkas, Albert G., and Frances Lomas Feldman, Professor of Social Policy and Health at the University of Southern California, authored the essay on this topic.

In Chap. 8, Kristen D. Seay, Kaela Byers, Megan Feely, Paul Lanier, Kathryn Maguire-Jack, and Tia McGill address the problem of scaling up promising interventions with fidelity. To retain the strong and important effects of any tested program, interventions need to maintain model fidelity at the individual and organizational level and faithfully replicate the content and process of the intervention's delivery system. Most agree on the importance of accurate and consistent replication. However, achieving a high level of fidelity and measuring the degree to which an evidence-based replication effort meets model standards is a challenging and complex undertaking. This chapter provides an overview of how monitoring program fidelity has been addressed in the child welfare system and assesses the current status of such efforts, detailing the development and use of fidelity monitoring systems within the context of two model interventions. Drawing on these examples, the chapter identifies the major questions and options facing practitioners, administrators, policymakers, and researchers as promising interventions are scaled up. Lucy Berliner, director of the Harborview Center for Sexual Assault and Traumatic Stress, University of Washington, authored the essay on this topic.

Chapter 9, by Tova B. Walsh, Sandra Nay McCourt, Whitney L. Rostad, Kaela Byers, and Kerrie Ocasio, addresses the opportunities presented by shifting the policy and practice perspective from risk avoidance to promoting protective factors and resilience. Increasingly, program planners and policymakers are incorporating this perspective in developing institutional policy and intervention focus. The chapter examines the development and implications of this paradigm shift within the context of child abuse prevention. The chapter includes several examples of innovative programming and research efforts that specifically focus on strengthening families by promoting protective factors and enhancing resilience. The authors conclude with a discussion of how a protective factors framework might be taken to scale and the research and policy initiatives currently underway that might inform this scale-up process. Bryan Samuels, executive director of Chapin Hall at the University of Chicago, authored the essay on this topic.

In the final chapter, Chap. 10, book editors Deborah Daro, Anne Cohn Donnelly, Lee Ann Huang, and Byron J. Powell summarize the key themes that emerge across the book from the perspective of understanding the issue and developing a more effective policy and practice response. While noting extraordinary progress on all these issues, the chapter underscores a number of areas in need of additional research. The chapter also addresses emerging strategies for building bridges and establishing common objectives with the potential for strengthening the linkages between those focused on treating the problem and those focused on preventing it. Finally, the chapter addresses the types of professional development opportunities that will be required going forward to build a deep and interdisciplinary workforce capable of sustaining the diverse and generative context needed to foster continued learning.

Conclusion

The issues covered in this book are not the only challenges facing the field, nor are they necessarily the thorniest. However, they represent areas that underscore the importance of embracing both empirical and practice perspectives in insuring continued learning. Research findings are best understood and most likely to be used when they are linked to an array of policy and practice opportunities. As the chapter authors have noted, none of these dilemmas are cast in stone or immutable. Notable advances have been made in how we conceptualize child maltreatment, understand its causal pathways, and determine the focus and scope of our interventions and public policy response. In presenting their viewpoints on these challenging issues, these emerging scholars are using their perspectives and innovative research skills to shape how these issues will be defined and addressed in the future.

Part I
The Child Maltreatment Landscape

Chapter 1
Reflections on Child Maltreatment Research and Practice: Consistent Challenges

Deborah Daro and Anne Cohn Donnelly

Overview

Over the past 50 years, the combined efforts of academic researchers, practitioners, public agency officials, child welfare advocates, and private philanthropists have created a robust field of academic study and professional practice around the causes, consequences, and appropriate response to child abuse and neglect. There has long been an understanding in the child maltreatment field of the importance of multiple perspectives in both defining and confronting the problem. Over time, however, these multiple perspectives have fractured along a number of dimensions, including a growing gap between those focusing on remediating the effects of maltreatment and those concerned with preventing its occurrence.

As observed in the most recent report on child maltreatment issued by the Institute of Medicine/National Research Council, an emphasis on trauma and trauma-informed care now dominate the strategies used to treat child maltreatment victims and perpetrators (IOM and NRC 2014). For example, the National Child Traumatic Stress Network (NCTSN), established by Congress in 2000 as part of the Children's Health Act, has grown from a collaborative network of 17 centers to over 150 funded and affiliate centers located across the nation. The network offers training, support, and resources to providers who work with children and families exposed to a wide range of traumatic experiences, including physical and sexual abuse; domestic, school, and community violence; natural disasters, terrorism, or military family challenges; and life-threatening injury and illness (Full description of the network available at: www.nctsnet.org). Those engaged in designing and

D. Daro (✉)
Chapin Hall at the University of Chicago, Chicago, IL, USA
e-mail: ddaro@chapinhall.org

A.C. Donnelly
Kellogg School of Management, Northwestern University, Evanston, IL, USA
e-mail: Annecohndonnelly@gmail.com

© Springer International Publishing Switzerland 2015
D. Daro et al. (eds.), *Advances in Child Abuse Prevention Knowledge*,
Child Maltreatment 5, DOI 10.1007/978-3-319-16327-7_1

evaluating treatment services are more focused on outcomes than causes and have developed "modular approaches that address multiple clinical outcomes rather than a single presenting problem" (IOM and NRC 2014, p. 248). As a result, clinicians working with victims or perpetrators of child maltreatment increasingly have more in common with professionals working with victims of other adversities such as domestic violence, community violence, or sudden and repeated changes in caretakers due to illness or abandonment than they might with those providing more generalized support to potential victims of adversity or those focusing on normative changes to reduce the likelihood of child maltreatment.

Prevention advocates, in turn, are focusing their research and program efforts on early childhood, developing and advocating for expanded services to support women during pregnancy or families at the time their infants are born. The increased emphasis child abuse prevention advocates place on supporting newborns and their parents have created a constellation of outcomes that find them more often aligned with those promoting healthy child development and school readiness than with those treating maltreatment victims. In some instances, those engaged in preventing child abuse have altered their message and operating frameworks to place greater emphasis on the behavioral and normative changes they are seeking in families and within the social fabric, explicitly avoiding the mention of abuse and its impacts on children (Kirkpatrick 2004; Patel and Goodman 2007; Committee on the Prevention of Mental Disorders 2009). Most recently, the Centers for Disease Control (CDC) adopted the promotion of safe, stable, and nurturing relationships between children and caregivers as its primary strategy for preventing child maltreatment (Centers for Disease Control 2013).

Such changes in a problem's formulation are to be expected as the understanding of and response to it matures. Decades of research on maltreatment has created a growing appreciation of the importance of context both in shaping an individual's behavior as well as sustaining high quality interventions (Daro and Benedetti 2014; IOM and NRC 2014). While the development and provision of interventions to both respond to and prevent child maltreatment remain important policy objectives, the most effective solutions are increasingly ones that embrace an array of strategies targeting all levels of the ecological framework. Equally important is creating opportunities for public institutions, be they health, education, or child welfare agencies to pool their resources in creating approaches that are mutually reinforcing (Kania and Kramer 2011). Indeed, many of the chapters in this volume emphasize child maltreatment's complexity and its co-occurrence with other adverse conditions and call for a more integrated public policy and research response.

Such thinking, while consistent with our current theoretical and empirical understanding of child maltreatment, may result in a system that fails to appropriately identify, target, and serve all families. Until robust systems are in place to assess the needs of all families and direct them to appropriate level of assistance, families unable to negotiate the patch-work of family support programs currently in place in many communities across the county may fail to receive the support needed to prevent abuse or neglect (Daro and Benedetti 2014). And those reported to child protective services who, while challenged but yet engaged in abuse or neglect, may receive nothing more than an assessment as evidenced by the 80 % of cases that are unsubstantiated every year (U.S. Department of Health and Human Services 2013). Indeed, the challenge of having one systemic response for all child maltreatment reports contributed to the development of differential response systems within child welfare that work to balance the need to support at-risk families with the responsibility to protect maltreated children from further harm (Waldfogel 2009). Developing and sustaining a robust and diversified set of supports that successfully integrates treatment, prevention, and protective factor frameworks may best be achieved not by embedding maltreatment in an array of child adversities but rather by invigorating interest in child abuse and neglect as a unique social dilemma.

In short, we have a problem whose successful resolution requires careful attention to its unique features as well as to the context in which it occurs. The problem may go unresolved if it is not specifically recognized as presenting a unique set of risks that impact how children develop and families function. Creating the knowledge base necessary to confront this dilemma will require collaborative thinking across disciplines and professions, drawing on the experiences of both treatment and prevention service planners, practitioners, and researchers.

The next generation of scholars that address issues of child welfare and child well-being will be entering a field needing interdisciplinary thinking and clear pathways linking its treatment and prevention functions. As noted by President Emeritus of the Carnegie Foundation, Lee Shulman, an important balance in any pursuit of knowledge is finding the "sweet spot" between "earlier traditions and sources" of a problem "while encouraging strikingly new ideas and courageous leaps forward" (Walker et al. 2007).

Given the role research has played in shaping the trajectory and substance of the child maltreatment field, this chapter highlights a number of seemingly intractable research and practice challenges surrounding the definition of and response to this thorny child welfare dilemma. Drawing on the findings and recommendations from two federally commissioned studies, conducted 20 years apart, the chapter identifies areas in which progress has been made and the contextual issues that limit further progress. One of these contextual challenges, the need for more intentional training and support for those beginning their research careers, is addressed in the final section of the chapter. The *Doris Duke Fellowships for the Promotion of Child Well-Being* offers one example of how young scholars interested in child maltreatment as a topic of study might be identified and engaged in a collaborative and interdisciplinary effort to examine both the basic and applied research questions challenging the field.

Historical Framework

As noted in our earlier work, efforts to address child maltreatment have moved through various stages: public and professional awareness and education, the development of various programmatic and policy options to prevent its occurrence or mitigate its consequences, and the adoption of conceptual and systemic frameworks to integrate diverse strategies into a coherent response (Daro and Cohn-Donnelly 2002). While increased knowledge of the problem brought with it calls for a more complex response, the first response to child maltreatment, while far reaching in its effects, centered on a single strategy—the development of a child abuse reporting system.

Early Research and Policy Efforts

Although several medical articles had appeared as early as the 1940s, describing outcomes suggestive of maltreatment, Henry Kempe's 1962 article in the *Journal of the American Medical Association* on the "battered child syndrome" was central in galvanizing political support for this strategy (Kempe et al. 1962). Kempe's work, in contrast to others in the medical community examining this issue, explicitly sought to link his research to specific policy options (Daro 1988). Kempe's national surveys of hospital emergency room X-rays and criminal cases involving injury caused by a parent or primary caretaker presented the public with a picture difficult to ignore. Hundreds, if not thousands, of children suffered physical and emotional trauma each year as a result of overburdened parents or caregivers using extreme forms of corporal punishment. Another source of trauma was the unavoidable consequence of young mothers, often single and suffering from depression or depressive symptoms unable or unwilling to meet their child's basic needs. At the time, no system existed for linking these cases to services that would protect the child from further harm or address the needs of those who had harmed them.

Using these data, Kempe and other advocates worked with legislative leaders to establish a formal system for accepting and responding to suspected cases of maltreatment, which all states enacted in some form between 1963 and 1967 (Nelson 1984). The first Federal legislation explicitly addressing child maltreatment, the Child Abuse and Neglect Prevention and Treatment Act (Public Law 93-274), was authorized in 1974. Over the years, several scholars have noted that while multiple factors contributed to this legislative accomplishment, Kempe's data and the burgeoning body of clinical case studies and academic research regarding the problem, contributed to this rapid and widespread public policy (Daro 1988; Myers 2006).

Once states established child abuse and neglect reporting laws, the number of identified cases increased exponentially. Between 1976 and 1980, reports to child protective services nearly doubled, from 413,000 to 788,000 (American Humane Association 1981). By the time the first federally mandated child abuse and neglect incidence study was issued in 1981, 17.8 per 1,000 children were identified as being reported for abuse. Almost half of these cases were identified and reported by non-professionals such as family members, neighbors, and friends (National Center on Child Abuse and Neglect and U.S. Department of Health and Human Services 1981). In response to this increase, an array of treatment programs emerged, generally applying the therapeutic interventions common at the time, including individual, family, and group counseling as well as an emerging field of self-help groups lead by such models as Parents Anonymous (Cohn 1979). Although such interventions changed parental practices and improved the ability of families to receive treatment and support, over one-third of the participants in these programs continued to mistreat their children while enrolled (Daro and Cohn 1987). The limitations of these early treatment programs, coupled with a continued increase in child abuse reports and foster care caseloads, fueled the interest among professionals and community advocates to adopt a more intentional focus on child abuse prevention with efforts targeting, as noted by Ray Helfer, "all levels" of the ecological framework (Helfer 1982).

Indeed, the 1980s represented a period of significant expansion for prevention services. Across the country, public agencies and nonprofit organizations developed myriad interventions to improve parents' understanding of child development and how best to nurture their children; to teach more appropriate discipline and child behavior management strategies as alternatives to corporal punishment; and to facilitate access to additional clinical services or informal supports for parents under stress or facing significant challenges (Daro 1988). As noted in an initial review of child abuse prevention services compiled by the National Committee to Prevent Child Abuse, early child abuse prevention strategies included, among others, services to new parents, general parenting education classes, parent support groups, family resource centers, and crisis intervention services such as hotlines and crisis nurseries (Cohn 1983). While most of these efforts targeted families with some identified level of risk, parenting education resources and public awareness messages targeting the general population were frequently adopted during this period. In the case of child sexual abuse, prevention education efforts designed to inform children how to respond to unwanted sexual touching or conduct were universal. These teachings were embedded within existing child service systems such as public schools, youth service organizations, and, in the case of young children, child care and early education centers (Daro 1994).

During this period, prevention strategies were frequently adopted more for their style than substance and evidence of impact. The program evaluations conducted during this period were generally conceptually weak both in terms of design and measurement with the vast majority of these efforts based solely on changes observed among the participants enrolled in prevention services. Minimal attention was paid to such issues as selection bias, pre-existing conditions, and external factors that might have accounted for suggested program effects (National Research Council 1993). Families often accessed an intervention not because it was the best fit for their needs but rather because it was the sole option available. And what was available across communities was far from consistent, making it difficult for families to know where to look for assistance or understand what help they might expect to receive. Simply providing a greater array of parenting support options to families proved insufficient. The prevention continuum had done a good job in creating a market of services which offered parents able to negotiate these diverse options an array of alternatives. However, it was far less successful in creating a system that could attract and retain families facing the greatest challenges (Daro 1993). Reaching these families required not just more services but services that understood how a diverse array of chronic and acute circumstances might influence parents' perception of their children, their role as parents, and their willingness to change.

The Shift to Early Intervention and Evidence-Based Practice

Support for a broad plethora of child maltreatment prevention programs began to wane in the 1990s as a result of at least two trends: neurological research documenting the critical impacts of early care on a child's development and life trajectory and an emphasis in directing prevention dollars to programs with evidence of success. In the first instance, new advances in neuroscience emerged which provided vivid imagery of the impact early trauma and lack of adequate emotional care had on an infant's developing brain (Perry 1994). Translated for popular consumption by the Carnegie Foundation's "Starting Points" report (1994) and special issues of *Time* and *Newsweek*, these images proved as powerful in generating public interest in the issue as Kempe's initial profiles in the 1960s. In response to this research, the child abuse prevention field, as well as the broader early childhood community, placed particular emphasis on developing strategies for and directing public investment to those approaches that would strengthen parent-child attachment and create environments that would promote healthy development (Shonkoff and Phillips 2000).

Economists assessing the return on investment (ROI) from early intervention programs noted that for the same level of investment at each age, the return is higher in human capital when a dollar is spent on the young than when it is spent on the old. This occurs, in part, because you have longer to reap benefits but also because "learning begets learning" (Heckman 2000). Investments in programs that could better create more robust and positive learning environments for young children were increasingly viewed as good for children and good for the economy.

Equally important in shifting the prevention emphasis during this period was the growing body of evidence that high-quality early intervention programs could actually make a difference in a child's developmental trajectory. Longitudinal studies on early intervention efforts implemented in the 1960s and 1970s found marked improvements in educational outcomes and adult earnings among children exposed to high-quality early intervention programs (Campbell et al. 2002; McCormick et al. 2006; Reynolds et al. 2001; Schweinhart 2004; Seitz et al. 1985). Most relevant for the child maltreatment field, David Olds and his colleagues began publishing the results of a randomized clinical trial of a nurse home visiting program implemented in Elmira, New York. His research was among the first to document the impact of such services on a range of child and parent outcomes, including a reduction in child maltreatment reports (Olds et al. 1986). Subsequent follow-up studies on the original population as well as additional randomized trials in Memphis and Denver continued to support the efficacy of this approach (Olds et al. 1994; Kitzman et al. 1997).

Drawing on these data, as well as the state of Hawaii's success in conducting universal screenings of all newborns in the state for the purposes of identifying those families in need of ongoing home visiting to help care for their infant, the U. S. Advisory Board on Child Abuse and Neglect, through a series of reports in 1990 and 1991, called for a universal system of home visitation for newborns and their parents. "Complex problems do not have simple solutions," the Board wrote. "While not a panacea, the Board believes that no other single intervention has the promise that home visitation has" (U.S. Department of Health and Human Services, U.S. Advisory Board on Child Abuse and Neglect 1991, p. 145). In response to this report, the National Committee to Prevent Child Abuse developed Healthy Families America and aggressively promoted this service model through its chapter network and the state Children's Trust and Prevention Funds. As HFA and other models such as Parents as Teachers, Parent-Child Home Program, HIPPY, and Early Head Start expanded, the notion of a "home visitation field" took shape. This was in part because of the evidence but also because states were now looking for ways to build the type of early intervention systems the Advisory Board had promoted (see *Future of Children*, 1993, 1999).

For over 20 years, home visiting has remained the flagship program of the child maltreatment field. Although a wide range of prevention services continue to be implemented across the country, some form of early home visiting is one of the most common components of any community's response to child maltreatment. The passage of the Maternal, Infant, and Early Childhood Home Visiting program (MIECHV), authorized as a part of the Affordable Care Act of 2010 (U.S. Department of Health and Human Services 2011), further raised the visibility of the strategy and underscored the public policy commitment to investing in evidence-based programs (Daro and Benedetti 2014). Despite uneven impacts within and across various home visiting models, home visiting is most likely to remain a core strategy for preventing child abuse for the foreseeable future.

Future Considerations

As the prevention field moves forward, emphasis on early intervention programs and directing public investments to interventions that have a strong evidence base is the dominant public policy. However, continued concern over the ability of prevention services to reach and effectively engage the most challenged populations and the inability of evidence-based programs to be replicated as designed suggest the need for new directions in both program development and research. With respect to program development, consideration is being given to interventions that adopt a community, or population-based, perspective on achieving change as opposed to a more limited focus on replicating services for individual participants (Daro and Dodge 2009). Growing out of the field's long standing commitment to a public health perspective, this paradigm encourages a policy response that explicitly seeks to alter both the individual and the context in which children are raised.

While sustaining a focus on replicating evidence-based interventions, this approach does so with the realization that context has an inescapable influence on how programs are implemented and the level of impact they will have on their participants (Boller et al. 2014).

Crafting a prevention framework that better aligns our programmatic efforts with the way in which we have come to understand the complexity of child maltreatment requires the policy, practice, and research communities to work collaboratively regardless of their specific role along the continuum of treatment to prevention. Improving the effectiveness of evidence-based programs, be they targeted to individuals or communities, requires attention to the way in which they are designed, implemented, and taken to scale (Daro and Benedetti 2014). In addition to understanding how best to implement programs, prevention planners need to consider, through rigorous research, how best to integrate these programs into a coordinated network of care. In contrast to the original continuum of prevention services, new prevention efforts will need to develop more intentional linkages to each other and work collaboratively to create an infrastructure to support this system. Research can assist program planners in achieving this type of integration by assessing the strategies used to improve collective planning and impact, noting the most efficient areas with respect to how resources are utilized and outcomes are achieved.

Persistent Challenges in Child Maltreatment

Over the past 50 years, numerous publications have documented trends in the child maltreatment field. Beginning with the initial publication of *The Battered Child*, edited by Kempe and Helfer (1968), the field's leading scholars have documented the history, new learning, and continued challenges facing those committed to identifying, treating, and preventing child abuse and neglect. The subsequent volumes, including four revised editions of *The Battered Child* (Kempe and Helfer 1974, 1980; Helfer and Kempe 1987; Helfer et al. 1997), three editions of *The APSAC Handbook on Child Maltreatment* (Briere et al. 1996; Myers et al. 2002; Myers 2011), and Korbin and Krugman's *Handbook of Child Maltreatment* (2014), cover a broad range of topics including advances in the definition and identification of child maltreatment, its causes and consequences, and the prevailing and most promising programmatic and policy responses.

In addition to these "internal" assessments conducted by those working in the field, the federal Administration for Children, Youth and Families has, from time to time, commissioned "state of the field" reports and recommendations regarding future research priorities from the broader scientific community. The first of these reviews was conducted in 1993 by a National Research Council (NRC) expert panel. Their report, *Understanding Child Abuse and Neglect*, found the state of child maltreatment research at the time to be "underdeveloped" in comparison to research in related fields such as child development, social welfare, and criminal violence. Overcoming the lack of broad and deep financial support and political demand for child maltreatment research was, in the panel's view, essential for building the type of knowledge base necessary to guide effective interventions and public policy. The panel concluded that the most generative research agenda for the field would focus on four objectives:

- Clarify the nature and scope of maltreatment by sharpening our definition of the problem and tracking its incidence.
- Deepen our understanding of the causes and consequences of maltreatment and use this new learning to inform practice and policy.
- Rigorously evaluate treatment and prevention programs in order to determine their efficacy and effectiveness.
- Develop a "science policy" for child maltreatment by fostering greater national leadership, human and fiscal resources, and institutional support for this work across multiple agencies (NRC 1993).

The NRC panel identified 17 specific research priorities to guide progress in all of these areas. As discussed in the previous overview, one of the panel's underlying themes, the importance of using research to guide policy and practice, did indeed take hold in the field, as reflected in more rigorous program evaluations and a commitment to evidence-based practice over the past several years.

Twenty years after the initial report, the Administration for Children, Youth and Families again funded the Institute of Medicine and National Research Council to review the panel's recommendations with an eye toward identifying areas in which progress had been made, highlighting areas in need of further attention, and recommending specific actions that would advance the field. The committee focused not only on identifying the key research questions that had been sufficiently addressed and those requiring additional study but also on articulating the type of infrastructure needed to initiate and sustain high quality research. The committee's report, *New Directions in Child Abuse and Neglect Research* (IOM and NRC 2014), confirmed many of the trends highlighted in the previous section and reflected in the initial NRC review. For every issue the committee addressed, they promoted a dual message—great progress has been made in the conceptualization, understanding, and response to child maltreatment but much remains unknown. Specific chapters in the report addressed seven key areas of research that have consistently challenged researchers and policy makers seeking to improve our ability to identify, understand and address child maltreatment (see Fig. 1.1). Underlying all of these issues is the prevailing challenge of understanding and integrating culture into the field's research and practice paradigms and an unwillingness or inability to pay adequate attention to the systemic barriers to change. As noted in the report, given the fact that child maltreatment has multiple causes, "tackling the problem strategically at multiple levels is the only way to make a substantial impact on the problem" (IOM and NRC 2014, p. 27).

In many respects, the research questions cited at the end of each section of the report reflect, in part, the field's progress in unraveling the complexity of the issue and the difficulty in identifying single-factor solutions for a multifactorial problem. In response to this emerging perspective, the committee called for a comprehensive,

- **Definitional issues**: While greater clarity exists in the field's ability to aggregate child abuse reporting data across all states, the research community continues to lack a uniform definition of the problem. This makes it difficult, in many cases, to develop meaningful patterns across research studies or track incidence rates over time.

- **Causality**: While there is evidence supporting the unique contributions certain interpersonal and environmental factors play in leading to child maltreatment, much remains unclear as to what causes a specific caretaker or adult to abuse or neglect a child in specific circumstances.

- **Consequences**: While ample evidence exists as to the devastating impact of maltreatment on a child's physical, emotional, and cognitive development, including the child's brain development, it remains unclear why these impacts are inconsistent across cases and how they interact with the impacts generated by other adversities a child may experience.

- **Interventions**: While treatment and prevention planners have myriad, well-supported, and evidence-based interventions to choose from in responding to child maltreatment victims and those at risk of maltreatment, all of these interventions face issues of implementation and replication across diverse contexts, limiting their ability, in many instances, to achieve consistent outcomes.

- **Child welfare system response**: While the number of children in foster care has declined and alternative response systems have afforded a greater number of families access to services, greater understanding is needed as to why the child welfare system lacks the organizational capacity to consistently implement evidence-based practices and interventions.

- **Policy**: While a plethora of state and federal legislation has been passed which elevates public recognition of child maltreatment, few of these policies have been systematically evaluated.

- **Building an effective research infrastructure**While the volume of child abuse research has increased exponentially, much of this research remains fragmented due to a continued lack of national leadership, fiscal resources and human capital.

Fig. 1.1 Persistent challenges in addressing child maltreatment

multidisciplinary approach to examining the issue. They added that the field "is lacking a core, national-level priority-setting body that can reach all of the many associated disciplines and that has the capacity to allocate resources necessary to develop a sustainable, accountable research infrastructure" (IOM and NRC 2014, p. 390). The committee identified four areas for investment in developing a coordinated research enterprise:

- Formulating a national strategic plan that would engage a wide range of federal, private, and academic institutions.
- Creating a National Surveillance System that would promote a more standardized use of definitions of maltreatment across agencies and researchers.

- Establishing a new generation of dedicated researchers committed to adopting an interdisciplinary and collaborative approach to their research.
- Encouraging evidence-based policy making by including support for evaluating the impacts on targeted objectives of all new federal and state child maltreatment legislation.

The committee identified child maltreatment as a unique and important social dilemma in need of unique and focused research, despite its frequent co-occurrence with other adversity and trauma that impacts social well-being. Rather than viewing this overlap as a problem, the committee viewed this situation as having potential benefit for advancing our understanding in other domains such as child development, child welfare, education, social work, pediatrics, and criminology (IOM and NRC 2014). Realizing this type of knowledge transfer, however, will require greater collaboration across disciplines and institutions as well as renewed investments in efforts to integrate the field's treatment and prevention activities.

New Leadership

As the complexity of child maltreatment becomes better documented, those engaged in examining the nature of the problem and the nature of the response must take greater care in developing a common understanding of how diverse disciplines and perspectives impact the issue. As the IOM committee noted, the complexity of child abuse and neglect requires a core body of individuals interested both in understanding the problem and in working across disciplines to engage in developing new knowledge. In commenting on this shift toward cross-discipline learning, a recent report by the Carnegie Initiative on the Doctorate (CID) observed that the most productive areas for advancing our understanding of diverse social problems may lie in the "border land between disciplines." The report goes on to note that maximizing the ability of young scholars to explore this territory will require a new approach to doctoral education, one which focuses on "building intellectual communities that have an intentional focus on diverse membership and multiple strategies for identifying new learning" (Walker et al. 2007, p. 3).

The *Doris Duke Fellowships for the Promotion of Child Well-Being* reflects much of this new thinking regarding doctoral education and training in its design and implementation plan. Established in 2010, the fellowship focuses on identifying and nurturing promising doctoral students from multiple disciplines to address emerging challenges in the field. From the onset, the fellowship recognized the challenges facing the child abuse prevention field and the importance of remaining open to innovation and new frameworks for conceptualizing the issue and crafting an effective response. Among the planning challenges the fellowship envisioned for the field were identifying more successful pathways to reach and engage the most troubled populations and most difficult communities; creating strategies to engage a diverse set of public and private institutions in the mission of prevention; and attracting top talent with the ability and interest in applying empirical evidence in discerning important practice and policy alternatives.

The fellowship's ongoing implementation is guided by three core operational objectives:

- Selecting individuals with the skills, passion, and institutional support necessary for sustaining long-term professional involvement in the field.
- Selecting cohorts of fellows that collectively represent a diverse group of scholars in terms of their backgrounds, disciplines, research interests, and technical expertise.
- Creating an active, self-generating learning network among the fellows through ongoing web-based conferences, annual meetings and other opportunities for informal meetings at related national conferences, and shared research projects.

From the onset, the most essential component for ensuring the program's success has been the quality of the fellows themselves. Over and above the obvious criteria of solid scholarship and productivity, fellow selection has carried the added burden of identifying those holding promise in the area of leadership. At its core, the initiative seeks fellows with human and intellectual capital who will make the type of sustained commitment to the field necessary to truly influence its trajectory. As such, the fellowship seeks out and supports individuals with the following attributes:

- Demonstrated initiative in fostering a network of like-minded scholars from diverse disciplines and active interest in building cross-disciplinary perspectives into their work.
- Active engagement in disseminating their findings through peer-reviewed publications, presentations at professional conferences, and discussions in various academic and stakeholder meetings.
- Active engagement and service to the field, as demonstrated by leadership in professional societies focusing on child maltreatment or elevating the profile of child maltreatment within the pool of discipline-specific professional societies.
- Presenting the findings of their research in a manner that maximizes the ability of program managers and policymakers to draw on this information to shape their practice and policy decisions.

During its initial 4 years, the fellowship has selected 60 young scholars from across the country for participation in this innovative approach to developing a new generation of leaders to improve the well-being of children and prevent child abuse. The continued evaluation activities have documented that both fellows and mentors place high "added value" on the fellowship's capacity to raise the visibility of the issue of child maltreatment, generate new avenues of research, and create new relationships within and across disciplines (Daro et al. 2013). This program—and fellowship programs in general—are but one strategy for supporting the development of new scholars. However, the Doris Duke Fellowship's commitment to strengthening learning across disciplines, creating opportunities for collaboration between fellows, and focusing on the link between research and practice offer important guidelines for others engaged in building leadership in their fields.

Conclusion

The emerging scholars contributing to this volume approach their research and the application of their findings through a lens shaped by their understanding of the problem's history and the role research and systematic inquiry plays in identifying new opportunities in the practice and policy domains. They bring unique skills in situating their interests within the child maltreatment landscape as defined by their discipline and training as well as the discipline and perspectives of their peers. As such, not all of the topics or research challenges facing the field are addressed in these chapters. Working collaboratively, and in many instances working across disciplines, the fellows crafted their own interpretation of emerging issues, placing greater emphasis on some than others. High priority questions for this group of scholars include balancing the co-occurrence of different forms of maltreatment and other trauma with opportunities to unravel how different types of maltreatment impact children; giving greater attention to the needs of adolescents and the opportunities this perspective offers in engaging diverse institutions in this work; and directly addressing the challenges associated with implementing, replicating, and taking evidence-based interventions to scale. Beyond these topical areas, the fellows offered new perspectives and frameworks for the field, including how to incorporate culture (in the broadest sense of the word) into how we perceive and respond to the issue and the potential of a protective factors framework to inform the prevention response. This type of recasting of old issues within the context of current challenges and learning offer the field clear opportunity for growth and for reconnecting its treatment and prevention elements.

References

American Humane Association (AHA). (1981). *National analysis of official child neglect and abuse reports*. Denver: The American Humane Association, Child Protection Division.

Boller, K., Daro, D., Del Grosso, P., Cole, R., Paulsell, D., Hart, B., et al. (2014). *Making replication work: Building infrastructure to implement, scale-up and sustain evidence-based early childhood home visiting programs with fidelity*. Washington, DC: Children's Bureau, Administration for Children and Families, U.S. Department of Health and Human Services.

Briere, J., Berliner, L., Bulkley, J., Jenny, C., & Reid, T. (1996). *The APSAC handbook on child maltreatment*. Thousand Oaks: Sage.

Campbell, F. A., Ramey, C. T., Pungello, E. P., Sparling, J., & Miller-Johnson, S. (2002). Early childhood education: Young adult outcomes from the Abecedarian Project. *Applied Developmental Science, 6,* 42–57.

Carnegie Task Force on Meeting the Needs of Young Children. (1994). *Starting points: Meeting the needs of our youngest children*. New York: Carnegie Corporation of New York.

Centers for Disease Control. (2013). Promoting safe, stable, and nurturing relationships: A strategic direction for child maltreatment prevention. www.cdc.gov/ViolencePrevention/pdf/CM_Strategic_Direction--OnePager-a.pdf. Accessed 30 Oct 2014.

Cohn, A. (1979). Effective treatment of child abuse and neglect. *Social Work, 24*(6), 513–519.

Cohn, A. (1983). *An approach to preventing child abuse*. Chicago: National Committee to Prevent Child Abuse.

Committee on the Prevention of Mental Disorders and Substance Abuse Among Children, Youth and Youth Adults. (2009). *Preventing mental, emotional, and behavioral disorders among young people*. Washington, DC: The National Academies Press.

Daro, D. (1988). *Confronting child abuse*. New York: The Free Press.

Daro, D. (1993). Child maltreatment research: Implications for program design. In D. Cicchetti & S. Toth (Eds.), *Child abuse, child development, and social policy* (pp. 331–367). Norwood: Ablex Publishing Corporation.

Daro, D. (1994). Prevention of child sexual abuse. *Future of Children, 4*(2), 198–223.

Daro, D., & Benedetti, G. (2014). Sustaining progress in preventing child maltreatment: A transformative challenge. In J. E. Korbin & R. D. Krugman (Eds.), *Handbook of child maltreatment* (pp. 281–300). New York: Springer.

Daro, D., & Cohn, A. (1987). Is treatment too late: What ten years of evaluative research tells us. *Child Abuse and Neglect, 11*(3), 433–442.

Daro, D., & Cohn-Donnelly, A. (2002). Charting the waves of prevention: Two steps forward, one step back. *Child Abuse and Neglect, 26*, 731–742.

Daro, D., & Dodge, K. (2009). Creating community responsibility for child protection: Possibilities and challenges. *Future of Children, 19*(2), 67–94.

Daro, D., Huang, L. A., & Benedetti, G. (2013). *Doris Duke fellowships for promoting child well-being: Annual report*. Chicago: Chapin Hall at the University of Chicago. Available at: www.chapinhall.org.

Future of Children. (1993). Home visiting. *3*(3).

Future of Children. (1999). Home visiting: Recent program evaluations. *9*(1).

Heckman, J. (2000). Policies to foster human capital. *Research in Economics, 54*, 3–56.

Helfer, R. (1982). A review of the literature on the prevention of child abuse and neglect. *Child Abuse and Neglect, 6*, 251–261.

Helfer, R. E., & Kempe, R. (Eds.). (1987). *The battered child* (4th ed.). Chicago: The University of Chicago Press.

Helfer, M. E., Kempe, R., & Krugman, R. D. (Eds.). (1997). *The battered child* (5th ed.). Chicago: The University of Chicago Press.

Institute of Medicine, & National Research Council. (2014). *New directions in child abuse and neglect research*. Washington, DC: The National Academies Press.

Kania, J., & Kramer, M. (2011). Collective impact. *Stanford Social Innovation Review, 9*(1), 36–41.

Kempe, C. H., & Helfer, R. E. (Eds.). (1968). *The battered child*. Chicago: The University of Chicago Press.

Kempe, C. H., & Helfer, R. E. (Eds.). (1974). *The battered child* (2nd ed.). Chicago: The University of Chicago Press.

Kempe, C. H., & Helfer, R. E. (Eds.). (1980). *The battered child* (3rd ed.). Chicago: The University of Chicago Press.

Kempe, C. H., Silverman, F., Steele, B., Droegemueller, W., & Silver, H. (1962). The battered child syndrome. *JAMA, 181*(17), 17–24.

Kirkpatrick, K. (2004). *Reframing child abuse and neglect for increased understanding and engagement: Defining the need for strategic reform*. Chicago: Prevent Child Abuse America. Available at: www.friendsnrc.org/reframing/PDF/WhitePaper1.pdf.

Kitzman, H., Olds, D., Henderson, C., Hanks, C., Cole, R., Tatelbaum, R., et al. (1997). Effects of prenatal an infancy home visitation by nurses on pregnancy outcomes, childhood injuries, and repeated childbearing: A randomized controlled trial. *JAMA, 278*(8), 644–652.

Korbin, J. E., & Krugman, R. D. (Eds.). (2014). *Handbook of child maltreatment*. New York: Springer.

McCormick, M., Brooks-Gunn, J., Buka, S., Goldman, J., Yu, J., Salganik, M., et al. (2006). Early intervention in low birth weight premature infants: Results at 18 years of age for the Infant Health and Development Program. *Pediatrics, 117*(3), 771–780.

Myers, J. E. B. (2006). *Child protection in America: Past, present, and future*. New York: Oxford University Press.

Myers, J. E. B. (Ed.). (2011). *The APSAC handbook on child maltreatment* (3rd ed.). Thousand Oaks: Sage.

Myers, J. E. B., Berliner, L., Briere, J., Hendrix, C. T., Jenny, C., & Reid, T. (2002). *The APSAC handbook on child maltreatment* (2nd ed.). Thousand Oaks: Sage.

National Center on Child Abuse and Neglect, & U.S. Department of Health and Human Services. (1981). *National Study of the Incidence and Severity of Child Abuse and Neglect: Study findings* (Publication No. OHDS 81-30325). Washington, DC: U.S. Department of Health and Human Services.

National Research Council. (1993). *Understanding child abuse and neglect*. Washington, DC: The National Academy Press.

Nelson, B. (1984). *Making an issue of child abuse: Political agenda setting for social problems*. Chicago: The University of Chicago Press.

Olds, D., Henderson, C., Chamberlin, R., & Tatelbaum, R. (1986). Preventing child abuse and neglect: A randomized trial of nurse home visitation. *Pediatrics, 78*(1), 65–77.

Olds, D., Henderson, C., & Kitzman, H. (1994). Does prenatal and infancy nurse home visitation have enduring effects on qualities of parental caregiving and child health at 25 to 50 months of life? *Pediatrics, 93*(1), 89–98.

Patel, V., & Goodman, S. (2007). Researching protective and promotive factors in mental health. *International Journal of Epidemiology, 36*, 703–707.

Perry, B. D. (1994). Neurobiological sequelae of childhood trauma: Post-traumatic stress disorders in children. In M. Murberg (Ed.), *Catecholamines in post-traumatic stress disorder: Emerging concepts* (pp. 253–276). Washington, DC: American Psychiatric Press.

Reynolds, A., Temple, J., Robertson, D., & Mann, E. (2001). Long-term effects of an early childhood intervention on educational achievement and juvenile arrest: A 15-year follow-up of low-income children in public schools. *JAMA, 285*(18), 2339–2346.

Schweinhart, L. (2004). The High/Scope Perry Preschool Study through age 40: Summary, conclusions and frequently asked questions. Retrieved from http://www.highscope.org/Research/PerryProject/PerryAge40SumWeb.pdf

Seitz, V., Rosenbaum, L., & Apfel, N. (1985). Effects of family support intervention: A ten-year follow-up. *Child Development, 56*, 376–391.

Shonkoff, J. P., & Phillips, D. (2000). *From neurons to neighborhoods: The science of early childhood development*. Washington, DC: National Academy Press.

U.S. Department of Health and Human Services. (2011). HHS announces $224 million to support evidence-based home visiting programs to help parents and children. News release.

U.S. Department of Health and Human Services. (2013). *Child maltreatment 2012*. http://www.acf.hhs.gov/sites/default/files/cb/cm2012.pdf. Accessed 18 Aug 2014.

U.S. Department of Health and Human Services, & U.S. Advisory Board on Child Abuse and Neglect. (1991). *Creating caring communities: Blueprint for an effective federal policy for child abuse and neglect*. Washington, DC: U.S. Government Printing Office.

Waldfogel, J. (2009). Prevention and the child protection system. *Future of Children, 19*(2), 195–210.

Walker, G. E., Golde, C. M., Jones, L., Bueschel, A. C., & Hutchings, P. (2007). *The formation of scholars: Rethinking doctoral education for the twenty-first century*. New York: The Carnegie Foundation for the Advancement of Teaching.

Deborah Daro is a senior research fellow at Chapin Hall at the University of Chicago. Dr. Daro's current research and written work focuses on developing effective early intervention systems to support all new parents and examining the impacts of reforms that embed individualized, targeted home-based interventions within universal efforts to alter normative standards and enhance community context. Reflecting her strong commitment to developing leadership in the area of child maltreatment prevention, she designed and directs the *Doris Duke Fellowships for the Promotion of Child Well-Being*. Dr. Daro has served as president of the American Professional Society on the Abuse of Children and as treasurer and Executive Council member of the International Society for the Prevention of Child Abuse and Neglect. Dr. Daro holds a Ph.D. in Social Welfare and a master's degree in City and Regional Planning from the University of California at Berkeley.

Anne Cohn Donnelly is a child abuse prevention researcher and lecturer at the Kellogg School of Management, Northwestern University. She is the founding director of the school's Board Fellows Program. Dr. Donnelly conducted the first national evaluation of child abuse treatment programs. Dr. Donnelly served for 17 years as the head of Prevent Child Abuse America where she launched the Healthy Families America Initiative. Prior to this, she served as a White House Fellow and a Congressional Science Fellow. Dr. Donnelly received a B.A. degree from the University of Michigan, an M.A. from Tufts University and both the M.P.H. and D.P.H. degrees in health administration and planning from the University of California (Berkeley) School of Public Health. She is a Fellow of the American Association for the Advancement of Science.

Part II
New Generation of Research: The Nature of the Problem

Chapter 2
Multiple Aspects of Maltreatment: Moving Toward a Holistic Framework

Amanda Van Scoyoc, Jessica S. Wilen, Kate Daderko, and Sheridan Miyamoto

Chapter 2 in Brief

Context

- Historically, different types of child maltreatment (physical abuse, sexual abuse, emotional abuse and neglect) have been considered discrete experiences; in truth, these actions frequently co-occur and overlap with other adversities (e.g., domestic violence, caregiver substance abuse, caregiver mental illness).
- This level of co-occurrence across maltreatment types complicates efforts to distinguish the unique impacts of certain parenting behaviors, which in turn has implications for the design of effective prevention programs.
- While more holistic approaches to designing child abuse prevention programs are warranted, certain types of maltreatment, such as sexual abuse and abusive head trauma, benefit from strategies that specifically address the pathways associated with these maltreatment experiences.

We would like to acknowledge Bart Klika's contribution to the writing of this chapter.

A. Van Scoyoc (✉)
University of Oregon, Eugene, OR, USA
e-mail: avanscoy@uoregon.edu

J.S. Wilen
Washington University in St. Louis, St. Louis, MO, USA
e-mail: jwilen@wustl.edu

K. Daderko
Penn Medicine, Philadelphia, PA, USA
e-mail: katedaderkophd@gmail.com

S. Miyamoto
University of California Davis, Davis, CA, USA
e-mail: Sheridan.miyamoto@ucdmc.ucdavis.edu

© Springer International Publishing Switzerland 2015
D. Daro et al. (eds.), *Advances in Child Abuse Prevention Knowledge*,
Child Maltreatment 5, DOI 10.1007/978-3-319-16327-7_2

Strategies for Moving Forward

- Utilize knowledge gained from research on individual forms of maltreatment to determine when targeted prevention approaches are likely to be most effective.
- Move towards a multi-tiered system of prevention that includes primary, secondary, and tertiary prevention efforts that collectively target a range of outcomes impacting all children.
- Balance prevention efforts that focus broadly on preventing all types of maltreatment (e.g., positive parenting programs) with prevention efforts that target a more narrow range of behaviors.
- Utilize evidence-based best practices in developing and implementing any prevention strategies.

Implications for Research

- Empirically define meaningful subpopulations of children with a common set of service needs and prevention supports by considering the wide range of adverse early experiences that impact early childhood outcomes.
- Conduct rigorous research to identify the most effective interventions for confronting maltreatment by better understanding how patterns of maltreatment experiences lead to different outcomes and how these interventions can be more fully integrated into a multi-tiered prevention system.
- Utilize Latent Class Analysis and other methodologies from a variety of disciplines to determine how patterns of maltreatment experiences lead to different outcomes thereby creating more empirically based subpopulations of maltreatment.

Introduction

The way that researchers define and categorize maltreatment experiences determines both the priorities and scope of scholarly work in the field. These critical decisions influence the way that researchers identify and collect information about who has or has not experienced abuse and neglect. Since the passage of the Child Abuse Prevention and Treatment Act of 1974 (CAPTA), federal legislation which addressed child abuse and neglect and authorized funds to help protect children from maltreatment, the field has largely considered the various forms of abuse and neglect (i.e., physical abuse, sexual abuse, emotional or psychological abuse, and neglect) as discrete experiences. This framework is reflected in the way researchers operationalize and study child abuse and neglect and in the design of child maltreatment prevention and intervention programs.

Despite this focus on individual forms of maltreatment, a growing body of research suggests that maltreated children are likely to experience a host of negative early experiences that impact their life trajectory. There is significant overlap in the various forms of abuse and neglect, suggesting that single forms occurring in isolation are rare (Teicher et al. 2006). For example, Herrenkohl and Herrenkohl (2009) found that rates of overlap among the various forms of child abuse and neglect ranged from 33 % to 94 %, depending upon which research studies were used. In addition to the overlap in maltreatment types, the Adverse Childhood Experiences Study demonstrates that children who experience abuse and neglect are at increased risk for being exposed to other adversity, including caregiver substance abuse, caregiver mental illness, witnessing intimate partner violence, divorce, and parental absence from the home (Dong et al. 2004). This body of work suggests the importance of considering the larger context in which adversity occurs.

In this chapter, we consider the current focus on discrete types of maltreatment and discuss moving prevention efforts beyond this limited focus to more broadly address the complex nature of adverse early experiences. We begin by considering the traditional approach before making recommendations for a holistic framework. Then we offer suggestions for addressing the spectrum of maltreatment experiences. We recommend that the field of child maltreatment prevention move toward a broader focus, with a goal of preventing a wide range of adverse experiences early in life and securing better outcomes for children.

To accomplish this goal, we consider two priorities for policy change and future research. First, we suggest there is a need for research identifying overlap in maltreatment experiences and discuss promising research methodologies for identifying how adverse experiences co-occur, as well as the different causes and consequences of these experiences. Second, we suggest the need for evidence-based, tiered prevention systems based on a public health model of primary, secondary, and tertiary prevention (Gordon 1983). Such a system will bolster families through universal programs, provide extra support to high-risk families, and include focused interventions when maltreatment is identified. Valuable knowledge obtained about individual forms of maltreatment can inform all levels of this tiered approach.

The Traditional Framework: Four Discrete Categories of Maltreatment

Definitions

The foundational steps in preventing child abuse and neglect are to clearly define maltreatment and to assess its scope and associated impact. Although attempts have been made to adopt and disseminate universal definitions of the four major maltreatment types, states and researchers have not reached consensus on these definitions. While there are no universal definitions across all states for the subtypes of maltreatment, the federal Child Abuse Prevention and Treatment Act provides minimum definition standards. This legislation defines maltreatment as "Any recent act or failure to act on the part of a parent or caretaker which results in death, serious physical or emotional harm, sexual abuse or exploitation." (CAPTA Reauthorization Act of 2010). Specifically, physical abuse refers to nonaccidental physical injury. Sexual abuse refers to a wide range of acts, including inappropriate touching or kissing, exposing children to adult sexuality, fondling, sexual assault (digital or oral penetration), and vaginal or anal rape. Emotional abuse is considered to be a pattern of behavior that impairs a child's emotional development or sense of self-worth, such as constant criticism, rejection, and withholding love. Finally, neglect is defined as a failure of a parent, guardian, or other caregiver to provide for a child's basic physical, medical, educational, and emotional needs.

Prevalence

Due to differences in definition, which lead to differences in tracking and surveillance, estimates of the prevalence of child abuse and neglect vary across systems. For example, the National Child Abuse and Neglect Data System (NCANDS) collects information annually from child protective services agencies in all 50 states and from the District of Columbia and Puerto Rico. In 2012, these 52 child protective service agencies received 3.4 million referrals for 6.3 million children. Of these reports, 62 % were investigated and 17.7 % of these were substantiated, resulting in a total of 686,000 unique victims of child abuse and neglect (U.S. Department of Health and Human Services 2013).

The Fourth National Incidence Study of Child Abuse and Neglect (NIS-4), which took place from 2005 to 2006, addresses the prevalence of maltreatment in the U.S. beyond relying on the count of children who are identified by child welfare systems (Sedlak et al. 2010). It is based on the assumption that cases that come to the attention of child welfare agencies represent only a proportion of children who are being harmed by maltreatment and thus the true prevalence is underestimated. The study includes data on children identified by child welfare agencies as well as on children who were not reported to the child protective system or who were screened out of child protective system without investigation. This additional information was collected by over 10,000 community professionals, called sentinels, from a national sample of 122 counties in the United States (Sedlak et al. 2010).

This study uses two different measurement standards: one which measures the number of children who experienced maltreatment and another which measures the number of children at risk for exposure to maltreatment. The former, called the Harm Standard, defines maltreatment as "an act or omission [that] result [s] in demonstrable harm" (Sedlak et al. 2010, p. 3). Using this definition, it was determined that over 1.25 million children experienced maltreatment during the study period. Thus, there is a discrepancy of almost 575,000 children between the NCANDS and the NIS-4 estimates.

The prevalence of the different forms of maltreatment varies, with substantiated reports indicating that the greatest number of children experience neglect. The most recent data collected from state child welfare administrative data systems indicates that 78.3 % of children with substantiated reports of maltreatment were neglected, 18.3 % were physically abused, 9.3 % were sexually abused, and 8.5 % were psychologically maltreated. Substantiated cases often involve multiple forms of maltreatment (U.S. Department of Health and Human Services 2013).

Trends

Tracking the prevalence of child abuse and neglect over time has indicated different trends in the four types of maltreatment. Using official child abuse reporting data gathered by the states, Finkelhor et al. (2013) observed a steady decline in rates of child sexual abuse and child physical abuse since the early 1990s (61 % and 55 % respectively), while rates of child neglect modestly decline (approximately 14 %). Findings from the NIS-4 comparing prevalence rates of the four different types of maltreatment at two data collection time points, 1993 and 2005–2006, identified a similar decrease in rates of physical and sexual abuse. These findings also identified increased rates of emotional neglect, indicating a failure to provide emotional support (Sedlak et al. 2010).

There is some question as to whether declines in child sexual abuse and physical abuse represent "real" declines or if other factors are responsible for these downward trends. Jones et al (2001) surveyed child welfare administrators to ascertain the reasons for the declines in child sexual abuse. While child welfare workers provided some indication of a real decline as a result of improved programming and more stringent prosecution for child sexual abuse crimes, the administrators pointed to changed policies within child protective services as being largely responsible for the declines. For example, changes in the threshold at which child sexual abuse becomes substantiated ("credible evidence" versus "preponderance of evidence") can influence rates of child sexual abuse. As more evidence is required to substantiate a case of child sexual abuse, fewer cases meet the substantiation threshold, resulting in fewer confirmed cases. While more work is needed to clearly understand the trends indicating a decrease in physical and sexual abuse, it is likely that at least some of the downward trend is a result of prevention and intervention programs. Whether these programs have separately or collectively influenced this decline has yet to be explored.

At the same time, the modest declines in child neglect and increases in emotional neglect are puzzling. This difference may reflect heightened attention to neglect as a form of maltreatment in recent decades that has led to increased reporting and case substantiation (Sedlak et al. 2010). One important consideration for why prevention and intervention programs may be more effective at addressing physical and sexual abuse than neglect is that the perpetrators of child neglect are frequently described as facing greater socio-economic adversity than those involved in other forms of maltreatment (Sedlak et al. 2010; U.S. Department of Health and Human Services 2013). Further, neglect is largely an act of omission (e.g., the lack of adequate food, shelter, or clothing) while sexual abuse and physical abuse are acts of commission (e.g., hitting and penetration). Perhaps our programs and interventions differentially target acts of commission, rather than acts of omission, resulting in decreased physical and sexual abuse reports. As a whole, these trends suggest that prevention efforts may have been more effective for some forms of maltreatment than for others. In the next section, we explore the unique nature of each form of child maltreatment.

Toward a New Framework

There is some utility in viewing child maltreatment as a set of distinct experiences. However, findings largely suggest that there are a host of risk factors and outcomes common to the four subtypes of maltreatment. For example, parent-child interaction characteristics (i.e., the parent perceiving the child as a problem), parent characteristics (i.e., anger or hyper-reactivity, low self-esteem, psychopathology, and depression), and child characteristics (i.e., low social competence and child externalizing behavior problems) all correlate with risk for both physical abuse and neglect (Stith et al. 2009). Additionally, research indicates that maltreatment generally is associated with poorer physical and mental health outcomes for children, including depression, anxiety, and chronic pain (Arnow 2004).

This categorization, however, does not fully represent the lived experience of children. As noted in this section, many, if not most, cases of maltreatment involve multiple forms of maltreatment and other adverse conditions. This level of co-occurrence complicates efforts to distinguish the unique impacts of certain parental behaviors and has implications on how prevention efforts are designed and implemented. In this section, we will explore ways in which highlighting the differences in maltreatment types can be both helpful and detrimental and then suggest a more holistic paradigm reflecting the reality of multi-type maltreatment.

The Challenge of Co-occurrence Across Types

Complicating the study of child abuse and neglect is the recent recognition that abuse and neglect is a multi-faceted problem that often overlaps in complex ways. Thus, studying one type of maltreatment in isolation does not account for other important traumatic experiences and does not reflect the complicated nature of early adversity.

A 2009 review of the literature found few studies directly researching this overlap. The studies that did analyze comorbidity between different maltreatment experiences varied considerably in their findings (Herrenkohl and Herrenkohl 2009). For example, the correlation of experiencing physical and emotional abuse ranged from $r = 0.206$ to $r = 0.694$. Given this variability, the authors suggest that the question of "which maltreatment types, singly and in combination, result in which outcomes and why" cannot clearly be answered given the current state of the literature (Herrenkohl and Herrenkohl 2009, p. 493). By not adequately accounting for overlap, the current literature remains murky at best, and at worst leads to inaccurate conclusions about predictors and outcomes associated with individual forms of maltreatment.

The research that does consider the overlap in maltreatment experiences strongly suggests that multitype maltreatment is common and is associated with greater long-term impairment than single forms of maltreatment or no maltreatment (Higgins and McCabe 2001). For example, Higgins and McCabe (2000b) found that four different types of maltreatment (sexual abuse, physical abuse, emotional abuse, and neglect) and witnessing family violence were all significantly correlated. The lowest correlation was between sexual abuse and witnessing family violence ($r = 0.24$, $p < 0.01$), with all other correlations ranging from $r = 0.42$ to $r = 0.74$ ($p < 0.001$). Researchers have responded to this known overlap in maltreatment experiences by highlighting the importance of researching and assessing multiple forms of maltreatment.

Other aspects of children's environment early in life that are often understudied in the maltreatment literature also have an important impact on adjustment. Aspects of the caregiving environment, including both risk and protective factors, should be considered alongside experiences of maltreatment when researching the context in which maltreatment occurs and the impact of early experiences on long-term outcomes. Higgins and McCabe (2000a) found that family characteristics (e.g., parental divorce, parental relationship satisfaction, family cohesion, parents having traditional values) predict maltreatment experiences and adjustment in adulthood.

Recent research also has focused on the cumulative impact of traumatic childhood experiences. There is a dose-response relationship between higher numbers of adverse experiences and future poor health outcomes, suggesting that the accumulation of stressful early experiences may be particularly damaging to the developing child (Anda et al. 2006). Specifically, a study by Turner and colleagues (2010) found that the extent of trauma symptomatology increased linearly for each incident of exposure to different types of violence until a child had experienced eleven types of exposure, at which point their risk of exhibiting trauma symptoms increased by approximately 250 %.

These and similar studies underscore the reality that individual types of child maltreatment do not always occur in isolation and that experiencing multiple types of maltreatment (and likely other risk factors) often leads to more detrimental outcomes than experiencing one (Arata et al. 2005, 2007; Edwards et al. 2003; Felitti et al. 1998). Although it can be helpful, in some contexts, to consider unique aspects of individual forms of maltreatment, having a singular focus on individual types of maltreatment runs the risk of delaying new developments and creating inefficiencies in the prevention field. While there are differences in the causes, co-occurring experiences and consequences of the four types of maltreatment, placing too much emphasis on addressing a given type of abuse when working with families exhibiting a range of poor parenting practices, and dealing with a range of environmental stressors all hamper our ability to develop robust prevention systems.

Embracing Co-occurrence

Two limitations of focusing on the unique patterns of individual forms of maltreatment include failing to adequately address the complex reality of adverse early experiences and focusing on the prevention of maltreatment experiences rather than on securing the best outcomes for all children.

The primary limitation of a research agenda that continues to focus solely on individual forms of maltreatment in isolation is that this narrow focus does not adequately address the reality of maltreated children's early life experiences. Rather, children who experience one form of maltreatment likely experience other forms of maltreatment and grow up in a stressful family environment with a multitude of other risk factors (Felitti et al. 1998; Higgins and McCabe 2000b). Furthermore, a focus on individual experiences as predictors of unique outcomes is not well supported in the current literature. Research on whether outcomes differ based upon particular constellations of maltreatment experiences has led to mixed and unclear results (Herrenkohl and Herrenkohl 2009). When taken as a whole, the literature suggests that the impact of different maltreatment experiences may be more similar than expected, and that the *accumulation* of risk may be the more salient predictor of child outcomes. A narrow focus on individual forms of maltreatment fails to adequately address the multitude of stressors and does not adequately predict child vulnerabilities, providing limited utility for preventative efforts (Herrenkohl and Herrenkohl 2009).

An additional benefit of embracing the complexity of the issue is that it shifts the goal of intervention from reducing the incidence of specific behaviors associated with one or more types of maltreatment to a more intentional focus on securing the best outcomes for all children. As we suggest in the next section, an alternate focus for child abuse prevention efforts would be operating within an integrated system in which broad support is provided to enhance well-being for all children. Then, more focused support is directed toward children at heightened risk for maltreatment as well as children who have already experienced maltreatment.

Considering Individual Types of Maltreatment, When Appropriate

While a more holistic approach to prevention services that recognizes the common factors at play across various types of maltreatment is an important avenue to pursue, equally important is identifying those cases in which a more targeted approach offers significant opportunities for addressing the problem. Two such cases include instances involving child sexual abuse and those involving abusive head trauma.

Among the four major types of maltreatment, cases of child sexual abuse present a different profile on many levels than cases involving physical abuse or neglect. Compared to these other forms of maltreatment, sexual abuse often is perpetrated by someone other than the child's primary caretaker. In approximately 60 % of cases, the perpetrator is an acquaintance or family friend who is able to gain access to the child (Finkelhor and Jones 2012). In contrast to physical abuse where infants and young children are at greatest risk, children 6 years of age and older are at increased risk for being sexual abused. Over 45 % of all substantiated cases of sexual abuse involve children between 12 and 17 years of age (U.S. Department of Health and Human Services 2013). Unlike serious physical abuse and neglect, in which male children are at increased risk of victimization (Bullock et al. 2009; Farst et al. 2013; Leventhal et al. 2012; Putnam-Hornstein et al. 2013; Stiffman et al. 2002; Welch and Bonner 2013), females are at greater risk for sexual abuse (Finkelhor et al. 2014).

Furthermore, sexual abuse has been consistently linked to sexual dysfunction in both childhood, when it is exhibited as sexual reactivity or precocious sexuality (Putnam 2003; Kendall-Tackett et al. 1993) and adulthood, when it often manifests as decreased sexual desire and contentment (Stephenson et al. 2012; Meston and Lorenz 2013). Additionally, when the perpetrator is a close family member or friend, there is a stronger negative impact on health outcomes (Edwards et al. 2012).

Reflecting these and other differences, research and public awareness efforts have been developed specifically around child sexual abuse. Prevention efforts addressing this form of maltreatment have taken the double-pronged approach of providing education for children and parents and strengthening laws against offenders. In terms of education, there are universal education programs aimed at educating children on appropriate versus inappropriate touching, "private zones," and seeking out a trusted adult when they feel uncomfortable (Martyniuk and Dworkin 2011). Multiple meta-analyses have shown that these programs are effective in increasing children's knowledge and skillset in this area (Daro and McCurdy 2007; Rispens et al. 1997; Zwi et al. 2008). Prevention efforts also focus on parent and teacher education, with some states mandating that teachers receive annual training on recognizing and responding to sexual abuse (Plummer and Klein 2013). At the same time, criminal punishment for offenders has become more severe, with some states implementing minimum sentencing provisions and eliminating or extending the statute of limitations. Federal legislation also has mandated that states create a sex offender registry (Whittier 2009). Although it is impossible to separate the individual and combined effects of these two approaches on decreased rates of child sexual abuse, the fact remains that prevention approaches, coupled with increased awareness, have led to a significant reduction in child sexual abuse reports (Jones et al. 2001).

Another example of how focusing preventative efforts on an individual maltreatment experience can be successful is efforts to reduce abusive head injury to infants. Abusive head injury is a type of injury resulting from physical abuse that leads to more fatalities and long-term poor outcomes than any other form of maltreatment, particularly for children under 1 year old (Duhaime et al. 1998). Understanding caregivers' actions that lead to this type of injury has led to prevention efforts specifically designed for abusive head injury. In infants, this type of injury often results from brief but violent shaking by a caregiver who is frustrated by inconsolable crying that persists despite the caregiver's efforts to soothe (Reece 2011). Universal prevention efforts administered to new mothers and fathers while they are in the hospital with their newborn have focused on educating caregivers about how to handle frustration when it arises because of persistent crying and also educates caregivers about the harm caused by shaking a baby. These efforts have been quite successful, with one program affecting a 47 % decrease in abusive head injuries to infants in the geographical region where the intervention was administered (Dias et al. 2005).

As the field of child abuse prevention moves forward, there are two main lessons to be learned from these success stories. First, identifying the dimensions of a form of maltreatment and increasing public knowledge can lead to effective prevention. Second, when there are clear, identifiable risk factors and causes of a specific form of maltreatment, prevention efforts that directly address these risks can be particularly effective. An effective child maltreatment system will be one that can balance the need for these types of targeted efforts with a more holistic approach, discussed in the following section.

Future Directions for Addressing the Spectrum of Maltreatment Experiences

In the following section, we offer two suggestions for prevention efforts that address the complex reality of adversity early in life. First, we suggest that identifying meaningful categorizations of maltreated children should be a priority. We will discuss a promising research methodology that identifies how multiple early adverse experiences overlap and impact outcomes. The impact of having multiple maltreatment experiences remains a murky area of the maltreatment literature, and we suggest that research in this area will inform prevention efforts that are both targeted and address a multitude of stressors.

Second, we suggest that policy efforts should focus on establishing a multitiered system of prevention for child maltreatment. This multitiered approach has the benefit of working toward optimal life trajectories for all children while targeting the needs of high risk and maltreated children. While we suggest this approach because it casts a broad net, addressing a range of early adverse experiences, we will discuss how knowledge about individual forms of maltreatment should inform prevention efforts within this multitiered system.

We believe that a commitment to these two priorities will move the field beyond a focus on individual types of maltreatment and will contribute to developing programs that prevent maltreatment before it occurs and procure the best outcomes for children who have already experienced maltreatment.

Developing Meaningful Sets of Subpopulations

Given the lack of clarity in the literature about the impact of multitype maltreatment, it may be beneficial for researchers to consider this area a priority. Novel research can identify the impact of overlapping types of maltreatment experiences, thus informing prevention strategies that target the needs of specific, high-risk subpopulations.

As discussed above, the concept of multitype child maltreatment has gained increasing attention in the research literature. This raises questions regarding the most appropriate methods for capturing the overlap in these experiences. A number of methods are used to quantitatively study subpopulations and overlap in experiences of child abuse and neglect. The cumulative approach relies on counting the number of different forms of child abuse and neglect that an individual is exposed to. For example, using this approach, a child who experiences physical abuse and sexual abuse would receive a maltreatment score of "2," as would a child who experiences emotional abuse and neglect. Using the maltreatment scores as a categorical variable (e.g., 0=no form of maltreatment, 1=one form of maltreatment, 2=two forms of maltreatment, and 3=three forms of maltreatment), researchers then examine differences in outcomes based upon the maltreatment categories. For example, Higgins and McCabe (2000a) found that, in comparison to those with one or two forms of child maltreatment, those with three or more forms of maltreatment reported increased levels of trauma symptomatology and self-deprecation.

A major limitation of the cumulative approach is that all forms and combinations of maltreatment are equally weighted. Using the cumulative approach, the combination of sexual abuse and physical abuse for example, is conceptually treated the same as the combination of neglect and emotional abuse. Such an approach limits researchers' capacity to identify the unique ways in which child abuse and neglect overlap and the risk and protective factors associated with unique combinations of maltreatment.

In contrast to the cumulative approach is the researcher-driven, or *a priori*, method of constructing maltreatment groups. Using this approach, researchers manually group individuals together based upon the types and combinations of maltreatment the individual experiences. For example, Moran, Vuchinich, and Hall (2004) explored the differences in substance use outcomes (i.e., tobacco, alcohol, and illicit drugs) for individuals who experienced physical abuse, emotional abuse, or sexual abuse. To explore multitype maltreatment, the research team created a group to include those individuals with physical abuse and sexual abuse. As hypothesized, all forms of abuse were related to later substance use outcomes, with the combination of physical abuse and sexual abuse having the strongest association.

While relatively simple to construct, researcher-driven methods are problematic for a number of reasons. First, few studies have sufficient sample sizes to adequately account for every type and combination of child abuse and neglect. Second, few studies collect data on all forms of child abuse and neglect (i.e., physical abuse, emotional abuse, sexual abuse, and neglect), forcing researchers to construct limited groupings of maltreatment types for future comparison. In the example above, child neglect was not included as a form of child maltreatment and the only combination of multitype maltreatment explored was physical abuse and sexual abuse. Third, if researchers examine all of the traditional forms of abuse and neglect (i.e., physical abuse, emotional abuse, sexual abuse, and neglect) in their research study, a researcher significantly increases the risk of inappropriately suggesting that a relationship between a specific maltreatment pattern and adverse outcome exists (known as a false positive) when comparing all forms and types of maltreatment in relation to predictors and outcomes.

In the last decade, a growing number of researchers have started utilizing mixed modeling techniques to examine questions regarding the overlap of child abuse and neglect (see, for example, Pears et al. 2008; Romano et al. 2006; Berzenski and Yates 2011; Armour et al. 2014; Nooner et al. 2010; Walsh et al. 2012; Hazen et al. 2009). Specifically, Latent Class Analysis (LCA) is a latent variable modeling technique well-suited for identifying subgroups within a population (Neely-Barnes 2010; Lanza and Rhoades 2013). LCA is an analytic approach which groups individuals into homogenous "classes" based upon response patterns to a set of observed variables. The goal of this research technique is to maximize within-class similarities and to maximize the uniqueness of each group. As is the case with other latent variable modeling approaches, the latent variable in LCA accounts for the correlation among a set of observed variables and allows the researcher to explicitly model measurement error. Unlike approaches such as factor analysis, which assumes a continuous latent variable (with factor loadings), the variable in LCA is categorical (with class probabilities). In studying child maltreatment, the categorical variable in LCA represents different combinations of child abuse and neglect.

Once latent classes have been identified, researchers can examine the predictors and outcomes associated with class membership. For example, Pears et al. (2008) identified four classes of child maltreatment in a sample of 117 children involved in the foster care system: (1) supervisory neglect and emotional maltreatment; (2) sexual abuse, emotional maltreatment, supervisory neglect, and physical neglect; (3) physical abuse, emotional maltreatment, supervisory neglect, and physical neglect; and (4) sexual abuse, physical abuse, emotional maltreatment, supervisory neglect, and physical neglect. The authors found differences among the classes on measures of cognitive functioning, internalizing behavior, and externalizing behavior.

Using similar maltreatment measures (i.e., physical abuse, emotional abuse, sexual abuse, emotional neglect, and physical neglect) Romano et al. (2006) identified two latent classes of maltreatment in their sample of 252 pregnant adolescent women: no maltreatment and multiple maltreatment experiences. While those in the multiple maltreatment group reported higher rates of conduct problems, there were no differences between the two groups on measures of depression.

Latent Class Analysis is a promising approach to the study of subpopulations of child abuse and neglect. Knowing that child abuse and neglect often occur in conjunction with other household adversities, it is important that researchers using this approach incorporate other risk factors into the estimation of latent classes. For example, the Adverse Childhood Experiences Study has made great strides in documenting the overlap and developmental impacts associated with early adversity, including, but not limited to, experiences of child abuse and neglect. What is less clear is whether certain combinations of adversity are more common than others (e.g., physical abuse and parental substance abuse) and whether these unique combinations of adversity have unique causal pathways in comparison to other combinations of adversity. Most, but not all, of the research utilizing an LCA approach has found that those who experience any combination of abuse and neglect will have worse outcomes as compared to those who do not experience any maltreatment. The data is less clear regarding whether particular combinations of abuse and neglect have unique risk profiles and whether certain combinations of maltreatment are more predictive of adverse outcomes than others. From a prevention standpoint, learning whether certain forms of adversity are more common than others and whether certain combinations of adversity have unique risk profiles can assist researchers and practitioners in determining when more targeted prevention and intervention strategies are indicated.

Multitiered Systems of Prevention Based on a Public Health Model

Our review of the research suggests a multitiered system based upon a public health prevention framework holds particular promise for promoting child well-being, particularly given the high number of instances of multiple types of maltreatment. Tiered systems have been a key aspect of public health disease prevention for decades (Gordon 1983). Increasingly, researchers and policymakers have recognized the importance of utilizing a public health framework for addressing child maltreatment (Covington 2012). This type of approach can impact entire populations by balancing universal support that benefits all families with increased support for children who are at greatest risk for maltreatment and poor outcomes. In adopting a multitiered approach to maltreatment, the primary level of prevention focuses on supporting all families regardless of risk status, enabling preventative programs and policies to provide universal benefit. At the secondary level, efforts focus on directing additional attention to children and families that are at an increased risk for maltreatment. Given that maltreatment tends to occur in the context of adversity early in life, prevention programs that focus on helping all families while directing additional resources to families with demonstrated need holds promise for decreasing overall rates of maltreatment. When toxic stress and maltreatment occur in spite of strong preventive efforts, programs and policies at the tertiary level address the needs of children who are experiencing the negative effects of growing up in a stressful early environment. This type of prevention approach can be conceptualized as a pyramid, with general preventative policy at the bottom and more targeted and specialized approaches at the top. These approaches at the top of the pyramid address the specific needs of children who have been maltreated or are at risk for maltreatment. Advocates of this approach argue that by directing resources to universal programs, there will be fewer incidents of maltreatment and less need for intervention at the top of the pyramid (Desair and Adriaenssens 2011).

Three-tiered frameworks, with their inherent emphasis on improving context and impacting positive outcomes, are particularly helpful in addressing situations in which children experience multiple types of maltreatment and adversity. The Centers for Disease Control and Prevention (CDC) developed a strategic, three-tiered framework for the prevention of child maltreatment called the Safe, Stable, and Nurturing Relationships and Environments Framework (Arias 2009; CDC 2013). This framework focuses on creating a physical and social environment for children aimed at reducing the occurrence of maltreatment and buffering the impact of adversity early in life. It is based upon the premise that safe, stable, and nurturing relationships and a safe and consistent living situation are key to healthy development. The CDC has also proposed an "Essentials for Childhood" framework which outlines steps communities can take to support essential, strong relationships (CDC 2013). Within this initiative, developing a healthy parent-child relationship is considered a key factor to securing children's well-being and is supported through prevention and intervention efforts at all three tiers as detailed below. (See Chap. 9 for a more detailed description of this framework and its related strategies).

Within a multitiered system of prevention, efforts at primary, secondary, and tertiary levels balance a broad focus on reducing adversity early in life and enhancing supportive environments across all types of maltreatment with specific initiatives informed by research on the prevention of individual forms of maltreatment. Both broad efforts and more targeted approaches are essential to maximizing prevention. In establishing a balance between these two approaches, a first step is identifying which maltreatment experiences lend themselves to targeted approaches and which maltreatment experiences can be effectively addressed through broader approaches.

Targeted approaches that focus on decreasing individual forms of maltreatment should be implemented at all three tiers. For maltreatment types that have clearly identifiable and unique risk factors, prevention efforts that focus on these risk factors are warranted, as in the cases of sexual abuse and head injury. At the secondary and tertiary levels, specific parenting practices and children's specific symptoms can be addressed through targeted interventions. At the secondary level, evidence-based parenting interventions, such as the Incredible Years, can help parents learn how to engage in child-directed play; provide praise and incentives; set limits; handle misbehavior; and be a social, emotional, and academic coach for their children (Webster-Stratton 2000). The Incredible Years program has been shown to reduce harsh discipline and child conduct problems with preschool-aged children, as well as increase positive parenting behaviors (Daro and McCurdy 2007; Webster-Stratton 1998).

At the tertiary level, for a child who is experiencing posttraumatic stress symptoms due to sexual abuse, trauma-focused cognitive behavioral therapy is likely to be a more successful intervention in improving child outcomes than a more broadly focused parent-child support program. This behavioral therapy was initially designed to address the needs of children who have experienced child sexual abuse, but has now been modified to address other traumatic experiences as well (Substance Abuse and Mental Health Services Administration 2013). This joint parent/child intervention leads to a decrease in symptoms of posttraumatic stress disorder, child sexual behaviors, depression, and anxiety (Cohen et al. 2005; Deblinger et al. 1999, 2006).

Alongside these targeted approaches, efforts that focus on bolstering protective factors in caregivers and their children hold particular promise for optimizing early environments while buffering against the risk of maltreatment. There currently is a strong research literature identifying aspects of child-caregiver relationships that are necessary for healthy development, including a focus on safe, stable, and nurturing relationships and the importance of "serve and return interactions." Identified by the Center for the Developing Child at Harvard University, "serve and return interactions" include instances when the caregiver notices a child's interest and responds to that interest. This back and forth interaction is a building block of healthy relationships and supports healthy brain development (Shonkoff et al. 2006). Strengths-based programs that promote healthy relationships are well suited for universal implementation as they benefit caregivers who exhibit a wide range of skills. However, efforts that focus on decreasing negative parenting behavior can feel critical and rejecting to caregivers and may lead to counterproductive results. Efforts that focus on building upon caregiver strengths can increase engagement and commitment to enhancing parenting practices (Kemp et al. 2013; Sykes 2011).

Conclusion

Child abuse and neglect research has historically focused on understanding the unique risk factors and consequences of distinct forms of maltreatment in isolation. There are benefits to this approach, and information gathered about individual forms of maltreatment should inform targeted preventative efforts, when appropriate. However, continuing to focus research and policy efforts on individual forms of maltreatment in isolation is insufficient based on our current understanding of the complexities of the multiple adversities faced by maltreated children. As such, we recommend focusing future research and practice initiatives on the following priorities: creating and understanding more useful subpopulations of at-risk children and developing and evaluating multitiered prevention approaches that can be applied across maltreatment types.

These proposed priorities will increase the breadth of prevention research by focusing on a wider range of adverse early experiences and adopting a public health framework (Gordon 1983). Furthermore, these efforts are designed to help balance the need to support all families and provide additional services to high-risk children and their families. A greater understanding of the cumulative impact of trauma and the identification of meaningful subpopulations of children will inform these efforts. In doing so, prevention efforts can better reflect the lived realities of maltreated children and target the needs of subpopulations of children who are most at risk for poor outcomes.

Reflection: Research on Subtypes of Child Maltreatment and Their Co-occurrence

Todd I. Herrenkohl
University of Washington, Seattle, WA, USA

Following researchers of an earlier generation, I have spent much of the past 20 years studying the life-course patterns of individuals who experienced child maltreatment, with a particular interest in how these individuals cope with and rebound from early adversity. Having been trained in prevention science, I have always held the belief that our primary objective as researchers should be to produce findings that translate very directly to actionable steps for program planning. It is through this lens that I review and critique others' research, and reflect on my own.

What follows is a brief essay on what we know about subtypes of child maltreatment, based largely on a review of literature in which colleagues and I point to inconsistencies in published studies. In our review, we looked at how other researchers approached the task of measuring and analyzing the different subtypes of child abuse (e.g., physical, emotional, and sexual) and neglect. We also looked at findings on the co-occurrence of these subtypes, or the degree to which they overlap. What we found is what most in the field now assume—and have come to understand from documented life histories of individuals who have grown up in abusive home environments—that subtypes do indeed overlap and the more severe and frequent the abuse of one or any form, the more damage inflicted on the individual. However, questions of how and to what extent subtypes overlap in the studies we reviewed are not simply answered. To some extent, what the findings communicated to us is that the answers depend on the choices made in the research process.

The numbers tell the story: In our review, we found that estimates of the co-occurrence of abuse subtypes ranged from around 33 % to 94 % across samples, even when data used in studies were culled from a single data source, such as child welfare records. When more than one data source was used, estimates of the co-occurrence among subtypes varied even more. How the subtypes were measured and whether the variables factored in qualities of an abusive experience—such as whether the abuse was more or less severe—added even more variability.

Another approach to examining questions about co-occurrence is to look at what percentage of individuals exposed to one form of abuse or neglect report exposure to another form. Dong and colleagues (2004) found that rate of co-occurrence varied considerably depending on which subtype was considered first. Among those who reported first that they had been emotionally abused, for example, over 80 % reported they had also been physically abused and about 59 % also reported being emotionally or physically neglected. Interestingly, when sexual abuse was considered first, the overlap with other forms of abuse was much lower—in the range of 20–40 %.

Pointing to the variability and apparent inconsistencies in the data sources and strategies used by researchers is not to imply the findings have no meaning or lack scientific rigor. It is more to suggest that what we know about issues like child abuse subtypes and their covariation is influenced sometimes notably by how researchers choose to study the issue. The take-home message in all of this, it then seems, is that rather than layering new findings on old, we need to first take a step back and ask fundamental questions about how best to study the issue—to question the choices behind a method and to assess whether the method aligns (or not) with those used in other studies. Ultimately, if the goal is to improve practice (as I believe it should be), new research findings are only helpful if they advance what we already know.

The more that is learned about how and to what extent subtypes of maltreatment add to the burden of risk for outcomes like adult depression and cardiovascular disease, which are costly yet increasingly preventable, the better positioned we in the field will be to tailor intervention programs to the very particular needs of individuals, families, and their ethnic and cultural groups. Researchers can help further that goal by continuing to drill down to the underlying patterns and mechanisms of risk that characterize the lived experiences of maltreated children, while all the time remaining mindful of the need to constantly refine, iterate, and standardize our research strategies so that results from studies, like those on child abuse subtypes, are more directly comparable, replicable, and usable in the real world.

References

Anda, R. F., Felitti, V. J., Bremner, J. D., Walker, J. D., Whitfield, C., Perry, B. D., et al. (2006). The enduring effects of abuse and related adverse experiences in childhood. A convergence of evidence from neurobiology and epidemiology. *European Archives of Psychiatry Clinical Neuroscience, 256*(3), 174–186.

Arata, C., Langhinrichsen-Rohling, J., Bowers, D., & O'Farril-Swails, L. (2005). Single versus multi-type maltreatment: An examination of the long-term effects of child abuse. *Journal of Aggression, Maltreatment & Trauma, 11*(4), 29–52.

Arata, C. M., Langhinrichsen-Rohling, J., Bowers, D., & O'Brien, N. (2007). Differential correlates of multi-type maltreatment among urban youth. *Child Abuse and Neglect, 31*(4), 393–415.

Arias, I. (2009). Preventing child maltreatment through public health. *Policy and Practice, 67*(3), 17–18.

Armour, C., Elklit, A., & Christofferson, M. N. (2014). A latent class analysis of childhood maltreatment: Identifying abuse typologies. *Journal of Loss & Trauma: International Perspectives on Stress & Coping, 19*, 23–39.

Arnow, B. A. (2004). Relationships between childhood maltreatment, adult health and psychiatric outcomes, and medical utilization. *Journal of Clinical Psychiatry, 65*(Suppl 12), 10–15.

Berzenski, S. R., & Yates, T. M. (2011). Classes and consequences of multiple maltreatment: A person-centered analysis. *Child Maltreatment, 16*(4), 250–261.

Bullock, D. P., Koval, K. J., Moen, K. Y., Carney, B. T., & Spratt, K. F. (2009). Hospitalized cases of child abuse in America: Who, what, when, and where. *Journal of Pediatric Orthopedics, 29*(3), 231–237.

Child Abuse Prevention and Treatment Act as amended by P.L. 111–320. The CAPTA Reauthorization Act of 2010, 42 U.S.C. § 5106(g).

CDC. (2013). *Essentials for childhood: Steps to create safe, stable, and nurturing relationships.* Atlanta: Centers for Disease Control and Prevention.

Cohen, J. A., Mannarino, A. P., & Knudsen, K. (2005). Treating sexually abused children: 1 year follow-up of a randomized controlled trial. *Child Abuse and Neglect, 29*(2), 135–145.

Covington, T. (2012). The public health approach for understanding and preventing child maltreatment: A brief review of the literature and a call to action. *Child Welfare, 92*(2), 21–39.

Daro, D., & McCurdy, K. (2007). Interventions to prevent child maltreatment. In L. S. Doll, S. E. Bonzo, J. A. Mercy, & D. A. Sleet (Eds.), *Handbook of injury and violence prevention* (pp. 137–155). New York: Springer Science + Business Media.

Deblinger, E., Steer, R. A., & Lippmann, J. (1999). Two-year follow-up study of cognitive behavioral therapy for sexually abused children suffering post-traumatic stress symptoms. *Child Abuse and Neglect, 23*(12), 1371–1378.

Deblinger, E., Mannarino, A. P., Cohen, J. A., & Steer, R. A. (2006). A follow-up study of a multi-site, randomized, controlled trial for children with sexual abuse-related PTSD symptoms. *Journal of the American Academy of Child Adolescent Psychiatry, 45*(12), 1474–1484.

Desair, K., & Adriaenssens, P. (2011). Policy toward child abuse and neglect in Belgium. In N. Gilbert, N. Parton, & M. Skivenes (Eds.), *Child protection systems: International trends and orientations*. New York: Oxford University Press.

Dias, M. S., Smith, K., DeGuehery, K., Mazur, P., Li, V., & Shaffer, M. L. (2005). Preventing abusive head trauma among infants and young children: A hospital-based, parent education program. *Pediatrics, 115*(4), 470–477.

Dong, M., Anda, R. F., Felitti, V. J., Dube, S. R., Williamson, D. F., Thompson, T. J., et al. (2004). The interrelatedness of multiple forms of childhood abuse, neglect, and household dysfunction. *Child Abuse & Neglect, 28*(7), 771–784.

Duhaime, A. C., Christian, C. W., Rorke, L. B., & Zimmerman, R. A. (1998). Nonaccidental head injury in infants—The "shaken-baby syndrome". *New England Journal of Medicine, 338*(25), 1822–1829.

Edwards, V. J., Holden, G. W., Felitti, V. J., & Anda, R. F. (2003). Relationship between multiple forms of childhood maltreatment and adult mental health in community respondents: Results from the adverse childhood experiences study. *American Journal of Psychiatry, 160*(8), 1453–1460.

Edwards, V. J., Freyd, J. J., Dube, S. R., Anda, R. F., & Felitti, V. J. (2012). Health outcomes by closeness of sexual abuse perpetrator: A test of betrayal trauma theory. *Journal of Aggression, Maltreatment & Trauma, 21*(2), 133–148.

Farst, K., Ambadwar, P. B., King, A. J., Bird, T., & Robbins, J. M. (2013). Trends in hospitalization rates and severity of injuries from abuse in young children, 1997–2009. *Pediatrics, 131*(6), e1796–e1802.

Felitti, V., Anda, R., Nordenberg, D., Williamson, D., Spitz, A., Edwards, V., et al. (1998). Relationship of child abuse and household dysfunction to many of the leading causes of death in adults: The Adverse Childhood Experiences (ACE) study. *American Journal of Preventive Medicine, 14*(4), 245–258.

Finkelhor, D., & Jones, L. (2012). Have sexual abuse and physical abuse declined since the 1990s? *Crimes Against Children Research Center.* http://www.unh.edu/ccrc/pdf/CV267_Have%20SA%20%20PA%20Decline_FACT%20SHEET_11-7-12.pdf. Accessed September 2014.

Finkelhor, D., Jones, L., Shattuck, A., & Saito, K. (2013). Updated trends in child maltreatment, 2012. *Crimes Against Children Research Center.* http://www.unh.edu/ccrc/pdf/CV203_Updated%20trends%202012_Revised_2_20_14.pdf. Accessed September 2014.

Finkelhor, D., Shattuck, A., Turner, H. A., & Hamby, S. L. (2014). The lifetime prevalence of child sexual abuse and assault assessed in late adolescence. *Journal of Adolescent Health, 55*(3), 329–333.

Gordon, R. S., Jr. (1983). An operational classification of disease prevention. *Public Health Reports, 98*(2), 107–109.

Hazen, A. L., Connelly, C. D., Roesch, S. C., Hough, R. L., & Landsverk, J. A. (2009). Child maltreatment profiles and adjustment problems in high risk adolescents. *Journal of Interpersonal Violence, 24*(2), 361–378.

Herrenkohl, R. C., & Herrenkohl, T. I. (2009). Assessing a child's experience of multiple maltreatment types: Some unfinished business. *Journal of Family Violence, 24*(7), 485–496.

Higgins, D. J., & McCabe, M. P. (2000a). Multi-type maltreatment and the long-term adjustment of adults. *Child Abuse Review, 9*, 6–18.

Higgins, D. J., & McCabe, M. P. (2000b). Relationships between different types of maltreatment during childhood and adjustment in adulthood. *Child Maltreatment, 5*(3), 261–272.

Higgins, D. J., & McCabe, M. P. (2001). Multiple forms of child abuse and neglect: Adult retrospective reports. *Aggression and Violent Behavior, 6*(6), 547–578.

Jones, L., Finkelhor, D., & Kopiec, K. (2001). Why is sexual abuse declining? A survey of state child protection administrators. *Child Abuse & Neglect, 25*, 1139–1158.

Kemp, S. P., Marcenko, M. O., Lyons, S. J., & Kruzich, J. M. (2013). Strength-based practice and parental engagement in child welfare services: An empirical examination. *Children and Youth Services Review*. Advance online publication. doi:10.1016/j.childyouth.2013.11.001.

Kendall-Tackett, K. A., Williams, L. M., & Finkelhor, D. (1993). The effects of sexual abuse on children: A review and synthesis of recent empirical findings. *Psychological Bulletin, 113*, 164–181.

Lanza, S. T., & Rhoades, B. L. (2013). Latent class analysis: An alternative perspective on subgroup analysis in prevention and treatment. *Prevention Science, 14*(2), 157–168.

Leventhal, J. M., Martin, K. D., & Gaither, J. R. (2012). Using U.S. data to estimate the incidence of serious physical abuse in children. *Pediatrics, 129*(3), 458–464.

Martyniuk, H., & Dworkin, E. (2011). Child sexual abuse prevention: Programs for children. *National Sexual Violence Resource Center*. Retrieved September 2014 from http://www.nsvrc.org/sites/default/files/Publications_NSVRC_Guide_Child-Sexual-Abuse-Prevention-programs-for-children.pdf

Meston, C. M., & Lorenz, T. A. (2013). Physiological stress responses predict sexual functioning and satisfaction differently in women who have and have not been sexually abused in childhood. *Psychological Trauma: Theory, Research, Practice, and Policy, 5*(4), 350–358.

Moran, P. B., Vuchinich, S., & Hall, N. K. (2004). Associations between type of maltreatment and substance use during adolescence. *Child Abuse & Neglect, 28*, 565–574.

Neely-Barnes, S. (2010). Latent class models in social work. *Social Work Research, 34*(2), 114–121.

Nooner, K. B., Litrownik, A. J., Thompson, R., Margolis, B., English, D. J., Knight, E. D., et al. (2010). Youth self-report of physical and sexual abuse: A latent class analysis. *Child Abuse & Neglect, 34*, 146–154.

Pears, K. C., Kim, H. K., & Fisher, P. A. (2008). Psychosocial and cognitive functioning of children with specific profiles of maltreatment. *Child Abuse & Neglect, 32*, 958–971.

Plummer, C., & Klein, A. (2013). Using policies to promote child sexual abuse prevention: What is working. http://www.vawnet.org/applied-research-papers/summary.php?doc_id=3554&find_type=web_desc_AR

Putnam, F. W. (2003). Ten year research update review: Child sexual abuse. *Journal of the American Academy of Child Adolescent Psychiatry, 42*(3), 269–278.

Putnam-Hornstein, E., Cleves, M. A., Licht, R., & Needell, B. (2013). Risk of fatal injury in young children following abuse allegations: Evidence from a prospective, population-based study. *American Journal of Public Health, 103*(10), e39–e44.

Reece, R. M. (2011). Medical evaluation of physical abuse. In J. E. B. Myers (Ed.), *The APSAC handbook on child maltreatment* (pp. 183–194). Thousand Oaks: Sage Publications.

Rispens, J., Aleman, A., & Goudena, P. P. (1997). Prevention of child sexual abuse victimization: A meta-analysis of school programs. *Child Abuse and Neglect, 21*(10), 975–987.

Romano, E., Zoccolillo, M., & Paquette, D. (2006). Histories of child maltreatment and psychiatric disorder in pregnant adolescents. *Journal of American Academy of Child & Adolescent Psychiatry, 45*(3), 329–336.

Sedlak, A. J., Mettenburg, J., Basena, M., Petta, I., McPherson, K., Greene, A., et al. (2010). *Fourth National Incidence Study of Child Abuse and Neglect (NIS–4): Report to Congress, executive summary*. Washington, DC: U.S. Department of Health and Human Services, Administration for Children and Families.

Shonkoff, J. P., Callister, G., & Oberklaid, F. (2006). *The science of early childhood development: Closing the gap between what we know and what we do*. National Scientific Council on the Developing Child (online publication). http://developingchild.harvard.edu/resources/reports_and_working_papers/science_of_early_childhood_development/. Accessed September 2014.

Stephenson, K. R., Hughan, C. P., & Meston, C. M. (2012). Childhood sexual abuse moderates the association between sexual functioning and sexual distress in women. *Child Abuse & Neglect, 36*(2), 180–189.

Stiffman, M. N., Schnitzer, P. G., Adam, P., Kruse, R. L., & Ewigman, B. G. (2002). Household composition and risk of fatal child maltreatment. *Pediatrics, 109*(4), 615–621.

Stith, S. M., Liu, T., Davies, L. C., Boykin, E. L., Alder, M. C., Harris, J. M., et al. (2009). Risk factors in child maltreatment: A meta-analytic review of the literature. *Aggression and Violent Behavior, 14*(1), 13–29.

Substance Abuse and Mental Health Services Administration. (2013). Trauma-focused cognitive behavioral therapy (TF-CBT). http://www.nrepp.samhsa.gov/viewintervention.aspx?id=135. Accessed 22 Mar 2013.

Sykes, J. (2011). Negotiating stigma: Understanding mothers' responses to accusations of child neglect. *Children and Youth Services Review, 33*(3), 448–456.

Teicher, M., Samson, J., Polcari, A., & McGreenery, C. (2006). Sticks, stones, and hurtful words: Relative effects of various forms of childhood maltreatment. *American Journal of Psychiatry, 163*(6), 993–1000.

Turner, H. A., Finkelhor, D., & Ormrod, R. (2010). Poly-victimization in a national sample of children and youth. *American Journal of Preventive Medicine, 38*(3), 323–330.

U.S. Department of Health and Human Services. (2013). *Child maltreatment 2012.* http://www.acf.hhs.gov/sites/default/files/cb/cm2012.pdf. Accessed 18 Aug 2014.

Walsh, J. L., Senn, T. E., & Carey, M. P. (2012). Exposure to different types of violence and subsequent sexual risk behavior among female sexually transmitted disease clinic patients: A latent class analysis. *Psychology of Violence, 2*(4), 339–354.

Webster-Stratton, C. (1998). Preventing conduct problems in Head Start children: Strengthening parent competencies. *Journal of Consulting and Clinical Psychology, 66*(5), 715–730.

Webster-Stratton, C. (2000). *Juvenile justice bulletin* (The incredible years training series). Washington, DC: Office of Juvenile Justice and Delinquency Prevention.

Welch, G. L., & Bonner, B. L. (2013). Fatal child neglect: Characteristics, causation, and strategies for prevention. *Child Abuse & Neglect, 37*(10), 745–752.

Whittier, N. (2009). *The politics of child sexual abuse: Emotion, social movement, and the state.* New York: Oxford University Press.

Zwi, K. J., Woolfenden, S. R., Wheeler, D. M., O'Brien, T. A., Tait, P., & Williams, K. W. (2008). Cochrane review: School-based education programmes for the prevention of child sexual abuse. *Evidence-Based Child Health: A Cochrane Review Journal, 3*(3), 603–634.

Amanda Van Scoyoc is a doctoral student in clinical psychology at the University of Oregon. Amanda's research focuses on promoting child well-being and preventing family disruption by addressing maternal addiction in pregnancy. Specifically, her doctoral research identifies pregnant women's common experiences and behavioral patterns while abusing substances in pregnancy. This project aims to identify protective behaviors that women engage in due to concerns about the developing fetus and determine whether these behaviors predict seeking treatment. Amanda has a documentary studies background and a strong interest in the dissemination of research findings beyond academia. Amanda received a B.A. in psychology from University of Pennsylvania and an M.S. in psychology from University of Oregon. Her research has been supported by the Doris Duke Charitable Foundation and the Lewis Hine Documentary Fellows Program.

Jessica S. Wilen currently coordinates special projects for the Office of the Vice Chancellor for Students at Washington University. In this role, she manages a university-wide sexual assault and relationship violence task force, develops and implements diversity and inclusion initiatives, and creates systems for at-risk students. Dr. Wilen received her doctoral degree in social work from Bryn Mawr College of Social Work and Social Research, where her research focused on treatment for adult survivors of childhood sexual abuse and research synthesis. Dr. Wilen's dissertation work was supported by the *Doris Duke Fellowships for the Promotion of Childhood Well-Being.* Previously, Dr. Wilen's worked as a clinical social worker with both survivors and perpetrators of sexual and domestic violence.

Kate Daderko is a postdoctoral fellow at Penn Medicine, where she provides treatment to children who have experienced trauma. She recently received her doctorate in school psychology from the

University of Washington. Kate's research and clinical interests are in child maltreatment, school-based mental health, and providing effective treatments for trauma.

Sheridan Miyamoto is a recent graduate of the Nursing Science and Health-Care Leadership doctoral program at the Betty Irene Moore School of Nursing at UC Davis. Prior to joining the School of Nursing, she was the clearance exam program coordinator at UC Davis Medical Center's Child and Adolescent Abuse Resource and Evaluation Diagnostic and Treatment Center, providing health and forensic services to children in Northern California. She also supported six rural sites through live telehealth sexual assault consultations, allowing children to receive quality care within their own community. Sheridan's research interests include merging administrative databases to improve risk tools to identify families at risk of recurrent subsequent serious maltreatment and the use of telehealth technology to improve forensic care for children in rural communities.

Jim—

Looking
forward to
working together
for years.

Lisa

Chapter 3
Preventing Adolescent Maltreatment: A Focus on Child Welfare, Juvenile Justice, and Sexual Exploitation

Carly B. Dierkhising, Jennifer Mullins Geiger, Tamara E. Hurst, Carlomagno Panlilio, and Lisa Schelbe

Chapter 3 in Brief

Context

- Little is known about the etiology, consequences, and circumstances related to adolescent maltreatment and how to prevent it.
- While self-report and population-based incidence studies suggest adolescents experience high rates of maltreatment, they are consistently less likely to be formally reported to child welfare agencies.

C.B. Dierkhising (✉)
School of Criminal Justice and Criminalistics, California State University, Los Angeles,
Los Angeles, CA, USA
e-mail: Carly.dierkhising@calstatela.edu

J.M. Geiger
Jane Addams College of Social Work, University of Illinois at Chicago, Chicago, IL, USA
e-mail: jmullins@asu.edu

T.E. Hurst
School of Social Work, The University of Southern Mississippi, Hattiesburg, MS, USA
e-mail: tamara.hurst@usm.edu

C. Panlilio
Department of Human Development and Quantitative Methodology, University of Maryland,
College Park, MD, USA
e-mail: panlilio@umd.edu

L. Schelbe
College of Social Work, Florida State University, Tallahassee, FL, USA
e-mail: Lschelbe@fsu.edu

© Springer International Publishing Switzerland 2015   43
D. Daro et al. (eds.), *Advances in Child Abuse Prevention Knowledge*,
Child Maltreatment 5, DOI 10.1007/978-3-319-16327-7_3

- Unlike younger children, adolescents are more likely to be abused outside the home in settings such as foster care and the juvenile justice system, suggesting that these residential settings present important opportunities for prevention.
- Child sexual exploitation is an increasingly recognized form of child maltreatment that disproportionately impacts adolescents.

Strategies for Moving Forward

- More consistently recognize and document adolescent maltreatment and its impact on adolescent development.
- Develop assessment protocols that effectively identify sexually exploited youth in a variety of service settings (e.g., mental health centers, juvenile detention facilities) and determine population overlap.
- Develop prevention programs that focus on pregnancy and parenting youth, pregnancy prevention, and youth in, and aging out of, foster care and the juvenile justice system.

Implications for Research

- Study the prevalence of repeating the cycle of abuse among youth who age out of foster care as well as the intersection of foster care, juvenile justice, and sexual exploitation since so many adolescents are involved in multiple systems.
- Conduct rigorous evaluations of initiatives focusing on preventing adolescent maltreatment and those focused on improving outcomes.
- Apply theoretical frameworks to policies regarding sexual exploitation to determine if and how they prevent maltreatment.
- Systematically identify the prevalence of pregnancy and parenting among youth and assess the efficacy of pregnancy prevention and parenting services available to at-risk youth.

Introduction

Much of the child maltreatment literature and much of child maltreatment prevention programming focuses on young children. Far fewer resources have been devoted to examining the etiology and circumstances related to maltreatment experienced by adolescents (Hoekstra 1984; Mersky et al. 2009). In contrast to trends observed in formal child abuse reporting data (U.S. Department of Health and Human Services 2013a), adolescents have been shown to experience higher rates of maltreatment when compared to younger children in population based surveys (Finkelhor et al. 2005). For instance, in a national prevalence study of child and adolescent victimization, children between the ages of 10 and 13 were four times more likely to experience physical assault or sexual abuse within a given year than children under the age of 1 (Finkelhor et al. 2009). Similarly, Everson and colleagues found prevalence rates 4–6 times higher for self-reported physical, sexual, and psychological abuse among adolescents when compared to the number of child welfare reports that involve an adolescent victim (Everson et al. 2008).

It is not clear why adolescent maltreatment has received less focused attention from the research and policy community. Some scholars have theorized that this may be related to the actual or perceived maturity of adolescents (Hoekstra 1984; Powers and Eckenrode 1988). Maturity, particularly physical maturity, may make it seem as though adolescents are more able than young children to protect themselves when faced with danger or remove themselves from dangerous situations. Adolescents also are often expected to independently seek out help from professionals (Hoekstra 1984). In some cases, adolescents may be perceived as "deserving" of punishment in cases where they act out or defy authority. Ryan and colleagues (2013) hypothesized that a perception of adolescents as "troublesome" rather than "troubled" (p. 462) occurs at the system response level (e.g., the juvenile justice system), adding a layer of complexity that makes it difficult for adolescents to receive needed attention (Ryan et al. 2013).

This chapter utilizes a developmental perspective which recognizes that adolescents experience maltreatment differently than younger children, due to changes in their bio-psychosocial capacities and developmental trajectory (Cicchetti and Rogosch 2002; Ryan et al. 2013). In fact, Ryan and colleagues posit that adolescent maltreatment may be a qualitatively different experience than maltreatment experienced by young children. For instance, conceptualizing neglect as an act of commission (e.g., locking an adolescent out) might be more accurate than conceptualizing neglect as an act of omission, as is typically done with younger children (Ryan et al. 2013). In addition, adolescent maltreatment is often masked as family conflict, with adolescents and their caregivers hitting or abusing each other (Hoekstra 1984). Importantly, the meaning adolescents attach to maltreatment experiences may also contribute to varying outcomes and consequences (Cicchetti and Rogosch 2002).

Central to an adolescent's development is a gradual increase in the time spent out of the home and the importance of peer relationships as opposed to family relationships. While much of the maltreatment reported to and addressed by child welfare agencies reflect acts occurring in the home and committed by parents, an adolescent may face greater risk for maltreatment outside the home. As such, researchers, policymakers, and practitioners concerned with adolescent maltreatment prevention need to consider alternative contexts where adolescent maltreatment might occur, such as foster care, the juvenile justice system, or the street. In considering these alternative pathways to maltreatment, it is important to examine the specific acts of maltreatment that adolescents might experience and how these acts may differ from the common perception of what constitutes child abuse and neglect.

This chapter discusses the prevalence of adolescent maltreatment, explores the need to develop interventions and prevention strategies for adolescent maltreatment within alternative contexts, and identifies emerging strategies and necessary next steps for improving the collective response to this problem.

The Context of Adolescent Maltreatment

Adolescents comprise approximately one-fifth (21 %) of official reports to child protective services across the country, although the rate and percentage of victimization decreases with age (U.S. Department of Health and Human Services 2013a). Although neglect and physical abuse are the most common reasons for reports across all age groups, adolescents more frequently report experiencing emotional and sexual abuse than do younger children (Raissian et al. 2014). In contrast to the story suggested by national child welfare reporting data, prevalence studies utilizing self-report data find that adolescents experience significantly more maltreatment, of all types, than younger children. When differences between specific types are examined, adolescents report significantly higher rates of physical abuse and emotional abuse than younger children (Finkelhor et al. 2005). Importantly, evidence suggests that maltreatment experienced in adolescence—or in both childhood *and* adolescence—has particularly detrimental effects on a variety of developmental domains (Thornberry et al. 2010). For instance, Thornberry and colleagues (2010) found that compared to maltreatment occurring only in early childhood, persistent maltreatment (maltreatment in both early childhood and adolescence) and maltreatment occurring only during adolescence had a broader and more consistent effect on delinquency, drug use, depression, risky sexual behavior, and both internalizing and externalizing problems in late adolescence.

Cumulative Risk

While the timing of maltreatment is salient in terms of later developmental outcomes, it is also essential to consider the experience of chronic or multiple types of maltreatment during early childhood and adolescence. An abundance of literature demonstrates that there is a dose-response relationship between the number of types of maltreatment in childhood and adolescence, as well as other traumatic experiences, with concurrent and long-term social, emotional, and health problems (Felitti et al. 1998; Finkelhor et al. 2011; Ford et al. 2011). Adolescents, compared to younger children, have been shown to experience significantly higher rates of experiencing multiple types of trauma (Finkelhor et al. 2007). This puts adolescents at greater risk for depression, posttraumatic stress, drug abuse, delinquency, and comorbid mental health disorders (Ford et al. 2010).

Crossover Youth Between Child Welfare and Juvenile Justice

Adolescent maltreatment and its associated outcomes are risk factors for involvement in foster care, the juvenile justice system, and sexual exploitation. Thus, it is not surprising that there is overlap in the youth experiencing contact with these agencies or these behaviors. True rates of overlap, or concurrent involvement, in these contexts among youth are largely unknown and somewhat unstable because of the dearth of research on sexual exploitation. However, there is an emerging area of research on crossover youth that provides some evidence on the frequency of involvement in both the child welfare or foster care system and the juvenile justice system (Herz et al. 2010). There are varying pathways from child maltreatment to delinquency and different levels of system involvement (Jonson-Reid and Barth 2000). Some crossover youth (also known as dually involved youth) move from the child welfare system (e.g., dependency court) into the juvenile justice system (e.g., delinquency court) while others experience the reverse sequence (Herz et al. 2010). In still other instances, maltreated youth who are never formally reported to child welfare or placed in foster care also frequently end up in the juvenile justice system (Dierkhising et al. 2013b). Nevertheless, studies have revealed that up to 42 % of justice-involved youth could be considered dually-involved or having official contact with both systems (Dierkhising et al. 2013b; Herz et al. 2010).

Crossover with Respect to Sexual Exploitation

Less is known about how many youth who have been involved in child welfare or the juvenile justice system also experience sexual exploitation. Youth with prior involvement in the child welfare system, in particular, have been found to be at risk for sexual exploitation (Shared Hope International 2009). In terms of their involvement with the justice system, sexually exploited youth who have had prior involvement in the juvenile justice system for other delinquent offenses are often treated as an offender rather than a victim on these charges, which may result in arrest and incarceration (Halter 2010). Efforts to distinguish "victim" from "offender" at the time a youth is arrest for a sexual offense are emerging but still in their infancy. For instance, Shared Hope International, a nonprofit agency based in Washington, DC, reports that while most states have enacted laws addressing human trafficking, there are vast disparities in how each state addresses victims and whether victims are subject to the state's prostitution law (Shared Hope International 2013).

Continued examination of the overlap among foster care, juvenile justice system, and sexual exploitation populations is needed to further understand the interaction between these populations and how best to target interventions and prevention efforts. Maltreated youth who enter the foster care system face a unique set of challenges and experience high rates of poor outcomes, particularly in those cases in which permanent placement is not identified and the youth "age out" of the system

(Courtney and Dworsky 2006). Similarly, adolescents in the juvenile justice system, who may also experience high rates of victimization during stays in residential facilities, face significant challenges once they exit this system (Beck et al. 2010; Mendel 2011; Sedlak and McPherson 2010). Finally, a recent Institute of Medicine report on sexual exploitation has described sexual exploitation as an "overlooked, misunderstood, and unaddressed form of child abuse" (Institute of Medicine 2013, p. 1). Collectively, all three of these populations face significant risk for continued mistreatment and poor life outcomes, making them appropriate and important targets for well-designed interventions.

Emerging Trends and New Perspectives

Despite the complexities in identifying and reaching these vulnerable adolescents, emerging research in all three domains suggest potential targets for prevention. This section considers these emerging trends and how practices and policies within the child welfare system, juvenile justice system, and the response to sexually exploited youth present opportunities for targeting and improving treatment and prevention efforts.

Adolescents and the Child Welfare System

As noted above, adolescents are less likely than younger children to be reported for maltreatment. However, once referred and accepted into the system, adolescents are more likely than young children to be placed in congregate care and residential settings versus family foster care or with relatives (U.S. Department of Health and Human Services 2013a), despite the fact that family and relative placements generally produce more favorable outcomes in terms of stability, support, and other positive traits (Barth et al. 2007). Somewhat predictable given their placement experiences, adolescents are more likely than younger children to leave care by aging out of foster care than through adoption, reunification with parents, or guardianship (U.S. Department of Health and Human Services 2013a). Although there are services to assist in the preparation for living independently, aging out of foster care often exacerbates many of the behavioral challenges and the emotional trauma associated with the maltreatment that first brought them into care (Antle et al. 2009; Goodkind et al. 2011).

Many of the poor psychosocial outcomes associated with aging out of foster care are highly correlated with child maltreatment risk factors, such as poor mental health, low educational attainment, unemployment, homelessness, and poverty. These risk factors place youth with a history of child maltreatment and child welfare system involvement at potentially greater risk of maltreating children, compared with others who have no history of maltreatment or child welfare system involvement (Geiger and Schelbe 2014).

In the last few decades, legislation has been adopted and implemented to address the needs of adolescents in the child welfare system as they prepare to leave care and become adults. For example, the Fostering Connections to Success and Increasing Adoptions Act of 2008 allows states to extend youths' stay in the child welfare system until age 21 and to let youth reenter care if needed. In addition, this legislation provides additional support for child welfare agencies to increase permanency support for all children in foster care through adoption or guardianship with relatives. It promotes educational stability and health care coordination, reinforcing the need for relationship building with youth in foster care often demonstrated in the literature (Ahrens et al. 2011; Goodkind et al. 2011; Jones 2013; Scott et al. 2012).

Evaluations of this legislative change has found that youth who remain in care or receive services (or both) until the age of 21 (versus the age of 18) tend to have better outcomes in several areas such as health insurance coverage (Dworsky et al. 2013), economic and housing stability, employment, and education (Courtney and Dworsky 2006). In addition, youth remaining in care longer have lower rates of unintended pregnancy and early parenting (Dworsky and Courtney 2010). In a study examining the services for pregnant and parenting youth in foster care, Dworsky and Decoursey (2009) found that 22 % of the sample was investigated for abuse or neglect of their child, with 11 % having a child placed in foster care. (The added risk this population faces with respect to the intergenerational transmission of child maltreatment is discussed in greater detail in Chap. 4).

The Juvenile Justice System's Role in Maltreatment Prevention

The juvenile justice system is rarely considered in relation to maltreatment prevention despite the fact that the majority of youth who become involved with the juvenile justice system have histories of trauma and maltreatment (Dierkhising et al. 2013b; Kerig and Becker 2010). Because of the extensive trauma histories of justice-involved youth, there is a growing focus on reforming the juvenile justice system at the federal and local levels (see, for example, National Research Council 2013; Newell and Leap 2013; U.S. Department of Justice 2012). Much of this work is based on empirical research, practice changes, and advocacy efforts that strive for trauma-informed juvenile justice systems (Dierkhising et al. 2013a; Griffin et al. 2012). A trauma-informed juvenile justice system is one that attempts to: ameliorate the impact of prior trauma through screening, assessment, and interventions; reduce further traumatization; and cultivate a safe environment of care (see Dierkhising et al. 2013a). In this section, we discuss the role specific system components, such as the quality of the environment, the rights of youth, and the role of oversight agencies, may play in contributing to youth outcomes.

Environment of Care

A critical component of maltreatment prevention is the quality of the environment youth experience during their stays in juvenile facilities. Not all youth who are arrested, even if they stand before a juvenile court judge, will be incarcerated in a residential juvenile facility. In fact, only a small minority of youth who are involved in the juvenile justice system spend time in these facilities. In 2011, nearly 1.5 million youth were arrested for a variety of crimes in the United States and in 2010, there were approximately 80,000 youth in juvenile facilities for committing juvenile crime (Puzzanchera 2013; Hockenberry 2013). In addition to youth who are housed in residential juvenile justice facilities, many more spend short stays in detention facilities following their arrest or while awaiting court dates. It is these two groups of youth for whom maltreatment is a particular concern, due to their increased risk of abuse during detainment or incarceration.

Recent national surveys of youth in juvenile facilities have overwhelmingly demonstrated that many youth are not safe while they are detained or incarcerated (Mendel 2011). Findings from the National Survey of Youth in Custody reveal that up to 10 % of youth report being sexually victimized by a staff member and the Survey of Youth in Residential Placement reveals that 28 % of youth experienced forceful restraint during their stay (Beck et al. 2010; Sedlak and McPherson 2010). In their efforts to examine the impacts of mistreatment on youth while in the juvenile justice system, Dierkhising and colleagues (2014) noted they were not able to control for whether such actions were recognized as legal (approved use of restraint, for example) or as an excessive use of force. While such a distinction has meaning for a legal perspective, the concept may have less value when considering the impact of such actions on a youth's social and emotional functioning. Other recent work also has shown that perceptions of the institutional experience, including safety, were related to other outcomes, such as recidivism (Schubert et al. 2012).

Similarly, Dierkhising and colleagues (2014) examined how abuse during incarceration is related to adjustment post release and found that witnessed, direct, and vicarious experiences of abuse (e.g., hearing about others being abused) were significantly related to increased posttraumatic stress, depression, and criminal involvement post release. Although more research is needed to shed light on the relationship between the environment of care and post release outcomes, these findings confirm that there is a relationship between these two constructs.

These statistics shed light on a pervasive but widely unrecognized context for child maltreatment prevention and are especially disturbing when considered along with the high rates of prior child maltreatment and victimization in this population. A study of over 600 youth involved in the justice system revealed that nearly half experienced prior emotional or psychological abuse, nearly two in five experienced prior physical abuse, and about a quarter experienced prior sexual abuse (Dierkhising et al. 2013b). Unfortunately, youth with prior maltreatment histories are at increased risk for abuse during incarceration (Beck et al. 2010; Dierkhising et al. 2014). For instance, a national survey of youth in juvenile facilities revealed that youth with prior sexual abuse histories were more than twice as likely to experience sexual abuse or assault during their stay in a juvenile facility (Beck et al. 2010).

Despite national prevalence studies, there is still limited existing research and information about what is actually happening to youth while they are incarcerated (rather than prior to incarceration) and how the environment of care may impact them post release. Having data on the relationship between how youth are treated during incarceration and post release outcomes might aid program planners and policymakers as they work to design appropriate preventive care environments.

Youth Rights

It is the legal and constitutional right of incarcerated youth to be free from abuse during incarceration (Burrell 1999; Dierkhising et al. 2014). Steps in providing a safe environment include informing youth of their rights, ensuring searches are as unintrusive as possible, staff receive appropriate training and supervision, and youth knowing who they can speak to if they are unsafe or experience abuse (Burrell 2013). Grievance policies, the typical method for reporting abuse, are important to have in place and should have clear guidelines. For instance, the Survey of Youth in Residential Placement revealed that one-third of youth had problems with grievance policies, such as not knowing how to file one or fear of retribution (Sedlak and McPherson 2010). Youth should also have multiple methods for reporting abuse, be assured that their complaint will receive attention, and not fear retribution for filing a grievance.

Oversight Committees

Local and federal policies also play an important role in ending the maltreatment of adolescents in juvenile facilities. The Prison Rape Elimination Act includes language for improving external oversight of facilities. It encourages increased access for advocates and stakeholders to the facilities and victims of sexual assault. A related policy was implemented by the presiding judge of Los Angeles Children's Court in 2011. The judge issued a controversial court order to open access to dependency court proceedings to the press, in hopes of bringing attention to critical issues faced by the court and the children it works to protect. While this practice no longer exists in Los Angeles, proponents of allowing access to court proceedings suggest that the policy can promote system reform by providing a more accurate picture of the system for legislators and the public and by increasing transparency and oversight of those who work in the system (Kapolko 2012). A similar policy for juvenile facilities could potentially lead to partnerships between community-based partners, researchers, and the juvenile court, and improve transparency and oversight of the system in order to prevent abuse.

Adolescents and Sexual Exploitation

Child sexual exploitation is a rapidly growing form of child maltreatment that disproportionately impacts adolescents, although there is limited research on its etiology and consequences (Institute of Medicine 2013). Indeed, the research on this population is far outpaced by the need for services and policies to protect children and adolescents from involvement in sexual exploitation. Despite this dearth of research, there is an emerging literature that illuminates the challenges associated with identifying and supporting victims of exploitation and provides important insights for practitioners and professionals who come in contact with this population.

Defining Terms

First, it is important to clearly define sexual exploitation and the scope of the population affected (Countryman-Roswurm and Bolin 2014). Child sexual exploitation is a form of child maltreatment commonly defined as an exchange of sex by a male or female under the age of 18 for tangible or intangible goods such as shelter, food, love, transportation, or money. Some adolescents may be more vulnerable to sexual exploitation because of homelessness, histories of child maltreatment, mental illness, substance abuse, low socio-economic status, or other risk factors (Estes and Weiner 2001). Sexual exploitation, for many adolescents, becomes a means to survive through obtaining basic necessities and has been noted as a pathway to commercial sexual exploitation (Roe-Sepowitz 2012). The commercial sexual exploitation of children typically involves a third party who reaps economic gains when children or adolescents exchange sex for tangible goods such as money or drugs. This third party is sometimes referred to as a "pimp" or "sex trafficker." In some instances, pimps or sex traffickers can be family members, peers, or acquaintances. In other cases, these parties are initially unknown to the youth.

Training Issues

Accurately identifying victims of sex trafficking is difficult and challenging even for highly trained and experienced helping professionals. Survivors of child sexual exploitation may not identify themselves as such out of fear or a lack of awareness that help is available (Macy and Graham 2012). Standard mental health protocols or youth assessment guidelines may be less effective with sexually exploited youth, who often feel threatened by their exploiters or feel compelled to protect them. Others may not discuss the circumstances surrounding the sexual exploitation, believing that trained professions are knowledgeable about the issue and therefore fully aware of what help they need. When these expectations go unmet, the lack of an appropriate response comingles with the youth's lack of trust in helping professionals, an outcome that has been documented in both empirical literature (Hurst 2013; Williams and Frederick 2009) and anecdotal literature (Lloyd 2011).

This combination of unmet expectations with a fundamental lack of trust can result in further alienating the youth from the very people who attempt to help.

Most states have recognized the need to address sexual exploitation in the laws that govern mandated reporters. These reporters are typically professionals such as medical personnel, educators, child welfare professionals, and law enforcement officials, and they are often the first to come into contact with youth who have been sexually exploited, whether commercially by third parties or as a means to survive. However, training mandated reporters to recognize youth sexual victimization through exploitive acts has been slow to develop and be disseminated. Many rural areas have little access to training, as most established programs are found in urban centers (e.g., My Life My Choice in Boston; Girls Education and Mentoring Services in New York; Breaking Free in Minneapolis; and Children of the Night in Los Angeles). Even with training, some professionals remain unable to identify child victims of sexual exploitation, indicating a need for program and training evaluations that can target areas for improved assessment capabilities and skill development (McMahon-Howard and Reimers 2013).

Challenges with victim identification combined with the absence of widespread training can be coupled with the notion that each professional or mandated reporter may have just one opportunity to recognize a child victim of sexual exploitation (Macy and Graham 2012). For example, a trafficked youth may appear at a health clinic one day and at a shelter the next. This allows mandated reporters a small window of time in which to identify a victim, build enough rapport to engage the youth, and provide resources. For this reason, it is clear that diverse groups of professionals must become knowledgeable about how to identify and respond to victims of child sexual exploitation and develop agency- or system-wide protocols specifically for sexually exploited youth.

Underlying a widespread lack of training is helping professionals' dualistic perspective of adolescents as either offenders of sexual solicitation laws or victims manipulated by those who buy or sell sex. Williams and Frederick (2009) studied the various relationships between youth and the social institutions and agencies with which youth come into contact. They noted professionals at agencies designed to help youth may also treat them as perpetrators of crimes rather than victims of exploitation. Other literature has also noted extreme variations in the treatment of sexually exploited adolescents by law enforcement officials, indicating a need for increased training on the dynamics of sexual exploitation (Finkelhor and Ormrod 2004; Halter 2010). Specifically, it has been suggested that law enforcement officials need training that reframes their concept of sexually trafficked youth as victims, rather than as offenders (Raphael et al. 2010).

This inconsistent treatment of adolescents may be due to a lack of education but scenarios described by survivors point to deeper social justice issues. These include the use of authority with a vulnerable population of sexually exploited youth and perhaps personal, subjective determinations of which youth might be deserving of protection (Hurst 2013). There is also an underlying notion that youth consider themselves neither "victim" nor "offender," but "survivor" (Williams 2010). The youth feel they have learned and applied survival skills to obtain basic human needs such as food and shelter, overcoming and enduring experiences of childhood maltreatment and victimization.

Treatment Needs

Although a willingness to assist sexually exploited youth seems apparent, there is an absence of specialized support services and a lack of direction among mandated reporters and other professionals. For example, sexually exploited youth may have experiences of complex trauma resulting from multiple forms of childhood maltreatment (e.g., physical, sexual, and emotional abuse or neglect), which likely increased their vulnerability to sexual exploitation (Hurst 2013; Roe-Sepowitz 2012). There are also few therapeutic housing options within the child welfare system designed for these youth, leading some to suggest the need for explicit partnerships between child welfare and those private agencies serving this population (Fong and Cardoso 2010). Unfortunately, there are very few private agencies serving sexually exploited youth with the skills and resources to serve these cases. Further, evaluations on the effectiveness of these programs are limited. Once in the foster care system, sexually exploited youth, like all youth taken into care, may experience a disruption in their education due to multiple placements and often lack family members who can participate in family treatment programs (Fong and Cardoso 2010).

Research thus far indicates that the prevention of sexual exploitation requires coordinated efforts and training of mandated reporters and other helping professionals. Difficulty with victim identification, lack of widely available effective training, limited response time, and a lack of therapeutic options hinder helping professionals and mandated reporters. Additionally, negative encounters with frontline personnel seem to exacerbate the extent of mistrust felt by youth who may have already experienced maltreatment or other traumas. The limited research on the identification and service provision for sexually exploited youth indicates that this is a unique population that requires targeted assessment and identification techniques, individualized services, and widespread training among professionals from a variety of agencies these youth may come in contact with.

Strategies Moving Forward: Implications for Practice and Policy

Recognizing Maltreatment Among Adolescents

Adolescents have different social and behavioral manifestations and reactions to maltreatment than younger children. For example, adolescents are more likely to express oppositional and reactive behaviors with adults and authority figures, run away, or engage in risky behaviors such as substance use and unprotected sex (Ford et al. 1999; National Child Traumatic Stress Network 2009; Putnam 2006). Adolescents' emotions and behaviors following maltreatment tend to attract the attention of law enforcement rather than child welfare professionals or other treatment providers (Lab et al. 2000). Practitioners and other mandated reporters (e.g., teachers) should consider adolescent behavior in context and respond with the most appropriate services and support.

It is also important to recognize that some adolescents who come to the attention of the juvenile justice system may be victims of sexual exploitation and should be treated as such. The response of the justice system to an adolescent involved in sexual exploitation, and a subsequent status determination of victim or delinquent, may depend upon law enforcement training and individual personal beliefs (Mitchell et al. 2010). Preventing further maltreatment might require an increase in law enforcement and juvenile court awareness of the etiology of sexual exploitation and a change in institutional policies to increase the identification of victims.

Placement Options for Youth in Foster Care

Practitioners and policymakers should work together to improve placement options for adolescents when placed in out of home care. Currently, almost 40 % of adolescents reside in group homes or residential facilities and institutions, compared with only 15 % of younger children (U.S. Department of Health and Human Services 2013b). Expanding the pool of available placements for adolescents required a more intentional effort to recruit and train foster parents with the interest and skills to meet the needs of adolescents. This process begins with understanding the challenges and benefits of being a foster parent as well as what factors are related to families' willingness to foster. For example, Geiger and colleagues found that the likelihood of foster parents choosing to foster an adolescent increases as the foster parent's age increases and if the foster parent had been fostered as a child (Geiger et al. 2014). Additionally, the authors found that this likelihood decreases in two-parent homes and homes with an annual income of more than $50,000. Based on open-ended responses to survey questions, the authors also found that foster parents feared problem behavior and were concerned about the negative impact on other children (Geiger et al. 2014). Having a better understanding of the reasons why foster families are fearful of fostering teens may provide the foundation for developing targeted recruitment and intervention strategies and ultimately increase the number and quality of foster homes available to youth in the child welfare system.

An additional strategy to improve the placement options for youth is to use evidence-based interventions to provide the education and support needed by foster parents (Barkan et al. 2014; Leve et al. 2012). The literature has several examples of evidence-based interventions that target specific mechanisms of change such as contextual, individual, and familial factors (Dozier and Fisher 2014; Leve et al. 2012). Multidimensional Treatment Foster Care is a family-based behavioral intervention for children in out of home placement. It is aimed at shifting family contexts in order to prevent or eliminate serious conduct problems (Gold and Healey 2012). A longitudinal study of this model by Harold et al. (2013) looked at 166 girls between ages 13 and 17 years old who had at least one juvenile justice referral in the past 12 months and were mandated to out of home care. Results showed that in addition to decreased recidivism, the application of Multidimensional Treatment Foster Care was significantly related to deceleration of depressive symptoms when compared with the care as usual group.

Foster Parents and Educational Achievement

Beyond the provision of a safe and stable placement, improving a youth's educational trajectory while in placement may serve as an important protective or mediating factor in reducing poor outcomes. McWayne et al. (2012) found that in addition to school quality, the quality of the home environment is important for the promotion of academic skills. Without stable placements, however, adolescents in care may not be in the necessary high quality home environment needed for success. This, in turn, negatively affects the stability of school attendance for adolescents (Zorc et al. 2013), as well as other indicators for academic success, such as grades and test performance (Stone 2007). Foster parents are well positioned to help mitigate negative cascading outcomes and promote academic success by intersecting with adolescents' education. Ensuring foster parents are able to play this role may require additional, focused training for foster parents on how to promote academic skills at home as well how to actively engage with their foster child's school (e.g., by serving as informal academic liaisons).

The Role of the Juvenile Justice System in Prevention Efforts

Juvenile justice systems are in a unique position to prevent maltreatment, improve youth safety, and improve the lives of adolescents. Recent federal policies and attention focused on juvenile justice reform, such as the Defending Childhood Initiative (U.S. Department of Justice 2012) and the National Research Council's report on reforming the juvenile justice system from a developmental perspective (National Research Council 2013), raise new perspectives and suggest priorities that can influence how the justice system responds to youth. An initial step moving forward is recognizing the justice system as a critical intervention and prevention point where youth safety and protection can be prioritized and addressed.

Reducing Juvenile Incarceration and Improving Community-Based Services

Improving the system's response to youth at various points of contact with the system, particularly during stays in juvenile facilities, can reduce adolescent maltreatment. We believe that reducing the number of youth that are incarcerated should be a priority moving forward. There are many programs that do not require incarceration that have been shown to prevent and reduce juvenile crime while also costing less (Mendel 2011). Unfortunately, because of the way funding is allocated, mental health services are often only available in a juvenile residential facility. Communities and courts should consider working collaboratively to enhance their community-based programs and mental health services so that residential facilities are not the only option for providing services to youth.

Focus on Prevention in Federal and State Policies for Sex Trafficking

Federal policy has been slow to recognize the needs of adult and juvenile victims of commercial sexual exploitation. The Trafficking Victims Protection Act in 2000 was a seminal piece of federal legislation that addressed prevention of sexual trafficking, protection for foreign national victims, and prosecution of offenders (U.S. Department of State 2000). The needs of domestic victims were not addressed until 2008 through the Trafficking Victims Protection Reauthorization Act (U.S. Department of State 2008). There are indications that these policies have been effective, at least at the federal level, in increasing the number of investigations, convictions, and prison sentences of offenders (Adams et al. 2010). However, funding mechanisms for prevention programs in this federal legislation required the development of public awareness campaigns highlighting children and teens who have already been victimized, rather than addressing prevention along indicated pathways to exploitation for adolescents such as juvenile delinquency, child maltreatment, or substance abuse (Reid 2011; Williams and Frederick 2009). Moving forward, more resources are needed to establish and evaluate prevention programming based on developmental pathways to sexual exploitation. In addition, the lack of resources and understanding of effective prevention programs in these areas likely leaves practitioners in fields such as juvenile justice and child welfare without direction as to best practices when encountering youth at risk for sexual exploitation.

Implications for Future Research

Foster youth, delinquent youth, and sexually exploited youth are often members of the same population, suggesting integrated efforts are needed in order to prevent further maltreatment of adolescents. Future research should consider the intersection of foster care, juvenile justice, and sexual exploitation when studying adolescent maltreatment prevention (see, for example, Harold et al. 2013). With so many adolescents involved in multiple systems, there needs to be a better understanding of how systems can identify and prevent maltreatment, including strategies that promote cross-system collaboration. The Center for Juvenile Justice Reform has developed a model for cross-system collaboration. The Crossover Youth Practice Model (Stewart 2013) aims to improve outcomes for youth that are known to both the child welfare and juvenile justice systems. While not focused on maltreatment prevention, programs similar to this model may be useful to replicate and build upon by including additional child-serving systems that adolescents are involved in (e.g., law enforcement and schools). Evaluation of the effectiveness of cross-system collaborations is needed and should include the absence of subsequent maltreatment and victimization as an indicator of success.

Federal and local initiatives that seek to prevent maltreatment or improve outcomes for maltreated adolescents should be empirically evaluated. Policy analyses on legislation such as the Fostering Connection for Success and Increasing Adoptions Act have shown preliminary success in improving outcomes for foster youth across various domains (Courtney and Dworsky 2006). In addition, the National Task Force Report on Children Exposed to Violence (U.S. Department of Justice 2012) outlines an extensive list of recommendations for changes in practice and policy to improve the response, identification, and treatment of children exposed to violence in these alternative contexts. These recommendations present a critical opportunity for researchers to evaluate their effectiveness in preventing exposure to violence and whether these changes can specifically prevent and reduce adolescent maltreatment.

The creation and enactment of federal and state legislation has far outpaced the generation of empirical evidence related to sexual exploitation prevention and intervention. Legislation that has been enacted or is being introduced provides calls for prevention programs, protection of victims, and prosecution of offenders; however, it is not apparent that the mechanisms which might support the effectiveness of such programs have been sufficiently explored or tested, particularly given a lack of data generated at the state level (Adams et al. 2010).

As policies are being enacted to prevent sexual exploitation, there is still a critical need for researchers to apply rigorous theoretical frameworks that might explain causal chains of events leading to adolescent involvement in sexual exploitation. A recent literature review noted a general lack of theoretical empirical studies (Hurst 2013). However, a few researchers have attempted to investigate the causes or pathways to sexual exploitation utilizing a theoretical lens. Reid (2011) applied the conceptual framework of general strain theory to sexually exploited victims. Reid posited that strain experienced by caregivers could lead to increased levels of juvenile delinquency, resulting in increased adolescent vulnerability to exploitation. For example, a caregiver who abuses alcohol may lash out at his or her child, causing the child to run away from home. This child then becomes vulnerable to an exploiter who may offer shelter or food to a homeless youth and then later require an exchange of sex between the youth and a third-party as payment for the offered resources. In another example of theory-based empirical studies, Williams and Frederick (2009) applied a life course perspective to adolescents at risk of sexual exploitation. Participants described a general lack of trust with persons in helping professions. The lack of trust was made worse by these participant's childhood experiences with maltreatment. Advancing our understanding of adolescent vulnerability to sexual exploitation will require similar theory-framed research.

An important element of future research on this topic is capturing the perspectives of youth, both in and aging out of the child welfare system, as well as their caregivers and service providers (Geiger and Schelbe 2014). Qualitative and ethnographic methods can be used to better understand the needs and experiences of youth aging out of foster care (Geiger and Schelbe 2014; Schelbe 2013). Participatory action research studies, such as those with youth being active members in the process of data collection, analysis, and program development, can ensure the relevance of the research (Geiger and Schelbe 2014).

Finally, child maltreatment prevention research should examine the role of inter-generational transmission of child abuse among foster youth, justice-involved youth, and sexually exploited youth (this topic is more fully explored in the following chapter of this volume). Subsequent interventions with youth involved in all of these contexts will likely need to address prior histories of child maltreatment, trauma, traumatic stress and other mental health problems, and relationship skills. In order to work towards breaking the cycle of child maltreatment within these groups as well as providing improved protections from adolescent maltreatment, a better understanding of the experiences of youth in these contexts can inform effective prevention and intervention techniques that can ultimately reshape and support healthy developmental trajectories.

Reflection: Adolescent Maltreatment

James Garbarino
Loyola University Chicago, Chicago, IL, USA

When I think about how things have changed regarding the issue of adolescent maltreatment in the 40 years that I have been involved in studying abuse and neglect issues, I focus on two developments: changes in the continuum of "sympathetic victimhood" and appreciation for the role of trauma and resilience in the dynamics of how adolescent maltreatment affects long-term development.

Looking back, I recall what I wrote in 1980 (in my book *Understanding Abusive Families*) about the simple "purity" of child victims vs. adolescent victims. I posited a circular continuum of victimization, a clock face in which children and the elderly are at the 1:00 and 11:00 points respectively, and adolescents and spouses are located at 4:00 and 7:00. At that time there was a sense that children and the elderly were more unambiguously "innocent" victims than adolescents and spouses, who were "suspect."

One was more likely to hear that adolescents and spouses who were subject to abuse "deserved," "asked for," and "chose" to be in and stay in abusive relationships. On the other hand, it was rare (but not unheard of) to find allegations that "difficult" children "caused" abuse because of their aversive behavior (e.g., crying) and that "cranky" elders invited abuse (particularly as a kind of payback from their offspring for the way they treated their own children when they were younger). I think decades of public awareness campaigns about domestic violence have succeeded in increasing sympathy for the abused spouse, but adolescents still lag behind spouses as "sympathetic" victims.

The second change is a dramatic shift in the way trauma is conceptualized as a factor in human development. This has important implications for the way we understand the developmental pathways that flow into and from adolescent maltreatment—most notably involvement in the foster care and justice systems. Understanding troubled and troubling adolescents as "untreated traumatized children inhabiting the bodies of teenagers" can reorganize policy and practice.

It can highlight the need for "trauma-informed therapy" for the most common developmental pattern: maltreated adolescents who come out of abuse and neglect in childhood. Their needs in detention (where a large majority have diagnosable mental health problems) or foster care (where foster parents and youth need therapeutic support and care that extends beyond the legal age of maturity—18 years old) are starkly evident within this trauma perspective. In addition, however, those kids who experience an onset of maltreatment when they *become* teenagers have mental health needs as well. But they are more likely to be the victims of "classic" single incident—acute trauma—and have more internal resources with which to deal with PTSD and find a path to resilience.

References

Adams, W., Owens, C., & Small, K. (2010). *Effects of federal legislation on the commercial sexual exploitation of children.* http://www.jcjrs.gov/pdffiles1/ojjdp/228631.pdf

Ahrens, K. R., DuBois, D., Garrison, M., Spencer, R., Richardson, L. P., & Lozano, P. (2011). Qualitative exploration of relationships with important non-parental adults in the lives of youth in foster care. *Children and Youth Services Review, 33*(6), 1012–1023.

Antle, B. F., Johnson, L., Barbee, A., & Sullivan, D. (2009). Fostering interdependent versus independent living in youth aging out of care through healthy relationships. *Families in Society: The Journal of Contemporary Social Services, 90*(3), 309–314.

Barkan, S., Salazar, A., Estep, K., Mattos, L., Eichenlaub, C., & Haggerty, K. (2014). Adapting an evidence-based parenting program for child welfare involved teens and their caregivers. *Children and Youth Services Review, 41*, 53–61. doi:10.1016/j.childyouth.2014.03.006.

Barth, R. P., Greeson, J. K., Guo, S., Green, R. L., Hurley, S., & Sisson, J. (2007). Changes in family functioning and child behavior following intensive in-home therapy. *Children and Youth Services Review, 29*(8), 988–1009.

Beck, A. J., Harrison, P. M., & Guerino, P. (2010). *Sexual victimization in juvenile facilities reported by youth, 2008–09.* Washington, DC: Bureau of Justice Statistics.

Burrell, S. (1999). Improving conditions of confinement in secure juvenile detention facilities. Baltimore: Annie E. Casey Foundation. http://www.aecf.org/KnowledgeCenter/Publications.aspx?pubguid=%7B5A809A92-841F-4E05-84D2-AC7FA3F0A2BA%7D

Burrell, S. (2013). *Trauma and the environment of care in juvenile institutions.* Los Angeles/Durham: National Center for Child Traumatic Stress.

Cicchetti, D., & Rogosch, F. A. (2002). A developmental psychopathology perspective on adolescence. *Journal of Consulting and Clinical Psychology, 70*(1), 6–20.

Countryman-Roswurm, K., & Bolin, B. L. (2014). Domestic minor sex trafficking: Assessing and reducing risk. *Child and Adolescent Social Work Journal* [serial online], 1–18. doi:10.1007/s10560-014-0336-6

Courtney, M. E., & Dworsky, A. (2006). Early outcomes for young adults transitioning from out-of-home care in the USA. *Child and Family Social Work, 11*, 209–219.

Dierkhising, C. B., Ko, S., & Halladay-Goldman, J. (2013a). *Trauma-informed juvenile justice roundtable: Current issues and new directions in creating trauma-informed juvenile justice systems.* Los Angeles/Durham: National Center for Child Traumatic Stress.

Dierkhising, C. B., Ko, S. J., Woods, B., Lee, R., Briggs, E. C., & Pynoos, R. S. (2013b). Trauma histories among justice-involved youth: Findings from the National Child Traumatic Stress Network. *European Journal of Psychotraumatology, 4*, 20274. doi:10.3402/ejpt.v4i0.20274.

Dierkhising, C. B., Lane, A., & Natsuaki, M. N. (2014). Victims behind bars: A preliminary study of abuse during incarceration and post-release social and emotional functioning. *Psychology, Public Policy, and Law, 2*, 181–190.

Dozier, M., & Fisher, P. (2014). Neuroscience enhanced child maltreatment interventions to improve outcomes. *Social Policy Report, 28*(1), 25–27.

Dworsky, A., & Courtney, M. E. (2010). The risk of teenage pregnancy among transitioning foster youth: Implications for extending state care beyond age 18. *Children and Youth Services Review, 32*, 1351–1356.

Dworsky, A., & DeCoursey, J. (2009). *Pregnant and parenting foster youth: Their needs, their experiences*. Chicago: Chapin Hall at the University of Chicago.

Dworsky, A., Ahrens, K., & Courtney, M. (2013). Health insurance coverage and use of family planning services among current and former foster youth: Implications of the Health Care Reform Law. *Journal of Health Politics, Policy and Law, 38*(2), 421–439.

Estes, R. J., & Weiner, N. A. (2001). The commercial sexual exploitation of children in the U.S., Canada and Mexico (pp. 260). Philadelphia: University of Pennsylvania, Center for the Study of Youth Policy.

Everson, M., Smith, J. B., Hussey, J. M., English, D., Litrownik, A. J., Dubowitz, H., et al. (2008). Concordance between adolescent childhood abuse and child protective service determinations in an at-risk sample of young adolescents. *Child Maltreatment, 13*, 14–26.

Felitti, V. J., Anda, R. F., Nordenberg, D., Williamson, D. F., Spitz, A. M., Edwards, V., et al. (1998). Relationship of childhood dysfunction to many of the leading causes of death in adults. *American Journal of Preventive Medicine, 14*(4), 245–258.

Finkelhor, D. D., & Ormrod, R. R. (2004). *Prostitution of juveniles: Patterns from NIBRS Juvenile Justice Bulletin*. Washington, DC: U.S. Department of Justice, Office of Justice Programs.

Finkelhor, D., Ormrod, R., Turner, H., & Hamby, S. L. (2005). The victimization of children and youth: A comprehensive, national survey. *Child Maltreatment, 10*, 5–25.

Finkelhor, D., Ormrod, R. K., & Turner, H. (2007). Revictimization patterns in a national longitudinal sample of children and youth. *Child Abuse & Neglect, 31*, 479–502.

Finkelhor, D., Turner, H. A., Ormrod, R. K., & Hamby, S. L. (2009). Violence, abuse, and crime exposure in a national sample of children and youth. *Pediatrics, 124*(5), 1–14.

Finkelhor, D., Turner, H., Hamby, S., & Ormrod, R. (2011). Polyvictimization: Children's exposure to multiple types of violence, crime, and abuse. *Juvenile Justice Bulletin, 1*–12. https://www.ncjrs.gov/pdffiles1/ojjdp/235504.pdf

Fong, R., & Cardoso, J. (2010). Child human trafficking victims: Challenges for the child welfare system. *Evaluation and Program Planning, 33*(3), 311–316. doi:10.1016/j.evalprogplan.2009.06.018.

Ford, J. D., Racusin, R., Daviss, W. B., Ellis, C. G., Thomas, J., Rogers, K., et al. (1999). Trauma exposure among children with oppositional defiant disorder and attention deficit–hyperactivity disorder. *Journal of Consulting and Clinical Psychology, 67*(5), 786–789.

Ford, J., Elhai, J., Connor, D., & Frueh, B. (2010). Poly-victimization and risk of posttraumatic, depressive, and substance use disorders and involvement in delinquency in a national sample of adolescents. *Journal of Adolescent Health, 46*(6), 545–552. doi:10.1016/j.jadohealth.2009.11.212.

Ford, J. D., Wasser, T., & Connor, D. F. (2011). Identifying and determining the symptom severity associated with polyvictimization among psychiatrically impaired children in the outpatient setting. *Child Maltreatment, 16*(3), 216–226. doi:10.1177/1077559511406109.

Geiger, J. M., & Schelbe, L. (2014). Stopping the cycle of abuse and neglect: A call to action to focus on pregnant and parenting foster youth. *Journal of Public Child Welfare, 8*(1), 1–26.

Geiger, J. M., Hayes, M. J., & Lietz, C. A. (2014). Providing foster care for adolescents: Barriers and opportunities. *Child & Youth Services, 35*(3), 1–18.

Gold, R., & Healey, C. V. (2012). Implementing multidimensional treatment foster care (MTFC). In A. Rubin (Ed.), *Programs and interventions for maltreated children and families at risk* (pp. 43–57). Hoboken: John Wiley & Sons Inc.

Goodkind, S., Schelbe, L. A., & Shook, J. J. (2011). Why youth leave care: Understandings of adulthood and transition successes and challenges among youth aging out of child welfare. *Children and Youth Services Review, 33*(6), 1039–1048.

Griffin, G., Germain, E. J., & Wilkerson, R. G. (2012). Using a trauma-informed approach in juvenile justice institutions. *Journal of Child and Adolescent Trauma, 5*(3), 271–283.

Halter, S. (2010). Factors that influence police conceptualizations of girls involved in prostitution in six U.S. cities: Child sexual exploitation victims or delinquents? *Child Maltreatment, 15*(2), 152–160.

Harold, G., Kerr, D., van Ryzin, M., DeGarmo, D., Rhoades, K., & Leve, L. (2013). Depressive symptom trajectories among girls in the juvenile justice system: 24-month outcomes of an RCT of Multidimensional Treatment Foster Care. *Prevention Science, 14*, 437–446.

Herz, D. C., Ryan, J. P., & Bilchik, S. (2010). Challenges facing crossover youth: An examination of juvenile justice decision making and recidivism. *Family Court Review, 48*, 305–321.

Hockenberry, S. (2013). *Juveniles in residential placement* (Juvenile offenders and victims: National report series). Washington, DC: U.S. Department of Justice.

Hoekstra, K. O. (1984). Ecologically defining the mistreatment of adolescents. *Children and Youth Services Review, 6*, 285–298.

Hurst, T. (2013). *Childhood emotional maltreatment and prevention of commercial sexual exploitation of children: A mixed methods study* (Doctoral dissertation). http://athenaeum.libs.uga.edu/xmlui/handle/10724/29846

Institute of Medicine. (2013). *Confronting commercial sexual exploitation and sex trafficking of minors in the United States: Briefing slides.* http://www.iom.edu/~/media/Files/Report%20Files/2013/Sexual-Exploitation-Sex-Trafficking/sextraffickingminors_slides.pdf. Accessed 21 May 2014.

Jones, L. L. (2013). The family and social networks of recently discharged foster youth. *Journal of Family Social Work, 16*(3), 225–242.

Jonson-Reid, M., & Barth, R. (2000). From maltreatment report to juvenile incarceration: The role of child welfare services. *Child Abuse & Neglect, 24*(4), 505–520.

Kapolko, J. (2012). *A watched system: Should journalists be granted access to juvenile dependency court proceedings?* San Francisco: Fostering Media Connections.

Kerig, P. K., & Becker, S. P. (2010). From internalizing to externalizing: Theoretical models of the processes linking PTSD to juvenile delinquency. In S. J. Egan (Ed.), *Posttraumatic stress disorder (PTSD): Causes, symptoms and treatment* (pp. 33–78). Hauppauge: Nova.

Lab, D. D., Feigenbaum, J. D., & De Silva, P. (2000). Mental health professionals' attitudes and practices towards male childhood abuse. *Child Abuse & Neglect, 24*, 391–402.

Leve, L. D., Harold, G. T., Chamberlain, P., Landsverk, J. A., Fisher, P. A., & Vostanis, P. (2012). Practitioner review: Children in foster care—Vulnerabilities and evidence-based interventions that promote resilience processes. *Journal of Child Psychology and Psychiatry, 53*(12), 1197–1211.

Lloyd, R. (2011). *Girls like us*. New York: Harper Collins Publishers.

Macy, R. J., & Graham, L. M. (2012). Identifying domestic and international sex-trafficking victims during human service provision. *Trauma, Violence, and Abuse, 13*(2), 59–76.

McMahon-Howard, J., & Reimers, B. (2013). An evaluation of a child welfare training program on the commercial sexual exploitation of children (CSEC). *Evaluation and Program Planning, 40*, 1–9.

McWayne, C. M., Hahs-Vaughn, D. L., Cheung, K., & Wright, L. E. G. (2012). National profiles of school readiness skills for Head Start children: An investigation of stability and change. *Early Childhood Research Quarterly, 27*, 668–683.

Mendel, R. A. (2011). *No place for kids: The case for reducing juvenile incarceration*. Baltimore: Annie E. Casey Foundation.

Mersky, J., Berger, L., Reynolds, A., & Gromoske, A. (2009). Risk factors for child and adolescent maltreatment: A longitudinal investigation of a cohort of inner-city youth. *Child Maltreatment, 14*(1), 73–88.

Mitchell, K., Finkelhor, D., & Wolak, J. (2010). Conceptualizing juvenile prostitution as child maltreatment: Findings from the National Juvenile Prostitution Study. *Child Maltreatment, 15*(1), 18–36. doi:10.1177/1077559509349443.

National Child Traumatic Stress Network, Justice Consortium. (2009). *Helping traumatized children: Tips for judges*. Los Angeles/Durham: National Center for Child Traumatic Stress.

National Research Council. (2013). *Reforming juvenile justice: A developmental approach.* Washington, DC: The National Academies Press.

Newell, M., & Leap, J. (2013). *Reforming the nation's largest juvenile justice system.* Children's Defense Fund/UCLA Luskin School of Public Affairs.

Powers, J. L., & Eckenrode, J. (1988). The maltreatment of adolescents. *Child Abuse & Neglect, 12*(2), 189–199.

Putnam, F. W. (2006). The impact of trauma on child development. *Juvenile and Family Court Journal, 57,* 1–11.

Puzzanchera, C. (2013). *Juvenile arrests 2011* (Juvenile offenders and victims: National report series). Washington, DC: U.S. Department of Justice.

Raissian, K. M., Dierkhising, C. B., Geiger, J. M., & Schelbe, L. (2014). Child maltreatment reporting patterns and predictors of substantiation: Comparing adolescents and younger children. *Child Maltreatment, 19,* 3–16.

Raphael, J., Reichert, J. A., & Powers, M. (2010). Pimp control and violence: Domestic sex trafficking of Chicago women and girls. *Women & Criminal Justice, 20*(1–2), 89–104.

Reid, J. A. (2011). Exploratory model of girls' vulnerability to commercial sexual exploitation in prostitution. *Child Maltreatment, 16,* 146–157.

Roe-Sepowitz, D. E. (2012). Juvenile entry into prostitution: The role of emotional abuse. *Violence Against Women, 18*(5), 562–579.

Ryan, J. P., Williams, A. B., & Courtney, M. E. (2013). Adolescent neglect, juvenile delinquency, and the risk of recidivism. *Journal of Youth and Adolescence, 42,* 454–465.

Schelbe, L. (2013). *"Some type of way": An ethnography of youth aging out of the child welfare system,* Doctoral dissertation, University of Pittsburgh, Pittsburgh.

Schubert, C. A., Mulvey, E. P., Loughran, T. A., & Losoya, S. H. (2012). Perceptions of institutional experience and community outcomes for serious adolescent offenders. *Criminal Justice and Behavior, 39*(1), 71–93. doi:10.1177/0093854811426710.

Scott, M. E., Moore, K., Hawkins, A. J., Malm, K., Beltz, M., & Child, T. (2012). *Putting youth relationship education on the child welfare agenda: Findings from a research and evaluation review. Executive summary.* Bethesda: Child Trends.

Sedlak, A. J., & McPherson, K. (2010). *Conditions of confinement: Findings from the survey of youth in residential placement.* Washington, DC: Office of Juvenile Justice and Delinquency Prevention. http://www.ncjrs.gov/pdffiles1/ojjdp/227729.pdf

Shared Hope International. (2009). *National report on domestic minor sex trafficking: America's prostituted children.* http://sharedhope.org/wp-content/uploads/2012/09/SHI_National_Report_on_DMST_2009without_cover.pdf. Accessed 21 May 2014.

Shared Hope International. (2013). *Protected innocence challenge: A legal framework of protection for the nation's children.* http://sharedhope.org/wp-content/uploads/2014/02/2013-Protected-Innocence-Challenge-Report.pdf. Accessed 19 Sept 2014.

Stewart, M. (2013). *Cross-system collaboration.* Los Angeles/Durham: National Center for Traumatic Stress.

Stone, S. (2007). Child maltreatment, out-of-home placement and academic vulnerability: A fifteen-year review of evidence and future directions. *Children and Youth Services Review, 29,* 139–161.

Thornberry, T., Henry, K., Ireland, T., & Smith, C. (2010). The causal impact of childhood-limited maltreatment and adolescent maltreatment on early adult adjustment. *Journal of Adolescent Health, 46*(4), 359–365. doi:10.1016/j.jadohealth.2009.09.011.

U.S. Department of Health and Human Services. (2013a). *Child maltreatment 2012.* http://www.acf.hhs.gov/sites/default/files/cb/cm2012.pdf

U.S. Department of Health and Human Services, Administration for Children and Families, Administration on Children, Youth and Families, Children's Bureau. (2013b). *The AFCARS report.* http://www.acf.hhs.gov/programs/cb/resource/afcars-report-20. Accessed 21 May 2014.

U.S. Department of Justice. (2012). *Report of the Attorney General's National Task Force on Children Exposed to Violence.* Washington, DC: GPO.

U.S. Department of State. (2000). Victims of Trafficking and Violence Protection Act of 2000. http://www.state.gov/j/tip/laws/61124.htm. Accessed 19 Sept 2014.

U.S. Department of State. (2008). Victims of Trafficking and Violence Protection Reauthorization Act of 2008. http://www.state.gov/j/tip/laws/113178.htm. Accessed 19 Sept 2014

Williams, L. M. (2010). Harm and resilience among prostituted teens: Broadening our understanding of victimization and survival. *Social Policy and Society, 9*(2), 243–254. doi:10.1017/S1474746409990376.

Williams, L. M., & Frederick, M. E. (2009). *Pathways into and out of commercial sexual victimization of children: Understanding and responding to sexually exploited teens.* Lowell: University of Massachusetts Lowell.

Zorc, C. S., O'Reilly, A. R., Matone, M., Long, J., Watts, C. L., & Rubin, D. (2013). The relationship of placement experience to school absenteeism and changing schools in young, school-aged children in foster care. *Children and Youth Services Review, 35*, 826–833.

Carly B. Dierkhising is an assistant professor at California State University, Los Angeles in the School of Criminal Justice and Criminalistics. She received her doctorate in developmental psychology from University of California, Riverside and her masters in clinical psychology from Pepperdine University. Previously, she was the special projects manager for juvenile justice activities in the Service Systems Program at the National Center for Child Traumatic Stress. Dr. Dierkhising's primary area of research is in trauma and juvenile justice with a focus on how to improve services for youth involved in juvenile courts and/or the juvenile justice system from both a practice and policy perspective.

Jennifer Mullins Geiger is a postdoctoral fellow at Arizona State University School of Social Work where she received her Ph.D. in social work in May 2014. Her research interests include child maltreatment prevention, issues facing youth aging out of foster care and transitioning into adulthood, pregnancy and parenting youth who are aging out, and foster family resilience and satisfaction. She was awarded a 2-year Fellowship for the Promotion of Child Well-Being from the Doris Duke Charitable Foundation in 2011. Dr. Geiger has worked on grant-funded projects aimed at improving children and adolescents' mental health outcomes and preventing child abuse.

Tamara E. Hurst earned her bachelor's and master's degrees in social work from Georgia State University. She earned her doctoral degree from The University of Georgia School of Social Work. Dr. Hurst is a licensed clinical social worker with 10 years of experience as a forensic social worker, and 8 years of experience as a forensic interviewer. She is currently an assistant professor at The University of Southern Mississippi School of Social Work where she teaches forensic social work, crisis intervention, along with other related courses. She is also a principal investigator on a grant funded project from the Mississippi Departments of Medicaid and Mental Health that provides statewide technical assistance to Mississippi agencies who offer services to families with children who require intensive behavioral and emotional support. Dr. Hurst frequently conducts presentations and trainings on topics related to child abuse and neglect and childhood sexual exploitation.

Carlomagno Panlilio is a doctoral candidate in the Department of Human Development and Quantitative Methodology at the University of Maryland, College Park. His area of specialization is in developmental science and holds a certificate in Education Measurement, Statistics, & Evaluation. Mr. Panlilio's research focuses on longitudinal analyses of early childhood school readiness domains for children with a history of maltreatment. More specifically, the role that emotion regulation, cognitive functioning, language, and context play on influencing later academic outcomes. He has a B.A. in psychology from the California State University at Long Beach and his Master of Science in Family Studies from the University of Maryland, College Park. Mr. Panlilio has also been in clinical practice as a licensed clinical marriage and family therapist since 2005 and continues to work in private practice. He has also worked as a family therapist in community agencies serving foster families, as well as children and families involved with Child Protective Services.

Lisa Schelbe is an assistant professor at Florida State University College of Social Work. She earned her doctorate from the University of Pittsburgh School of Social Work where she was a recipient of the *Doris Duke Fellowships for the Promotion of Child Well-Being*. Dr. Schelbe received her Master in Social Work from the George Warren Brown School of Social Work at Washington University in St. Louis. Her research primarily focuses on the experiences of youth aging out of the child welfare system. She is interested in how youth aging out negotiate the transition out of care and how services impact youth aging out during the transition. Dr. Schelbe is currently examining the educational experiences of youth aging out. Her diverse social work practice experience includes work with survivors of family and intimate partner violence and of natural disasters. Dr. Schelbe has background in program development, grant writing, and political advocacy.

Chapter 4
Intergenerational Transmission of Maltreatment: Ending a Family Tradition

Jennifer Mullins Geiger, Lisa Schelbe, Megan J. Hayes, Elisa Kawam, Colleen Cary Katz, and J. Bart Klika

Chapter 4 in Brief

Context

- While it is commonly assumed that individuals with a history of child maltreatment may be at an increased risk of maltreating their own children, this process is poorly understood and far from self-evident.
- Theoretical frameworks, such as attachment, social learning, risk and resilience, and ecological frameworks have been used to understand the cycle of abuse.

J.M. Geiger (✉)
Jane Addams College of Social Work, University of Illinois at Chicago, Chicago, IL, USA
e-mail: jmullins@asu.edu

L. Schelbe
College of Social Work, Florida State University, Tallahassee, FL, USA
e-mail: Lschelbe@fsu.edu

M.J. Hayes
School of Social Work, Arizona State University, Phoenix, AZ, USA
e-mail: Megan.J.Hayes@asu.edu

E. Kawam
Robert Stemper College of Public Health and Social Work, Florida International University, Miami, FL, USA
e-mail: ekawam@gmail.com

C.C. Katz
Silberman School of Social Work, Hunter College, New York, NY, USA
e-mail: Colleen.Katz@hunter.cuny.edu

J.B. Klika
School of Social Work, University of Montana, Missoula, MT, USA
e-mail: bart.klika@mso.umt.edu

© Springer International Publishing Switzerland 2015
D. Daro et al. (eds.), *Advances in Child Abuse Prevention Knowledge*,
Child Maltreatment 5, DOI 10.1007/978-3-319-16327-7_4

- Research suggests the cycle is most likely to occur among those maltreated children who are raised in families with limited social support, have experienced other trauma including intimate partner violence, or have aged out of the foster care system.
- Safe, stable, and nurturing relationships and environments have been shown to reduce the occurrence of child maltreatment and may be useful in breaking this cycle of violence.

Strategies for Moving Forward

- Use child welfare administrative data to examine intergenerational links of child maltreatment within families.
- Train child welfare professionals about the unique challenges in addressing the abuse cycle.
- Develop interventions that explicitly consider parents' histories of child abuse and neglect, experiences of trauma, and unaddressed mental health issues, including teaching parents effective skills on how to create safe, stable, and nurturing environments.

Implications for Research

- Identify clear patterns of child maltreatment across generations and how these patterns may differ among specific subgroups or vulnerable populations.
- Use more consistent definitions and measures of violence, trauma, and maltreatment as they relate to the intergenerational transmission of child abuse.
- Include the examination of both protective and risk factors in developing models to better understand the cycle of violence and how these factors work across the various ecological levels.
- Incorporate epigenetics and biomarkers in identifying stressors and the effect of trauma on parenting ability, family bonding, and attachment.

Introduction

Parental history of abuse or neglect is considered a major risk factor for child maltreatment. Eighty-one percent of children reported for maltreatment in the United States are maltreated by a parent (U.S. Department of Health and Human Services 2012). Studies have shown that between 25 % and 35 % of parents who have been maltreated will likely continue a cycle of maltreatment with their own children (Belsky 1993; Dixon et al. 2005; Egeland et al. 1988; Kim 2009; Li et al. 2011;

Pears and Capaldi 2001). While not fully predictive of subsequent parent behavior, having experienced maltreatment as a child is viewed by many as a substantive risk factor for repeating the cycle. However, this body of research is not without its critics. Concerns have been raised regarding methodological rigor and design elements such as small sample sizes, samples limited to high risk participants, a focus on mothers only, and inadequate definitions of maltreatment or distinctions of the type of maltreatment being examined (Ertem et al. 2000; Kim 2009; Newcomb and Locke 2001; Thornberry et al. 2012).

Although there is a higher risk for parents who were maltreated as children to perpetuate the cycle of violence, most researchers examining this issue identify many who break the cycle; abuse is not inevitable (Kaufman and Zigler 1987; Widom 1989; DuMont et al. 2007). Indeed, researchers have identified several protective factors associated with individuals who have not gone on to continue the cycle of child maltreatment and violence. For example, women with a history of maltreatment who did not continue the cycle of abuse have demonstrated a higher likelihood to have had positive relationships with a caring adult during their childhood and to have been involved in therapy (Egeland et al. 1988). Consistent and nurturing relationships between intimate partners and between parents and children also have been associated with breaking the cycle of abuse (Jaffee et al. 2013). In addition to high levels of social support, Li and colleagues (2011) identified education and marriage as protective factors against child maltreatment.

These competing bodies of evidence underscore, at a minimum, the need to identify clear patterns of child maltreatment across generations with specific subgroups and individuals in order to maximize the contribution of this line of research to program and policy planning. In addition to identifying risk and co-occurring factors, researchers can further contribute to effective program development by identifying the protective factors most frequently associated with individuals and families who do not go on to maltreat their own children. Drawing on these data, researchers will be in a stronger position to determine the utility of existing theories that examine this phenomenon as well as create new and innovative theories.

This chapter begins with a summary of the existing research and theory that is frequently used to identify the pathways that lead those who have been maltreated to continue the behavior with their own children. The chapter then focuses on the unique roles intimate partner violence, poverty, foster care placement, and other trauma that co-occur with child maltreatment can play in contributing to this cycle of violence and neglect. While these are not the only contexts and populations to consider in unraveling the intergenerational transmission of maltreatment (parental substance abuse, mental illness, and criminal activity may also co-occur with child maltreatment), these four population groups are particularly important to consider in targeting promising intervention and prevention strategies. Building on this discussion, the chapter identifies emerging topics and research, including the increasing role epigenetics and biomedical research can play in assessing the impacts trauma has on the intergenerational transmission of child maltreatment. The chapter concludes with an outline of recommendations and strategies for practice, policy, and research.

Theories Pertaining to the Intergenerational Transmission of Child Maltreatment

Social learning theory, attachment theory, ecological, and risk and resilience frameworks have been widely used to contribute to the understanding of the intergenerational transmission of child maltreatment. These theories vary about the mechanisms of how abuse and neglect are passed down through generations, which may prove useful in understanding the complexity and contributing factors of the intergenerational transmission of child maltreatment.

Social Learning Theory

Social learning theory suggests transmission of parenting practices reflects observational or experiential learning (Bandura 1977; Conger et al. 2003; Patterson 1998). Children raised in a particular manner may come to believe the style in which they were raised is appropriate and utilize it when they parent. Children learn parenting practices (healthy and unhealthy) through observation. For example, children who are exposed to corporal punishment as a means of physical discipline may learn to believe that this is an acceptable form of discipline and be more inclined to use it with their own children.

Attachment Theory

Bowlby's attachment theory, explains how a child's relationship with the child's primary caregiver influences development and stability, and forms the foundation for future relationships (Bowlby 1969). The primary functions of protection and well-being that are promoted through secure attachments are often missing in cases of child maltreatment. In addition to the broken or weakened attachment, the child may also miss out on specific developmental experiences necessary to coordinate verbal and nonverbal skills. Broken and weakened attachments may follow children into adolescence and even into adulthood. Insecure attachment can create difficulties in parent-child relationships as well as complications in adult relationships, which may be transferred to their own children (Crittenden and Ainsworth 1989).

Ecological Frameworks

Ecological frameworks posit that there is no single mechanism to explain child maltreatment, but, instead, that maltreatment is the result of various factors occurring on multiple, interacting levels (Bronfenbrenner 1979). Indeed, this theory is particularly useful in examining the intergenerational transmission of child maltreatment. The theory integrates predisposing risk factors, as well as the interaction of protective factors, in nested domains of individual characteristics (personality traits), family factors (strong parent-child relationships), social factors (social support), culturally transmitted parenting beliefs, societal influences (family supportive policies and legislation), and socially acceptable child-rearing behaviors (Belsky 1993; Kotch et al. 1995).

Resilience and Protective Factors

Much research has been conducted on the interplay between risk and protective factors related to the occurrence of child maltreatment and level of risk present for children and families. (For example, see Chap. 9 in this volume.) More recently, researchers have shifted their interest to an explicit examination of the strategies and resources individuals draw on in breaking the cycle of violence. The concept of resilience was developed through an examination of individuals and groups who were able to "overcome the odds" and do well in light of adversity (see, for example, Masten et al. 1990; Werner and Smith 1992). Similarly, protective factors are "conditions or attributes in individuals, families, communities, or the larger society that, when present, mitigate or eliminate risk in families and communities that, when present, increase the health and well-being of children and families" (U.S. Department of Health and Human Services 2014).

Several factors that protect against child maltreatment and the intergenerational transmission of abuse and neglect have been identified. For example, a study by Dixon and colleagues (2009) found that financial stability and social support were associated with reducing the likelihood of child maltreatment in the first 13 months of the child's life. Li and colleagues (2011) found that marriage, education, and higher levels of social support served as protective factors. Egeland and colleagues (1988) had similar findings in that mothers with more emotional support and stable and satisfying relationships were less likely to maltreat their own children. More recently, in a special issue of the *Journal of Adolescent Health* on breaking the cycle of maltreatment, Jaffee and colleagues (2013) sought to identify contextual and interpersonal factors that distinguish families exposed to a history of child abuse or neglect. They found that low levels of partner violence, supportive and trusting relationships with partners, and high levels of maternal warmth were factors associated with fewer incidences of child maltreatment. Studies in the same issue concur with the findings of Jaffee and colleagues (2013) that safe, stable, and nurturing relationships are indeed able to act as protective factors in breaking the cycle of child maltreatment (Conger et al. 2013; Schofield et al. 2013; Thornberry et al. 2013).

All of these theories point to myriad factors with the potential to interrupt the cycle of violence toward children. Depending on the framework used, intervention and prevention efforts may be targeted differently, with varying outcomes. Based on this research, prevention and intervention programs targeting families affected by a history of child maltreatment might include strategies to develop formal and informal social support, relationship skills building, parenting skills, family planning, counseling to address early trauma, and the promotion of formal education and professional opportunities.

Factors with High Probability of Increasing Intergenerational Maltreatment

In this section, we discuss four risk factors that have been shown to be particularly relevant in contributing to the intergenerational transmission of child maltreatment: intimate partner violence, poverty, aging out of foster care, and experiencing multiple forms of trauma. As noted in our discussion, all of these experiences can have a major impact on one's thoughts, beliefs, and behavior. In addition, these conditions can contribute to a pattern of unsafe, unstable and unhealthy relationships, parenting, and family circumstances. Many factors affect outcomes; however, having a deeper understanding of how intimate partner violence, poverty, aging out of foster care and other trauma impact a child's perceptions and development offers unique opportunities to improve our ability to design and better target prevention and intervention programs and system reforms.

Intimate Partner Violence

Research demonstrates that victims of child abuse and neglect are at increased risk for being exposed to intimate partner violence, highlighting the need to consider both forms of violence exposure when attempting to examine the intergenerational transmission of abuse (Appel and Holden 1998; Moffitt and Caspi 2003; Dong et al. 2003). For example, in their meta-analytic review, Appel and Holden (1998) found the rate of overlap between child abuse and neglect and intimate partner violence was approximately 40 % (Edleson 1999; Jouriles et al. 2008; Hazen et al. 2009; Osofsky 2003; Cox et al. 2003; Rumm et al. 2000; Tajima 2000; Dixon et al. 2007). Due to the wealth of research documenting the overlap, some have argued that intimate partner violence should be conceptualized as a form of emotional abuse (Gewirtz and Edleson 2007).

Violence in the family, in the form of abuse, neglect, and exposure to intimate partner violence, creates what Cicchetti and Toth (2005) term a "pathogenic relational environment." As noted by Holt, Buckley, and Whelan (2008), intimate partner violence may increase the risk for mental health problems for the survivor (such as depression and posttraumatic stress disorder, or PTSD), which may in turn impact a parent's ability to respond in a caring and nurturing way to the developing child. Parents may withdraw from their children as a result of mental health challenges or may respond to their children in overly controlling or aggressive ways.

Children who are exposed to intimate partner violence are at increased risk for relational violence in the adolescent and adulthood years. For example, Smith et al. (2011) found that youth exposed to intimate partner violence were at increased risk for relational violence in early adulthood (between ages 21 and 23) after accounting for early experiences of child abuse. Early adulthood relational violence mediated the association between youth intimate partner violence exposure and intimate partner violence perpetration between ages 29 and 31. It is possible that exposure to intimate partner violence sets in motion a pattern of hostile interactions that last into adulthood and may be transmitted to future generations in the forms of direct abuse or exposure to intimate partner violence.

Poverty

Children living in poverty or lower socio-economic conditions are more likely to be maltreated and involved in the child welfare system (Berger 2004; Slack et al. 2004; Drake and Pandey 1996; Jonson-Reid et al. 2009). The Institute of Medicine and National Research Council's (2014) report on child maltreatment describes insufficient evidence for poverty *causing* maltreatment. However, the report clearly states that poverty is a risk factor for abuse and neglect, with neglect being most strongly associated with poverty, followed by physical abuse. Although a strong association exists between poverty and child maltreatment, the relationship is not fully understood. Drake and Jonson-Reid (2014) argue that there is no single explanation for why poverty and maltreatment are connected. Rather, there likely are multiple ways to understand the relationships between these two complex phenomena. For example, some have posited that parents' individual factors (education, family structure, age, substance abuse) contribute directly to both poverty and maltreatment. Others cite structural factors (access to resources) as contributing to poverty, thereby impacting parents' ability to provide care for their children, causing maltreatment. (For a more detailed review of research and a discussion of poverty and child maltreatment, see Drake and Jonson-Reid 2014). It is important to remember that while poverty is a risk factor for child maltreatment, not all children living in poverty are abused or neglected. Many scholars have stressed that in order to develop more effective responses, it is necessary to better understand which children in poverty are maltreated and under what circumstances (Institute of Medicine and National Research Council 2014; Drake and Jonson-Reid 2014).

Empirical studies on the intergenerational transmission of child maltreatment largely have not incorporated variables related to poverty, although recent studies have controlled for socioeconomic status (Thornberry et al. 2013; Conger et al. 2013). Poverty is an important contextual factor to consider when examining the intergenerational transmission of child maltreatment for many of the same reasons it is important to consider it in formulating child abuse prevention programming and research priorities. The fact that socioeconomic status, like the intergenerational transmission of child maltreatment, is transmitted across generations makes it especially pertinent (see, for example, Conger and Donnellan 2007). Having parents with lower socioeconomic status was a predictor of financial stress for children in adulthood, and socioeconomic level was related to how the children were parented as well as how they parented their children (Thornberry et al. 2003). Similarly Conger et al. (2009) describe how quality of parenting can be negatively impacted by variables related to poverty, including neighborhood quality, life stress, socioeconomic disadvantage, and parents' age at birth.

In addition to examining the relationship between poverty and child maltreatment at the family level, it can also be examined at the neighborhood or community level. It is well understood that the larger environment impacts child well-being and that living in a poor community is a risk factor for several public health concerns, including child maltreatment (Coulton et al. 1995; Drake and Pandey 1996). Eckenrode and colleagues (2014) found higher income inequality at the county level was associated with higher rates of child maltreatment. Studies examining the intergenerational transmission of child maltreatment have not typically incorporated neighborhood poverty rates, the exception being Thornberry and colleagues (2013), who did use neighborhood poverty rates as control variables.

Youth Aging Out of Foster Care

Of the estimated 28,000 youth who "age out" of the child welfare system each year (U.S. Department of Health and Human Services 2012), most face a broad range of challenges associated with achieving independence and self-sufficiency (Courtney and Dworsky 2006; Pecora et al. 2003). Common outcomes include poor mental health, low educational attainment, unemployment, homelessness, instability and poverty (Courtney and Dworsky 2006; Pecora et al. 2003). In addition, these youth have been shown to have significantly higher rates of pregnancy (Dworsky and Courtney 2010; King et al. 2014; Matta Oshima et al. 2013) and repeat pregnancies (Dworsky and Courtney 2010) than the general population. In a study examining the services for pregnant and parenting youth in foster care, Dworsky and DeCoursey (2009) found that 22 % of their sample was investigated for abuse or neglect of their child, with 11 % having a child placed in foster care.

The importance of focusing prevention efforts on foster youth who become parents while in care is further supported by the general risk for maltreatment observed across all teen parents (Stevens-Simon et al. 2001; Whitson et al. 2011). Some estimates indicate children of adolescent mothers are twice as likely to be maltreated as children of older mothers (Stevens-Simon et al. 2001). Although it may be difficult to identify the cause, several factors have been linked to the relationship between early parenting and child maltreatment, many of which are common among youth aging out of care. Young parents may lack the cognitive functioning that helps them identify their child's needs. They may also lack knowledge about child development, resulting in inappropriate expectations of the child (Bavolek and Keene 1999). Teen parents are more likely to be unemployed, have lower incomes, and lower levels of education (Afifi 2007). Young parents are more likely to be single parents and unmarried, exposed to poverty, and to have fewer supports (Lee and Goerge 1999). These are all variables associated with child maltreatment and all characteristics frequently found among youth aging out of care.

Trauma

It is useful to consider what is known about populations who have experienced trauma and its impact on the intergenerational transmission of maltreatment. Events that are potentially traumatic include child maltreatment, physical assault, sexual assault, kidnapping, torture, severe car accidents, or illness (American Psychiatric

Association 2013). Even without a history of trauma, parenting can be a stressful experience. As such, a history of trauma or child maltreatment can further complicate an already tenuous and highly stressful situation (Belsky et al. 2009). If there is a parental history of child maltreatment, becoming a parent can itself be re-traumatizing (Berlin et al. 2011; Neppl et al. 2009). With trauma, parents may be less responsive to their children's needs and play time may be mechanistic and routine (Belsky et al. 2009).

Over time, parents may actually adopt an avoidant or even aggressive parenting style and the child can learn to distrust the caregivers (Cohen et al. 2008). The child may learn to self-soothe, where they learn to self-regulate emotions, becoming quiet and appearing calm. At first glance, this reaction may seem positive. However, such behaviors often signal a broken or weakened attachment, with the child seeking ways to become isolated and protected from future maltreatment (Bakermans-Kranenburg et al. 2011; Kwako et al. 2010). If these children become parents, they may be more likely to continue the cycle of maltreatment with their own children, demonstrating the importance of intervening with families as early as possible (Ammerman et al. 2009).

New and Emerging Research

New and emerging topics related to the intergenerational transmission of child maltreatment are being examined in an effort to prevent child maltreatment through policy and practice innovations. However, there is still much to be discovered about these contexts to address the transmission of child maltreatment across generations. The following is a discussion of new and emerging research within these contexts.

New Topics of Interest in the Transmission of Intimate Partner Violence

Scholars continue to advance the field of interpersonal violence transmission by asking critically important questions and examining it in new ways. This section explores advances in the understanding of interpersonal violence that are related to gender, same-sex relationships, measurement and methodological advancements, and theoretical developments.

Understanding the Relationship Between Interpersonal Violence and Gender

Intimate partner violence perpetration in adolescence and young adulthood is not limited to one gender or another (O'Keefe 1997; Palmetto et al. 2013). Girls are perpetrating violence as frequently and sometimes more than boys (Cascardi et al. 1994; Courtney et al. 2011). As such, scholars must ask how exposure to violence in childhood affects girls, boys, and transgendered youth and how these different experiences relate to violence perpetration. Timmons Fritz et al. (2012) found partial support for their belief that transmission of aggression across generations was gender-specific; men tended to imitate their fathers' violence more than women did. However, the models examining mothers' violence did not support a similar pattern.

Understanding Intimate Partner Violence in Same Sex Relationships

It is necessary to begin to explore the relationship between violence exposure in childhood and violence perpetration in same-sex relationships. While there has been significant research on intimate partner violence in same-sex romantic relationships, practically no research exists on the link between previous violence exposure and subsequent perpetration in these relationships. The field would be enhanced by studying violence transmission in individuals involved in same-sex relationships to determine if the patterns are comparable to those observed in heterosexual relationships.

Measurement and Methodological Advances Related to Violence Exposure

As with research on multiple forms of maltreatment, many have observed that children often experience a combination of child maltreatment and parental intimate partner violence (Herrenkohl and Herrenkohl 2007). The importance of this type of approach is supported by research by Franklin et al. (2012) who reported that experiencing both forms of family-of-origin violence (child maltreatment and parental intimate partner violence) makes it 1.73 times more likely the child will perpetrate adult intimate partner violence. This approach is also supported by the work of Park et al. (2012) who report that experiencing both forms of family-of-origin violence increases the risk of some antisocial outcomes. This line of research may contribute to a better understanding of how various forms of violence and child maltreatment are transmitted intergenerationally.

A growing number of scholars are focusing on how the personal history of each partner may affect the occurrence of interpersonal violence. These researchers are examining how the maltreatment histories of both partners influence relationship behavior and subsequent violence with each other and their children. These scholars are employing samples and models that include both partners of a relationship, often calling upon Kenny's actor-partner interdependence model (Kenny 1996, see also Capaldi et al. 2003; Timmons Fritz and Smith Slep 2009; O'Leary and Smith Slep 2003). Recently, Timmons Fritz, Smith Slep, and O'Leary conducted a couple-level analysis supporting intergenerational transmission and assessed both partners' intimate partner violence histories and family of origin aggression (2012). Findings indicate that although both respondents' and their partners' histories of aggression within their family of origin generally predicted physical intimate partner violence victimization and perpetration, couples where both partners had family of origin histories of violence were not at increased risk for intimate partner violence. However, the factors most predictive of intimate partner violence were respondents' witnessing aggression between parents and their partners' having parents who perpetrated aggression.

Theoretical Advances

Scholars investigating the intergenerational transmission of violence and maltreatment are also beginning to employ theories that expound upon the links between cognition, emotion. and behavior. Early perspectives outlined by Huesmann and Guerra (1997) suggested that cognitive processes link observational learning and aggressive behavior. They stated that cognitive schema, the internal framework an individual uses to make sense of the world, mediate the relationship between an input (stimuli) and an output (aggression). Aggressive youth tend to have aggressive schema if they have observed more aggression and believe it is an appropriate and effective problem solving option (Huesmann and Guerra 1997; Guerra et al. 2003).

Early violence exposure appears to contribute to beliefs about "acceptability" of violence (Franklin and Kercher 2012). Building on Huesmann and Guerra's work, Jouriles and colleagues (2011) have developed a theory to examine youths' exposure to family violence (both child maltreatment and intimate partner violence) and subsequent dating violence perpetration. The theory, which has not been thoroughly tested, examines "explicit beliefs" and "implicit knowledge structures" that may facilitate aggression and "executive functioning" to explore the role of cognition along with trauma, emotion regulation, and rejection sensitivity (Jouriles et al. 2012). In a recent study, Jouriles and his colleagues (2013) found that explicit beliefs justifying aggression and knowledge structures contributed significantly to between-subject differences in teen dating violence. The study also showed that only explicit beliefs justifying aggression contributed significantly to within-subject differences in the same sample. Understanding the nuances of the impact of youths' exposure to family violence has the potential to inform interventions and treatment. Findings such as these support the need for trauma informed care as well as cognitive-based therapies.

New Topics of Interest Among Foster Care Youth and Youth Aging Out

There are only a few studies examining the intergenerational transmission of child maltreatment to children and youth who have been in foster care. For example, one study found that parents who have a history of child welfare system involvement as children experienced more risk factors and were less likely to be reunified with their children than parents who were not in the system as children (Marshall et al. 2011). There is a lack of documentation regarding child welfare system involvement among children of parents who are or who have spent time in foster care. Indeed, we know little about the relationship between child welfare system involvement as a child and again as a parent.

Foster Care Impacts on Youth Development

Removal from the care of an abusive or neglectful parent or caregiver, and subsequent child welfare system involvement among children and adolescents, involves advantages and disadvantages. Ideally, when a child is removed from an abusive or neglectful environment, the risk of harm decreases and the child receives treatment and services to address the traumatic experiences associated with child maltreatment. Services are offered to the parent and family to improve parent-child interactions, increase family home stability and resources, and reduce the likelihood of future incidence of child maltreatment. However, a child placed in foster care may also be exposed to other risks and adverse circumstances, such as child maltreatment by a care provider and instability in placement, school, and social groups and networks (Crosse et al. 1993; Magunson and Shager 2010). In addition, children may experience trauma when removed from their home (Bruskas 2008; Liotti 2004). Therefore, it is necessary to evaluate policies and practices related to the removal of children, and to consider whether or not removal is the best option or if an alternative intervention would enhance the family's stability and reduce the risk for future maltreatment.

Impacts on Mental Health

The experience of child maltreatment has the potential to create behavioral and emotional difficulties that profoundly affect a child's development and life course, with long-term consequences impacting not only the children experiencing maltreatment but also their families, future relationships, and society (Crosse et al. 1993; Liotti 2004; Magunson and Shager 2010). Likely due to traumatic experiences of abuse and neglect, youth involved in the foster care system with a history of maltreatment have an increased likelihood of developing behavioral and emotional problems relative to youth of comparable backgrounds. There are estimates of between 37 % and 80 % of youth in child welfare systems exhibiting mental health distress as compared to between 10 % and 26 % of the general population (dos Reis et al. 2001; McMillen et al. 2005; Merikangas et al. 2010; Raghavan et al. 2005; Zima et al. 2000).

Although mental health symptoms among maltreated youth often continue after they age out of systems of care (Pecora et al. 2009), research also suggests that mental health service utilization decreases dramatically after leaving care (Courtney et al. 2005; McMillen and Raghavan 2009). The elevated levels of psychological distress and lack of appropriate intervention and services related to mental health are important factors to consider in the context of future relationships and parenting.

Young adults with impaired psychological functioning may become parents who then have trouble providing developmentally appropriate and responsive care to their children (Kotch et al. 1995). Parents with a history of maltreatment who are also struggling with psychological distress may be at higher risk than other parents of abusing or neglecting their children (Dixon et al. 2005; Marshall et al. 2011). Although not all maltreated children with mental health issues will perpetuate the cycle of abuse and neglect, it is an important factor to consider in research and practice.

Impacts on Youth Aging Out

Studies have repeatedly shown that youth aging out experience significant difficulties in adjusting to living on their own. Youth aging out have overall poorer outcomes than those who have never been in foster care, in the domains of employment, housing, education, justice system involvement, mental health, substance use, physical health, and early parenting (Courtney and Dworsky 2006; Courtney et al. 2011; Reilly 2003). Youth aging out are a particularly vulnerable group and future research needs to consider their needs and experiences in order to develop tailored interventions and preventive programs to stop the cycle of maltreatment. Interventions should take into consideration the youths' history of maltreatment; experiences in foster care; relationships, networks, and supports; and their transition from foster care. More research on youth aging out and their pregnancy and parenting, attitudes, outcomes, and experiences is needed (Geiger and Schelbe 2014). Research regarding the challenges and successes from the pregnant and parenting youths' perspective is also being pursued to better inform the circumstances and experiences of youth that may influence the familial transmission of child maltreatment (Schelbe et al. 2014).

New Research on Trauma

Trauma and Epigenetics

Recent developments in the field of epigenetics and trauma have brought attention to the ways in which the social environment and family dynamic may create biochemical changes in the body (Ogden et al. 2006). A person's epigenetic profile, or vulnerability to developing an illness or disorder when specific genes are present, is directly connected to the experiences of family members in past generations (Perry 2009). What happens to children's parents and grandparents influences the way that the children's brains form and develop; it is possible that when parents and grandparents have histories of untreated trauma (specifically child maltreatment), their children are born primed to cope in ways that are both child abuse and trauma influenced (Anda et al. 2006; Ammerman et al. 2009; 2010). As with an increased risk for cancer, diabetes, and heart disease, it is now hypothesized that trauma can be passed down from generation to generation, resulting in maladaptive coping skills. Investigating the etiology of these maladaptive coping mechanisms and the traumatic experiences that underlie them may be a key to actually breaking the cycle of child maltreatment (Belsky et al. 2009).

Multiple generations of families that have endured child abuse and neglect and who have experienced some of the aforementioned risk factors may have markedly different gene expressions (Debellis et al. 2010; Perry et al. 1995; Shonkoff and Phillips 2000). When this occurs, these expressed genes are then passed down to later generations; in essence, the events of the past are realized in future generations of children.

Trauma and Developing Interventions

Children who are born into families affected by intergenerational maltreatment may not only have their direct environment effected (for example, via drug use, mental illness, intimate partner violence), but also may be born primed to respond to stress much differently than their peers not raised in homes affected by intergenerational maltreatment. This premise locates intergenerational maltreatment and traumatic event exposure in a manner that provides depth and breadth of the effects over time and proscribes quite a different approach to assessment and treatment. Given what is known about how epigenetics and cumulative exposure to stress can influence the risk of child abuse and neglect, it is believed that habits and traits may become permanent genetic states over time (Perry et al. 1995). Therefore, it is necessary to utilize a approach to social service provision and prevention programming that takes into account the full life span. Researchers and practitioners alike must realize the effect multigenerational exposure to child maltreatment and violence have on the developing brain. They also must meet the needs of each family differently, while being cautious of triggers of trauma and traumatic event memories (Foa et al. 2009). While previously the gene expression changes were believed to be permanent, new research suggests that enrichment of the environment and pharmaceuticals may reverse the changes in the brain (Yang et al. 2013; Weder and Kaufman 2011).

Trauma and Gender Differences

Traumatic events affect men and women differently and add to the complexity of understanding trauma through a child welfare-related lens. Men tend to respond to a traumatic event with increased aggression and impulsiveness whereas women tend to respond to a traumatic even with increased relational dysfunction as well as decreased communication (Ogden et al. 2006). Recent work in brain development has posited that women may perceive stress more intensely and more vividly than men due to hormonal differences (Appleyard et al. 2011; Cicchetti and Cohen 2006). Research focusing on brain development has demonstrated that women may perceive stress more intensely and more vividly than men due to this hormonal difference (Appleyard et al. 2011; Cicchetti and Cohen 2006). Some researchers have noticed that due to these different, gender-based responses to trauma, traumatized men are more likely to commit crimes like assault and homicide, increasing their chances for placement in the criminal justice system. On the other hand, traumatized women tend have an increased representation in the child welfare system due to offenses related to child maltreatment (Friedman et al. 2007; Ogden et al. 2006).

Summary

Pathways are needed to further examine the use of innovative evidence-based, trauma-informed methods of practice with specific groups such as youth from the foster care system and individuals and families experiencing intimate partner violence and trauma. By employing methods that allow for a more comprehensive and holistic examination of risk and resiliency in intergenerational maltreatment research, more innovative, testable, and effective interventions will emerge, leading to a reduction in child maltreatment and violence.

Strategies for Moving Forward

Advances in child maltreatment prevention require action from researchers, educators, practitioners, and policymakers. Individuals, couples, families, and communities are affected by child maltreatment, intimate partner violence, and trauma. It is critical to incorporate a holistic approach to understanding and preventing child maltreatment while continuing to work towards a better understanding of the risk and protective factors that influence the occurrence of child maltreatment. A holistic approach to understanding the intergenerational transmission of child maltreatment should also be incorporated in order to inform policies, programs, and future research. The following are suggestions of strategies for professionals and researchers working with individuals, families, and communities as they relate to education and assessment, focus of intervention, and directions for research.

Education and Assessment

All professionals who interact with the child welfare population, including doctors, lawyers, social workers, and behavioral health clinicians, should have explicit training in conducting comprehensive assessments. Every client in the system should be approached as though they may have experienced trauma and, as a result, may be affected genetically, biochemically, cognitively, and socially. As part of a proper assessment, professionals should be trained to examine both present circumstances as well as past experiences. During the assessment process, providers should apply a trauma-informed systems perspective and pay careful attention to past traumatic events, triggers, and symptoms.

It is also important for practitioners and researchers to focus on both the cognitive and the emotional mechanisms that link childhood maltreatment and later violence perpetration. Jouriles and colleagues' (2011) comprehensive conceptual model takes a variety of cognitive and emotional mediators into consideration; it will be important to test this model as it may contribute to the development of effective evidence-based interventions.

Focus of Intervention

Currently, there are several approaches to intervention that show promise in working with families presenting a history of trauma, child abuse or neglect, and other forms of violence. Promising efforts include trauma-focused cognitive behavioral therapy and narrative-based therapies that utilize support groups and safety planning to help stabilize individuals (Cohen et al. 2005; Foa et al. 2009). Although child welfare workers do not typically treat (but rather assess, stabilize, and refer), the engagement, rapport building, and communication concepts embedded in these models are still applicable in most child welfare contexts.

Youth aging out of foster care are a particularly vulnerable population and at high risk for the intergenerational transmission of maltreatment. During the aging out process, there are unique opportunities for interventions to help youth learn about parenting and access services to assist with resolving their experiences with trauma. These services can be provided along with the independent living skills that are currently offered to youth transitioning out of foster care. Intervention and prevention efforts should also focus not only on teaching effective parenting skills to foster youth who are already parents, but also creating the conditions and contexts where children and families can thrive.

Directions for Research

In order to continue to move the field forward, researchers should continue to identify and examine protective factors and those factors affecting individuals who break the cycle of child maltreatment. Specifically, researchers should consider the contexts of intimate partner violence and poverty when examining the presence or absence of intergenerational transmission of child maltreatment.

Researchers should consider focusing on the influence of multiple forms of maltreatment and exposure to violence rather than, or in addition to, attempting to tease apart the unique effects of various forms of maltreatment when predicting later outcomes and the intergenerational transmission of child maltreatment. Often, children experience more than one form of maltreatment or violence exposure and these experiences interact. Using techniques such as latent class and latent profile analysis allows one to take interactions into consideration and can identify categories of individuals for further study. (For more detail about targeting subpopulations, see Chap. 2).

Robust theories explaining intergenerational transmission of child maltreatment are lacking. Developing a better theoretical understanding of the phenomenon benefits both researchers and practitioners. As thinking about the cycle of maltreatment is refined, researchers can improve models for further testing. Likewise, practitioners may develop higher quality interventions based upon new theories.

Finally, researchers and practitioners should continue to seek to understand how psychological distress and mental health service utilization impact long-term outcomes, future relationships, and parenting for those having experienced child maltreatment. Continued education and awareness of the consequences of child maltreatment which incorporates context and a holistic approach to maltreatment prevention provides insight and direction for research, policy, and practice in future generations.

Reflection: Intergenerational Transmission of Child Maltreatment

Cathy Spatz Widom
John Jay College and the Graduate Center,
City University of New York, New York, NY, USA

As someone who has been struggling with the challenges of conducting research in the field of child maltreatment for almost 30 years, I believe there is more awareness of the barriers preventing greater forward movement in understanding the causes of maltreatment and, in particular, the intergenerational transmission of child maltreatment. Indeed, it is fairly common now to find critical reviews of the existing literature that catalogue the limitations and point out the few studies that are exceptions. Nonetheless, the challenges are enormous and, I believe, have increased over time.

Conducting this type of research is challenging. It is difficult to recruit samples and navigate the ethical and legal requirements regarding reporting suspected maltreatment. Institutional Review Boards (IRBs) have become more legalistic and sensitive to the conduct of research in this area and have made it more difficult for studies to be approved. For example, if IRBs require the researcher to obtain permission from parents of the child (who are potentially or allegedly the perpetrator) to discuss potential maltreatment with their children, how does this affect your ability to interview children who may be most vulnerable? Because of mandatory reporting, researchers from other fields who now recognize the importance of these early childhood experiences are afraid to include child abuse and neglect in their studies, fearing that they may lose participants by asking about these sensitive topics.

Determining causality remains one of the field's greatest challenges. In contrast to other areas, I believe we have made relatively little progress in understanding causes. We have learned about some of the individual and contextual factors that increase the risk of child abuse and neglect. These findings, while important, are not analogous to knowing what *causes* maltreatment. What do we need? Longitudinal studies enrolling participants before the birth of the child would allow more controlled studies of who does and does not abuse or neglect their children and allow us to better specify with what individual, family, or community characteristics contribute to these outcomes. Prospective longitudinal designs provide an opportunity to determine the correct temporal order of risk factors and child maltreatment, to adjust for social and individual confounding factors as they happen, and minimize reliance on recall and the selection of participants on the basis of outcomes. Such designs are rare because they are expensive and take time to mature. Some of us have argued for the inclusion of child maltreatment in the National Children's Study. This large-scale study would have allowed us to better assess causes and consequences of child abuse and neglect, but we met resistance, in large part for many of the reasons described above.

Where should research go in the future? Many of us work on an ecological model that assumes that behavior is complex and multiply determined by characteristics of the individual, parent and family, and neighborhood and community and that behavior changes over time, not necessarily in a linear manner. Thus, snapshots of children, adolescents, or adults at any one point in time will only reflect that data point. Most of the existing literature still involves retrospective studies and cross-sectional designs. There is a need to move beyond correlational studies and analyses to test causal models.

Another question is whether we should focus exclusively on parents who abuse their children or should expand our studies to include parents with histories of abuse who put their children at risk for abuse by others. Studies of early neglect with animal models, particularly rats and mice, may also offer opportunities to understand the causes of child maltreatment, including intergenerational processes that affect behavior. Animal analogue studies provide a way to manipulate characteristics of parents to determine whether some of the candidate risk factors identified by research in humans lead to animal versions of abuse and neglect. Finally, researchers need to ask whether there are differences or similarities in the causes of child maltreatment based on cultural context, sex, race, and ethnicity of parents. We have made little progress in understanding the "common and divergent pathways in etiologies of different forms of child maltreatment for diverse populations." Hopefully in the future we will do better.

References

Afifi, T. O. (2007). Child abuse and adolescent parenting: Developing a theoretical model from an ecological perspective. *Journal of Aggression, Maltreatment, and Trauma, 14*(3), 89–105.

American Psychiatric Association. (2013). *Diagnostic and statistical manual of mental disorders* (5th ed.). Arlington: American Psychiatric Publishing.

Ammerman, R., Putnam, F., Margolis, P., & Van Ginkel, J. (2009). Quality improvement in child abuse prevention programs. In K. Dodge & D. Coleman (Eds.), *Preventing child maltreatment.* New York: Guilford.

Ammerman, R., Putnam, F., Bosse, N., Teeters, A., & Van Ginkel, J. (2010). Maternal depression in home visitation: A systematic review. *Aggression and Violent Behavior, 15*(3), 191–200.

Anda, R., Filetti, V., Bremner, J., Walker, J., Whitfield, C., Perry, B., et al. (2006). The enduring effects of abuse and related adverse experiences in childhood: A convergence of evidence from neurobiology and epidemiology. *European Archives of Psychiatry and Clinical Neuroscience, 256*(3), 174–186.

Appel, A. E., & Holden, G. W. (1998). The co-occurrence of spouse and physical child abuse: A review and appraisal. *Journal of Family Psychology, 12*(4), 578–599.

Appleyard, K., Berlin, L., Rosanbalm, K., & Dodge, K. (2011). Preventing early child maltreatment: Implications from a longitudinal study of maternal abuse history, substance use problems, and offspring victimization. *Prevention Science, 12*(2), 139–149.

Bakermans-Kranenburg, M. J., Steele, H., Zeanah, C. H., Muhamedrahimov, R. J., Vorria, P., Dobrova-Krol, N. A., et al. (2011). Attachment and emotional development in institutional care: Characteristics and catch-up. Children without permanent parents: Research, practice, and policy. *Monographs of the Society for Research in Child Development, 76*(4), 62–91.

Bandura, A. (1977). *Social learning theory*. Englewood Cliffs: Prentice-Hall.

Bavolek, S. J., & Keene, R. G. (1999). *Adult-Adolescent Parenting Inventory (AAPI-2) administration and development handbook*. Park City: Family Development Resources, Inc.

Belsky, J. (1993). Etiology of child maltreatment: A developmental-ecological analysis. *Psychological Bulletin, 114*(3), 413–434.

Belsky, J., Conger, R., & Capaldi, D. (2009). The intergenerational transmission of parenting: Introduction to the special section. *Developmental Psychology, 45*(5), 1201–1204.

Berger, L. M. (2004). Income, family structure, and child maltreatment risk. *Children and Youth Services Review, 26*(8), 725–748.

Berlin, L. J., Appleyard, K., & Dodge, K. A. (2011). Intergenerational continuity in child maltreatment: Mediating mechanisms and implication for prevention. *Child Development, 82*(1), 162–176.

Bowlby, J. (1969). *Attachment and loss* (Attachment, Vol. 1). New York: Basic Books.

Bronfenbrenner, U. (1979). *The ecology of human development: Experiments by nature and design*. Cambridge, MA: Harvard University Press.

Bruskas, D. (2008). Children in foster care: A vulnerable population at risk. *Journal of Child and Adolescent Psychiatric Nursing, 21*(2), 70–77.

Capaldi, D. M., Shortt, J. W., & Crosby, L. (2003). Physical and psychological aggression in at-risk young couples: Stability and change in young adulthood. *Merrill-Palmer Quarterly, 49*(1), 1–27.

Cascardi, M., Avery-Leaf, S., & O'Leary, K. (1994) Building a gender sensitive model to explain adolescent dating violence. Paper presented at the 102nd Annual Meeting of the American Psychological Association, Los Angeles.

Cicchetti, D., & Cohen, D. (2006). *Developmental psychopathy* (2nd ed., Vol. 2). New York: Wiley.

Cicchetti, D., & Toth, S. L. (2005). Child maltreatment. *Annual Review of Clinical Psychology, 1*, 409–438.

Cohen, J., Deblinger, D., & Mannarino, A. (2005). *Trauma-focused cognitive-behavioral therapy*. New York: Guilford Press.

Cohen, L. R., Hien, D. A., & Batchelder, S. (2008). The impact of cumulative maternal trauma and diagnosis on parenting behavior. *Child Maltreatment, 13*(27), 27–38.

Conger, R. D., & Donnellan, M. B. (2007). An interactionist perspective on the socioeconomic context of human development. *Annual Review of Psychology, 58*, 175–199.

Conger, R. D., Neppl, T., Kim, K. J., & Scaramella, L. (2003). Angry and aggressive behavior across three generations: A prospective, longitudinal study of parents and children. *Journal of Abnormal Child Psychology, 31*(2), 143–160.

Conger, R. D., Belsky, J., & Capaldi, D. M. (2009). The intergenerational transmission of parenting: Closing comments for the special section. *Developmental Psychology, 45*(5), 1276–1283.

Conger, R. D., Schofield, T. J., Neppl, T. K., & Merrick, M. T. (2013). Disrupting intergenerational continuity in harsh and abusive parenting: The importance of a nurturing relationship with a romantic partner. *Journal of Adolescent Health, 53*(4), S11–S17.

Coulton, C. J., Korbin, J. E., Su, M., & Chow, J. (1995). Community level factors and child mal-treatment rates. *Child Development, 66*(5), 1262–1276.

Courtney, M. E., & Dworsky, A. (2006). Early outcomes for young adults transitioning from out-of-home care in the USA. *Child and Family Social Work, 11*, 209–219.

Courtney, M. E., Dworsky, A., Ruth, G., Keller, T., Havlicek, J., & Bost, N. (2005). *Midwest evaluation of the adult functioning of former foster youth: Outcomes at age 19.* Chicago: Chapin Hall at the University of Chicago.

Courtney, M. E., Dworsky, A., Brown, A., Cary, C., Love, K., & Vorhies, V. (2011). *Midwest evaluation of the adult functioning of former foster youth: Outcomes at age 26.* Chicago: Chapin Hall at the University of Chicago.

Cox, C. E., Kotch, J. B., & Everson, M. D. (2003). A longitudinal study of modifying influences in the relationship between domestic violence and child maltreatment. *Journal of Family Violence, 18*(1), 5–17.

Crittenden, P. M., & Ainsworth, M. D. (1989). Child maltreatment and attachment theory. In D. Cicchetti & V. Carlson (Eds.), *Child maltreatment: Theory and research on the causes and consequences of child abuse and neglect* (pp. 432–463). Cambridge, UK: Cambridge University Press.

Crosse, S. C., Kaye, E., & Ratnofsky, A. C. (1993). *A report on the maltreatment of children with disabilities.* Washington, DC: National Center on Child Abuse and Neglect.

Debellis, M. D., Hooper, S. R., Wooley, D. P., & Shenk, C. E. (2010). Demographic, maltreatment, and neurobiological correlates of PTSD symptoms in children and adolescents. *Journal of Pediatric Psychology, 35*(5), 570–577.

Dixon, L., Browne, K., & Hamilton-Giachritsis, C. (2005). Risk factors of parents abused as chil-dren: A meditational analysis of the intergenerational continuity of child maltreatment (Part I). *Journal of Child Psychology and Psychiatry, 46*(1), 47–57.

Dixon, L., Hamilton-Giachritsis, C., Browne, K., & Ostapuik, E. (2007). The co-occurrence of child and intimate partner maltreatment in the family: Characteristics of the violent perpetra-tors. *Journal of Family Violence, 22*(8), 675–689.

Dixon, L., Browne, K., & Hamilton-Giachritsis, C. (2009). Patterns of risk and protective factors in intergenerational cycle of maltreatment. *Journal of Family Violence, 24*, 111–122.

Dong, M., Anda, M. R., Dube, S. R., Giles, W. H., & Felitti, V. J. (2003). The relationship of expo-sure to childhood sexual abuse to other forms of abuse, neglect, and household dysfunction during childhood. *Child Abuse & Neglect, 27*(6), 625–639.

dos Reis, S., Zito, J. M., Safer, D. J., & Soeken, K. L. (2001). Mental health services for youths in foster care and disabled youths. *American Journal of Public Health, 91*, 1094–1099.

Drake, B., & Jonson-Reid, M. (2014). Poverty and child maltreatment. In J. Korbin & R. D. Krugman (Eds.), *Handbook of child maltreatment* (pp. 131–148). Dordrecht: Springer.

Drake, B., & Pandey, S. (1996). Understanding the relationship between neighborhood poverty and specific types of child maltreatment. *Child Abuse & Neglect, 20*(11), 1003–1018.

Dumont, K. A., Widom, C. S., & Czaja, S. J. (2007). Predictors of resilience in abused and neglected children grown-up: The role of individual and neighborhood characteristics. *Child Abuse & Neglect, 31*, 255–274.

Dworsky, A., & Courtney, M. E. (2010). The risk of teenage pregnancy among transitioning foster youth: Implications for extending state care beyond age 18. *Children and Youth Services Review, 32*, 1351–1356.

Dworsky, A., & DeCoursey, J. (2009). *Pregnant and parenting foster youth: Their needs, their experiences.* Chicago: Chapin Hall at the University of Chicago.

Eckenrode, J., Smith, E. G., McCarthy, M. E., & Dineen, M. (2014). Income inequality and child maltreatment in the United States. *Pediatrics, 133*(3), 454–461.

Edleson, J. L. (1999). The overlap between child maltreatment and woman battering. *Violence Against Women, 5*(2), 134–154.

Egeland, B., Jacobitz, D., & Sroufe, L. A. (1988). Breaking the cycle of abuse. *Child Development, 59*, 1080–1088.

Ertem, I. O., Leventhal, J. M., & Dobbs, S. (2000). Intergenerational continuity of child physical abuse: How good is the evidence? *The Lancet, 356*, 814–819.

Foa, E. B., Keane, T. M., Friedman, M. J., & Cohen, J. A. (2009). *Effective treatments for PTSD*. New York: Guilford Press.

Franklin, C. A., & Kercher, G. A. (2012). The intergenerational transmission of intimate partner violence: Differentiating correlates in a random community sample. *Journal of Family Violence, 27*(3), 187–199.

Franklin, C. A., Menaker, T. A., & Kercher, G. A. (2012). Risk and resiliency factors that mediate the effect of family-of-origin violence on adult intimate partner victimization and perpetration. *Victims & Offenders, 7*(2), 121–142.

Friedman, M., Keane, T., & Resick, P. (2007). *Handbook of PTSD: Science and practice*. New York: Guilford.

Geiger, J. M., & Schelbe, L. A. (2014). Stopping the cycle of child abuse and neglect: A call to action to focus on pregnant and parenting youth in and aging out of the foster care system. *Journal of Public Child Welfare, 8*(1), 1–26.

Gewirtz, A. H., & Edleson, J. L. (2007). Young children's exposure to intimate partner violence: Towards a developmental risk and resilience framework for research and intervention. *Journal of Family Violence, 22*, 151–163.

Guerra, N. G., Rowell Huesmann, L., & Spindler, A. (2003). Community violence exposure, social cognition, and aggression among urban elementary school children. *Child Development, 74*(5), 1561–1576.

Hazen, A. L., Connelly, C. D., Roesch, S. C., Hough, R. L., & Landsverk, J. A. (2009). Child maltreatment profiles and adjustment problems in high-risk adolescents. *Journal of Interpersonal Violence, 24*(2), 361–378.

Herrenkohl, T. I., & Herrenkohl, R. C. (2007). Examining the overlap and prediction of multiple forms of child maltreatment, stressors, and socioeconomic status: A longitudinal analysis of youth outcomes. *Journal of Family Violence, 22*(7), 553–562.

Holt, S., Buckley, H., & Whelan, S. (2008). The impact of exposure to domestic violence on children and young people: A review of the literature. *Child Abuse & Neglect, 32*, 797–810.

Huesmann, L. R., & Guerra, N. G. (1997). Children's normative beliefs about aggression and aggressive behavior. *Journal of Personality and Social Psychology, 72*, 408–419.

Institute of Medicine and National Research Council. (2014). *New directions in child abuse and neglect research*. Washington, DC: The National Academies Press.

Jaffee, S. R., Bowes, L., Ouellet-Morin, I., Fisher, H. L., Moffit, T. E., Merrick, M. T., et al. (2013). Safe, stable, and nurturing relationships break the intergenerational cycle of abuse: A prospective nationally representative cohort of children in the United Kingdom. *Journal of Adolescent Health, 53*(4), S4–S10.

Jonson-Reid, M., Drake, B., & Kohl, P. L. (2009). Is the overrepresentation of the poor in child welfare caseloads due to bias or need? *Children and Youth Services Review, 31*(3), 422–427.

Jouriles, E. N., McDonald, R., Smith Slep, A. M., Heyman, R. E., & Garrido, E. (2008). Child abuse in the context of domestic violence: Prevalence, explanations, and practice implications. *Violence and Victims, 23*(2), 221–235.

Jouriles, E. N., Grych, J. H., Rosenfield, D., McDonald, R., & Dodson, M. C. (2011). Automatic cognitions and teen dating violence. *Psychology of Violence, 1*(4), 302–314.

Jouriles, E. N., McDonald, R., Mueller, V., & Grych, J. H. (2012). Youth experiences of family violence and teen dating violence perpetration: Cognitive and emotional mediators. *Clinical Child and Family Psychology Review, 15*(1), 58–68.

Jouriles, E. N., Rosenfield, D., McDonald, R., Kleinsasser, A. L., & Dodson, M. C. (2013). Explicit beliefs about aggression, implicit knowledge structures, and teen dating violence. *Journal of Abnormal Child Psychology, 41*(5), 789–799.

Kaufman, J., & Zigler, E. (1987). Do abused children become abusive parents? *American Journal of Orthopsychiatry, 57*(2), 186–192.

Kenny, D. A. (1996). Models of non-independence in dyadic research. *Journal of Social and Personal Relationships, 13*(2), 279–294.

Kim, J. (2009). Type-specific intergenerational transmission of neglectful and physically abusive parenting behaviors among young parents. *Children and Youth Services Review, 31*, 761–767.

King, B., Putnam-Hornstein, E., Cederbaum, J. A., & Needell, B. (2014). A cross-sectional examination of birth rates among adolescent girls in foster care. *Children and Youth Services Review, 36*, 179–186.

Kotch, J. B., Browne, D. C., Ringwalt, C. L., Stewart, P. W., Ruina, E., Holt, K., et al. (1995). Risk of child abuse or neglect in a cohort of low-income children. *Child Abuse & Neglect, 19*(9), 1115–1130.

Kwako, L., Noll, J., Putnam, F., & Trickett, P. (2010). Childhood sexual abuse and attachment: An intergenerational perspective. *Clinical Child Psychology and Psychiatry, 15*(3), 407–422.

Lee, B. J., & Goerge, R. M. (1999). Poverty, early childbearing, and child maltreatment: A multinomial analysis. *Children and Youth Services Review, 21*(9/10), 755–780.

Li, F., Godinet, M. T., & Arnsberger, P. (2011). Protective factors among families with children at risk of maltreatment: Follow up to early school years. *Children and Youth Services Review, 33*, 139–148.

Liotti, G. (2004). Trauma, dissociation, and disorganized attachment: Three strands of a single braid. *Psychotherapy: Theory, Research, Practice, Training, 41*, 472–486.

Magunson, K., & Shager, H. (2010). Early education: Progress and promise for children from low income families. *Children and Youth Services Review, 32*, 1186–1198.

Marshall, J. M., Huang, H., & Ryan, J. P. (2011). Intergenerational families in child welfare: Assessing needs and estimating permanency. *Children and Youth Services Review, 33*, 1024–1030.

Masten, A. S., Best, K. M., & Garmezy, N. (1990). Resilience and development: Contributions from the study of children who overcome adversity. *Development and Psychopathology, 2*(4), 425–444.

Matta Oshima, K. M., Narendorf, S. C., & McMillen, J. C. (2013). Pregnancy risk among older youth transitioning from foster care. *Children and Youth Services Review, 25*(10), 1760–1765.

McMillen, J. C., & Raghavan, R. (2009). Pediatric to adult mental health service use of youth in the foster care system. *Journal of Adolescent Health, 44*, 7–13.

McMillen, J. C., Zima, B. T., Scott, L. D., Auslander, W. F., Munson, M. R., Ollie, M. T., et al. (2005). Prevalence of psychiatric disorders among older youths in the foster care system. *Journal of the American Academy of Child & Adolescent Psychiatry, 44*(1), 88–95.

Merikangas, K. R., He, J. P., Burstein, M., Swanson, S. A., Avenevoli, S., Cui, L., et al. (2010). Lifetime prevalence of mental disorders in U.S. adolescents: Results from the National Comorbidity Survey Replication–Adolescent Supplement (NCS-A). *Journal of the American Academy of Child & Adolescent Psychiatry, 49*(10), 980–989.

Moffitt, T. E., & Caspi, A. (2003). Preventing the intergenerational continuity of antisocial behaviour: Implications of partner violence. In D. P. Farrington & J. W. Coid (Eds.), *Early prevention of adult antisocial behaviour* (pp. 109–129). Cambridge, UK: Cambridge University Press.

Neppl, T., Conger, R., Scaramella, L., & Ontai, L. (2009). Intergenerational continuity of observed early parenting behavior: Mediating pathways and child effects. *Developmental Psychology, 45*(5), 1241–1256.

Newcomb, M. D., & Locke, T. F. (2001). Intergenerational cycle of maltreatment: A popular concept obscured by methodological limitations. *Child Abuse & Neglect, 25*(9), 1219–1240.

O'Keefe, M. (1997). Predictors of dating violence among high school students. *Journal of Interpersonal Violence, 12*(4), 546–568.

O'Leary, K. D., & Smith Slep, A. M. (2003). A dyadic longitudinal model of adolescent dating aggression. *Journal of Clinical Child and Adolescent Psychology, 32*(3), 314–327.

Ogden, P., Minton, K., & Pain, C. (2006). *Trauma and the body: A sensorimotor approach to psychotherapy.* New York: W.W. Norton & Company.

Osofsky, J. D. (2003). Prevalence of children's exposure to domestic violence and child maltreatment: Implications for prevention and intervention. *Clinical Child and Family Psychology Review, 6*(3), 161–170.

Palmetto, N., Davidson, L. L., Breitbart, V., & Rickert, V. I. (2013). Predictors of physical intimate partner violence in the lives of young women: Victimization, perpetration, and bidirectional violence. *Violence and Victims, 28*(1), 103–121.

Park, A., Smith, C., & Ireland, T. (2012). Equivalent harm? The relative roles of maltreatment and exposure to intimate partner violence in antisocial outcomes for young adults. *Children and Youth Services Review, 34*(5), 962–972.

Patterson, G. (1998). Continuities—A search for causal mechanisms: Comment on the special section. *Developmental Psychology, 34*, 1263–1268.

Pears, K. C., & Capaldi, D. M. (2001). Intergenerational transmission of abuse: A two generational prospective study of an at-risk sample. *Child Abuse & Neglect, 25*, 1439–1461.

Pecora, P. J., Williams, J., Kessler, R., Downs, A., O'Brien, K., Hiripi, E., et al. (2003). *Assessing the effects of foster care: Early results from the Casey National Alumni Study*. Seattle: Casey Family Programs.

Pecora, P. J., White, C. R., Jackson, L. J., & Wiggins, T. (2009). Mental health of current and former recipients of foster care: A review of recent studies in the USA. *Child and Family Social Work, 14*, 132–146.

Perry, B. (2009). Examining child maltreatment through a neurodevelopmental lens: Clinical applications of the neurosequential model of therapeutics. *Journal of Loss and Trauma, 14*(4), 240–255.

Perry, B., Pollard, R., Blakley, T., Baker, W., & Vigilante, D. (1995). Childhood trauma, the neurobiology of adaptation, and "use-dependent" development of the brain: How "states" become "traits". *Infant Mental Health Journal, 16*(4), 271–291.

Raghavan, R., Zima, B. T., Anderson, R. M., Leibowitz, A. A., Schuster, M. A., & Landsverk, J. (2005). Psychotropic medication use in a national probability sample of children in the child welfare system. *Journal of Child and Adolescent Psychopharmacology, 15*(1), 97–106.

Reilly, T. (2003). Transition from care: Status and outcomes of youth who age out of foster care. *Child Abuse and Neglect, 82*(6), 727–746.

Rumm, P. D., Cummings, P., Krauss, M. R., Bell, M. A., & Rivara, F. P. (2000). Identified spouse abuse as a risk factor for child abuse. *Child Abuse & Neglect, 24*(11), 1375–1381.

Schelbe, L., Geiger, J. M., & Phillips, C. (2014, January). Parenting under pressure: Struggles with parenting faced by youth aging out of the child welfare system. Paper presented at the Society for Social Work and Research Annual Conference, San Antonio.

Schofield, T. J., Lee, R. D., & Merrick, M. T. (2013). Safe, stable, and nurturing relationships as a moderator of the intergenerational continuity of child maltreatment: A meta-analysis. *Journal of Adolescent Health, 53*, S32–S38.

Shonkoff, J., & Phillips, D. (Eds.). (2000). *From neurons to neighborhoods: The science of early childhood development*. Washington, DC: National Academy Press.

Slack, K. S., Holl, J. L., McDaniel, M., Yoo, J., & Bolger, K. (2004). Understanding the risks of child neglect: An exploration of poverty and parenting characteristics. *Child Maltreatment, 9*(4), 395–408.

Smith, C. A., Ireland, T. O., Park, A., Elwyn, L., & Thornberry, T. P. (2011). Intergenerational continuities and discontinuities in intimate partner violence: A two-generational prospective study. *Journal of Interpersonal Violence, 26*(18), 3720–3752.

Stevens-Simon, C., Nelligan, D., & Kelly, L. (2001). Adolescents at risk for mistreating their children: Part II: A home- and clinic-based prevention program. *Child Abuse & Neglect, 25*(6), 753–769.

Tajima, E. A. (2000). The relative importance of wife abuse as a risk factor for violence against children. *Child Abuse & Neglect, 24*(11), 1383–1398.

Thornberry, T. P., Freeman-Gallant, A., Lizotte, A. J., Krohn, M. D., & Smith, C. A. (2003). Linked lives: The intergenerational transmission of antisocial behavior. *Journal of Abnormal Child Psychology, 31*(2), 171–184.

Thornberry, T. P., Knight, K. E., & Lovegrove, P. J. (2012). Does maltreatment beget maltreatment? A systematic review of the intergenerational literature. *Trauma, Violence & Abuse, 13*(3), 135–152.

Thornberry, T. P., Henry, K. L., Smith, C. A., Ireland, T. O., Greenman, S. J., & Lee, R. D. (2013). Breaking the cycle of maltreatment: The role of safe, stable, and nurturing relationships. *Journal of Adolescent Health, 53*(4), S25–S31.

Timmons Fritz, P. A., & Smith Slep, A. M. (2009). Stability of physical and psychological adolescent dating aggression across time and partners. *Journal of Clinical Child & Adolescent Psychology, 38*(3), 303–314.

Timmons Fritz, P. A., Slep, A. M. S., & O'Leary, K. D. (2012). Couple-level analysis of the relation between family-of-origin aggression and intimate partner violence. *Psychology of Violence, 2*(2), 139–153.

U.S. Department of Health and Human Services. (2012). *Child maltreatment 2010*. Washington, DC: U.S. Department of Health and Human Services, Administration for Children and Families, Administration on Children, Youth, and Families, Children's Bureau.

U.S. Department of Health and Human Services. (2014). *Protective factors*. Child Welfare Information Gateway. Retrieved 28 Apr 2014 from https://www.childwelfare.gov/can/factors/protective.cfm

Weder, N., & Kaufman, J. (2011). Critical periods revisited: Implications for intervention with traumatized children. *Journal of the American Academy of Child and Adolescent Psychiatry, 50*(11), 1087–1089.

Werner, E. E., & Smith, R. S. (1992). *Overcoming the odds: High risk children from birth to adulthood*. Ithaca: Cornell University Press.

Whitson, M. L., Martinez, A., Ayala, C., & Kaufman, J. S. (2011). Predictors of parenting and infant outcomes for impoverished adolescent parents. *Journal of Family Social Work. 14*(4), 284–297. doi.org/10.1080/10522158.2011.587173.

Widom, C. S. (1989). Does violence beget violence? A critical examination of the literature. *Psychological Bulletin, 106*(1), 3–28.

Yang, B. Z., Zhang, H., Ge, W., Weder, N., Douglas-Palumberi, H., Perepletchikova, F., et al. (2013). Child abuse and epigenetic mechanisms of disease risk. *American Journal of Preventive Medicine, 44*(2), 101–107.

Zima, B. T., Bussing, R., Freeman, S., Yang, X., Belin, T. R., & Forness, S. R. (2000). Behavior problems, academic skill delays and school failure among school-aged children in foster care: Their relationship to placement characteristics. *Journal of Child and Family Studies, 9*, 87–103.

Jennifer Mullins Geiger is a postdoctoral fellow at Arizona State University School of Social Work where she received her Ph.D. in Social Work in May 2014. Her research interests include child maltreatment prevention, issues facing youth aging out of foster care and transitioning into adulthood, pregnancy and parenting youth who are aging out, and foster family resilience and satisfaction. She was awarded a 2-year Fellowship for the Promotion of Child Well-Being from the Doris Duke Charitable Foundation in 2011. Dr. Geiger has worked on grant-funded projects aimed at improving children and adolescents' mental health outcomes and preventing child abuse.

Lisa Schelbe is an assistant professor at Florida State University College of Social Work. She earned her doctorate from the University of Pittsburgh School of Social Work where she was a recipient of the *Doris Duke Fellowships for the Promotion of Child Well-Being*. Dr. Schelbe received her Master in Social Work from the George Warren Brown School of Social Work at Washington University in St. Louis. Her research primarily focuses on the experiences of youth aging out of the child welfare system. She is interested in how youth aging out negotiate the transition out of care and how services impact youth aging out during the transition. Dr. Schelbe is currently examining the educational experiences of youth aging out. Her diverse social work practice experience includes work with survivors of family and intimate partner violence and of natural disasters. Dr. Schelbe has background in program development, grant writing, and political advocacy.

Megan J. Hayes is a doctoral candidate in the School of Social Work at Arizona State University. She received a master's degree in social work at Arizona State University and a bachelor's degree in biopsychology from Nebraska Wesleyan University. Megan's research interests include youth aging out of the child welfare system, pediatric to adult mental health system transitions, and the intergenerational transmission of child maltreatment. She has worked on research grant projects related to child welfare training and child abuse prevention and her professional experience includes program supervision and administration in behavioral health and foster care group homes. Megan was awarded a 2-year *Doris Duke Fellowships for the Promotion of Child Well-Being* in 2013.

Elisa Kawam is a Ph.D. candidate in the School of Social Work at Arizona State University. She obtained her Bachelors of Social Work in 2007 and a Masters of Social Work in 2008. During her masters, she chose to specialize in policy, advocacy, and community aspects of social work and obtained a graduate certificate in child welfare. She previously worked as an investigator for Child Protective Services in South Phoenix and also supervised a transitional housing facility for pregnant and parenting teenage mothers. Her research interests include the prevention of child maltreatment and the intersectionality of trauma symptomology, epigenetics, attachment, policy, and intergenerational cycles of violence.

Colleen Cary Katz is an assistant professor at Silberman School of Social Work, Hunter College. She earned her doctorate at the University of Chicago School of Social Service Administration and her MSW at Columbia University School of Social Work. Dr. Katz is interested in how children and adolescents experience trauma, particularly those youth who have been placed in the foster care system as a result of parental maltreatment. She has focused her research on supporting the needs of this population and minimizing the risks associated with the experience of maltreatment in youth. Some of this research was funded by the *Doris Duke Fellowships for the Promotion of Child Well-Being* that Dr. Katz received in 2013. She has a background in clinical social work, providing assessment and psychotherapy to youth who have experienced trauma and/or parental maltreatment.

J. Bart Klika is an assistant professor in the School of Social Work at the University of Montana. He completed his doctoral degree from the School of Social Work at the University of Washington where he was a recipient of the *Doris Duke Fellowships for the Promotion of Child Well-Being* (inaugural cohort). Bart completed his master's degree at the School of Social Service Administration at the University of Chicago. During his doctoral studies, Bart worked as a research assistant on the Lehigh Longitudinal Study, a prospective study examining the developmental consequences associated with various forms of family violence. His research focuses on understand the etiology of child maltreatment, the long-term consequences of child maltreatment, and the ways in which some maltreated children develop well despite early experiences of maltreatment.

Chapter 5
Cultural Considerations in Refining Intervention Designs

Megan Finno-Velasquez, Elizabeth A. Shuey, Chie Kotake, and J. Jay Miller

Chapter 5 in Brief

Context

- Culture is often defined monolithically using physically evident characteristics such as race and ethnicity. However, culture is a fluid construct that is formulated by assimilation of cultural tools from successive generations and a family's individual needs, experiences, and interpretation.
- Families from cultural minority groups are often disproportionately represented in the child welfare system.
- The role of culture in parenting and child maltreatment may be best understood when examined through an interdisciplinary, multi-dimensional lens, and through its intersection with race and ethnicity, social stratification, ecological context and individual family experiences.
- Insufficient attention is paid to the role an individual family's social and economic context and experiences (e.g., immigration experiences) play in shaping parenting behaviors and risk for child maltreatment.
- Culture is not sufficiently examined in the development, implementation, and evaluation of prevention programs.

M. Finno-Velasquez (✉)
School of Social Work, University of Southern California, Los Angeles, CA, USA
e-mail: finno@usc.edu

E.A. Shuey • C. Kotake
Eliot-Pearson Department of Child Study and Human Development, Tufts University, Medford, MA, USA
e-mail: elizabeth.shuey@tufts.edu; chie.kotake@tufts.edu

J.J. Miller, PhD, MSW, CSW
College of Social Work, University of Kentucky, Lexington, KY, USA
e-mail: Justin.Miller1@uky.edu

© Springer International Publishing Switzerland 2015
D. Daro et al. (eds.), *Advances in Child Abuse Prevention Knowledge*,
Child Maltreatment 5, DOI 10.1007/978-3-319-16327-7_5

Strategies for Moving Forward

- Consider culture and its impacts on parenting behaviors, beliefs and choices in designing and implementing prevention services
- In professional education and in practice, present culture as a fluid and dynamic construct to facilitate the ability of service providers, researcher and others to better understand and respect families' heritage and tools in forming the service relationship.
- Increase the number and visibility of culturally diverse leaders in child maltreatment prevention research, policy, and practice.

Implications for Research

- Consider culture as a central organizing concept.
- Integrate the work of those examining family characteristics and ecological contexts and those exploring cultural values and beliefs.

Introduction

Child maltreatment occurs in families all around the world, as well as in families from all cultures in the United States. The definition and meaning of child maltreatment, particularly physical and sexual abuse, is fairly consistent across cultures, but the way in which these definitions are operationalized and applied to families can vary tremendously (Cyr et al. 2013). Moreover, less consistency in the definition and meaning of child neglect and shifting norms around corporal punishment in the United States also contribute to the need for considering child maltreatment within cultural context (Durrant 2008).

This chapter focuses on culture and parenting as a frame for understanding diverse families' experiences with the U.S. child welfare system. Our goal is to discuss and give context to the past and current disproportional involvement with child welfare systems for certain subgroups and populations. We will also provide suggestions for moving research, policy, and practice forward in a way that is attentive to variations in parenting and culture. The ideas presented here are rooted in an interdisciplinary perspective, as we attempt to discuss the roles of culture, parenting, practice, and policy at multiple levels using concrete examples.

We begin by defining culture and then use that definition as an orienting concept to understand child maltreatment at three levels: societal, program, and individual. Building on these definitional issues, we recommend strategies for improving the child maltreatment prevention field's capacity to promote child well-being in culturally diverse families and communities. These strategies include: (1) improving the definition and measurement of culture and cultural competence in research; (2) strengthening research to identify risks for and protective factors against maltreatment in different cultural groups; (3) increasing cultural diversity in the workforce; and (4) developing and advancing interventions that are culturally responsive.

Defining Culture in Research, Practice, and Policy Related to Child Maltreatment

Culture is a heterogeneous construct that is defined and operationalized in multiple ways (see Small et al. 2010), too often without attention paid to practical meaning and applications. For the purposes of clarity and grounding our discussion, we rely on the definition of culture provided by Le and colleagues, who describe culture as "a dynamic phenomenon" that "represents ways of living that have been developed by a group of people to meet their biological, psychological, and emotional needs" (Le et al. 2008, p. 164). To further understand the groups of people referred to in this definition, we draw loosely on the framework proposed by Hays (2001) to understand cultural identity as a multidimensional construct informed by individuals' gender, age, religion, ethnicity and race, socioeconomic status, sexual orientation, national origin, heritage, and disability status. We also use the theory of intersectionality (see McCall 2005). In addition, we discuss culture consistent with Rogoff's model (2003), based in sociocultural theory, to understand how culture may serve to mitigate or exacerbate risk factors for child maltreatment.

At the heart of these conceptualizations is the idea that culture is neither static nor easily distilled into one or two core elements. Often, culture is treated as a *cause* of individual behaviors (Rogoff 2003), whereas our definition draws attention to the fluid aspects of culture and the contributions that individuals themselves bring to the development of culture (Institute of Medicine and National Research Council 2013; Korbin 2002). Cultural tools and knowledge are inherited by successive generations, but at the same time, these tools and knowledge are interpreted, transformed, and adapted by families and individuals within a particular socio-economic and political context to fit their own needs. For example, a young, recently migrated family may be accustomed to a communal style of child rearing in which many adults are responsible for ensuring the child's well-being. This approach to child care is seldom a viable option in the United States, but parents may find that a child care center, where many adults are present to supervise children, fits well with their child rearing goals and beliefs (Obeng 2007). In this manner, parents shape their children's experience of culture by joining elements of typical child care from the US and their home country. In addition, the culture of the child care center, and perhaps its employees and other families, is reciprocally shaped by interactions with this new family.

Recognition of culture as a shared and dynamic process that involves mutual influences between an individual and the environment allows a more nuanced and effective understanding of the role culture plays in child maltreatment. Truly understanding the role of culture in any form of parenting necessitates an examination of myriad factors that may influence the mutual constitution of culture and family functioning. Explicit attention should be given to our assumptions about shared elements of culture for diverse families. For instance, two mothers may both have been raised in Catholic households, but if only one of the mothers considers herself to be Catholic, the meaning of this aspect of culture will be different for children in the two households. If the mother who considers herself Catholic is also Mexican American, she may teach her children to celebrate particular religious holidays and saints' days, consistent with the traditions she learned as a child. She may do this even if she does not, for example, pray in Spanish or subscribe to other traditional cultural practices that may differ between children in Mexican and European Americans families. Fluid considerations of culture allow us to discuss practically how prevention and intervention programs adapt to diverse families.

Unfortunately, in much research and applied work in the area of child maltreatment, cultural groups are frequently portrayed as uniform communities, typically with emphasis on easily visible shared characteristics and features (Rogoff 2003). This limited representation of culture is particularly evident in literature that attempts to explain cultural differences using ethnicity and race alone. Such an approach fails to recognize other cultural experiences that are critical to individual behaviors, masking great heterogeneity in experiences, beliefs, and practices within ethnic minority groups. Moreover, limited or overgeneralized conceptualizations of culture potentially dilute the effectiveness of cultural adaptations for child maltreatment prevention and intervention programs. These conceptualizations fail to address the many nuances of culture. Ignoring aspects of culture distinct from race and ethnicity results in researchers and practitioners alike conflating social stratification, particularly by race or ethnicity and socioeconomic status, with culture (Institute of Medicine and National Research Council 2013), limiting our understanding of parenting similarities and differences across diverse families.

The need to move beyond race and ethnicity in our conceptualization of culture does not diminish the historical, social, and political contexts that have resulted in significant disadvantages and disproportionate representation of racial and ethnic minority families in the child welfare system. These disparities are evident throughout the child welfare system, from prevention to intervention, and include rates of maltreatment reporting and investigation, substantiation of maltreatment allegations, and foster care entry and exits (Drake et al. 2009; Fluke et al. 2003; Harris and Skyles 2008; Hill 2004; Hines et al. 2004; Knott and Donovan 2010; Lu et al. 2004; Needell et al. 2003; Putnam-Hornstein et al. 2013). Several explanations for this disproportionality have been offered in the extant literature, and experiencing a combination of factors likely contributes to the greater problem. First, differential rates of maltreatment reporting and victimization for ethnic minority children may be largely explained by differences in poverty and the associated increased risk of maltreatment (Putnam-Hornstein et al. 2013). More nuanced analyses further suggest that certain races, ethnicities, or cultures are not inherently more or less likely to maltreat their children, but rather, are differentially exposed to common risk factors for child maltreatment beyond poverty (i.e., lack of health insurance; see Putnam-Hornstein 2011; Putnam-Hornstein et al. 2013).

In addition to this stratification in exposure to risk factors for child maltreatment, some experts have argued that policies implemented over the past century have disproportionately affected racial and cultural minorities. These policies incrementally move away from helping the poor and marginalized to protect their children and toward increasing social and economic deprivation and heightening risk of removal from parents (Roberts 2002). Another widely accepted explanation for the lopsided representation of racial minority children in the child welfare system, most notably African Americans, is racism and bias in reporting and processing of these children in the child welfare system (Fluke et al. 2011; Wells et al. 2009). A recent literature review suggests that discriminatory practices and policies within child welfare agencies continue to exist, as does heightened surveillance in African American communities. Both of these likely contribute to higher levels of child maltreatment reports for minority groups (Fluke et al. 2011).

Considerable debate continues over how to reduce these racial and ethnic disparities in the child welfare system (e.g., Bartholet 2009). Some experts support implementing prevention initiatives that include more progressive social welfare policies to reduce maltreatment among racial and cultural minorities disproportionately affected by poverty, substance abuse, and fragmented family structures. Others advocate for increasing awareness of both racial and cultural biases among professionals, as well as eliminating barriers faced by culturally diverse families that lead them to receive less effective services (Harris and Hackett 2008; Stevenson et al. 1992). Both of these approaches have resulted in a focus on enhancing the cultural competence of systems, interventions, and professionals by incorporating specific strategies into policy formation and service delivery, training, and practice (Cross et al. 1989; Pierce and Pierce 1996).

We do not wish to downplay or discount the disproportional representation of ethnic and racial minority families in the child welfare system. Nonetheless, we wish to expand the dialogue around culture, parenting, and child maltreatment. We also want to recognize that families and communities of different racial and ethnic backgrounds, historically treated as monolithic groups, in fact have varied cultural histories, beliefs, and experiences that intersect with other factors and contribute to child well-being in different ways. The remainder of the chapter explicitly focuses on culture rather than race and ethnicity. This approach is consistent with a growing awareness in the field of child maltreatment prevention that has led to a call for more direct examination of the interaction of culture with social stratification, ultimately to better understand and address the role of culture in developing and implementing effective child maltreatment prevention and intervention initiatives (Institute of Medicine and National Research Council 2013). We divide our presentation of culture and parenting into three broad levels, moving from macro to micro as we discuss culture and parenting at the societal level, then the program level, and finally at the individual level. In each section we provide expanded, more applied definitions of culture, as well as examples, in an effort to add clarity to these discussions.

Culture, Parenting, and Child Maltreatment in Societal Context

Parenting is a complex issue from a societal and policy perspective, centering on the roles, rights, and responsibilities of individuals versus the collective. As a concept itself, Faircloth and colleagues suggest that "parenting" is a cultural construction, emerging from language of twentieth century psychologists and sociologists in North America (Faircloth et al. 2013). Still, general agreement among scholars of parenting and culture suggests that parents have always been a primary source of cultural transmission across generations and societies rely on parents to teach children common social values and promote positive social engagement (Bornstein and Lansford 2010; Faircloth et al. 2013). For societies such as the United States, where individualism is prized, parents hold primary, if not sole, responsibility for child care and rearing; however, in many societies throughout the world, these responsibilities are much more collective (Rogoff 2003).

Laws protecting children from maltreatment draw a line between parents' rights and state responsibilities, dictating at what point parental behaviors fall outside of socially sanctioned practices. Despite evidence that parents' definitions of child abuse are fairly consistent across a wide range of cultures (Cyr et al. 2013; Lubell et al. 2008; Maiter et al. 2004), specific parental behaviors may take on different meaning in different societal contexts. Although child neglect is perceived as serious mistreatment of children across cultures (Garbarino and Ebata 1983), what constitutes neglectful behavior is culturally and contextually grounded (Rose and Meezan 1996). Defining and identifying neglect has been a difficult task, with European American middle-class values and perceptions shaping most research and policy in the U.S. Many parents from ethnic and cultural minorities perceive extended family members, and even their children, as partly responsible for providing family support in the forms of financial assistance and child care. This practice may be viewed as neglect by practitioners trained in the dominant U.S. cultural practices (Dykeman et al. 1996; Lum 1992; Tower 1996). Immigrant parents who are unfamiliar with U.S. customs and laws also are vulnerable to allegations of neglect, especially those who are newly arrived and may leave children unattended for short periods, delay medical attention while using traditional folk remedies, or fail to have a child immunized (Dettlaff 2008). Furthermore, punitive immigration policies and enforcement activities that have systematically deported hundreds of thousands of parents over the past decade have created widespread fear and mistrust of government entities among marginalized immigrant groups (Immigration Policy Center 2012). This mistrust has resulted in parents removing children from school and losing access to needed support services (Chaudry et al. 2010). These practices may be alleged to be either neglectful or protective of family unity, depending on the lens used.

Corporal punishment is yet another parenting behavior that can challenge societal definitions of child abuse. Despite the fact that corporal punishment remains a normative parenting tool in the United States (Hawkins et al. 2010), it is losing ground as a socially sanctioned parenting practice as researchers and practitioners advocate for nonviolent discipline strategies (Gershoff 2013). Such a shift in cultural norms for parenting highlights the need for researchers, practitioners, and policy-makers to attend to the meanings and contexts of parenting behaviors among diverse families in order to effectively prevent child maltreatment, as well as intervene when child maltreatment occurs.

Culture, Parenting, and Child Maltreatment at the Program Level

At the program level, research and dialogue around the influence of culture on parenting and child well-being have focused on two main areas. First, the design of evidence-based intervention and prevention programs increasingly considers family background and culture. Similarly, research on uptake of and outcomes from evidence-based programs often include elements of culture. Second, there has been much emphasis on training programs and workplace policies in child and family serving systems that contribute to developing organizational and workforce capacity to sensitively respond to the needs of diverse families served. We will discuss each of these aspects of program-level approaches to recognizing the diverse cultural background of children and parents.

Parenting programs that have demonstrated some degree of effectiveness through randomized controlled trials are considered the most robust evidence-based programs; however, in many cases, the initial development and testing of the program or its evaluation are rooted in dominant values and norms of the European American middle-class majority culture, raising concern over with whom such programs are effective. Lower rates of program enrollment and completion among ethnic minorities relative to European Americans, controlling for other background characteristics, could suggest a mismatch between program goals and the goals of families with diverse cultural backgrounds (Broman 2012; Lau 2006). Yet questions remain regarding the necessity of evidence-based programs tailored for specific cultures. Those raising such questions cite evidence of the effectiveness of such programs with diverse families whether or not they have been specifically adapted. Indeed, many programs targeted at different levels of prevention and intervention for child maltreatment have promising results with diverse children and families. These range from the Safe Child Program (Kraizer et al. 1989), which teaches children about preventing abuse, to programs such as Systematic Training for Effective Parenting (STEP; Huebner 2002) and Parents as Teachers (Wagner et al. 2002) that have been successfully used with parents of diverse races, ethnicities, and countries of origin. Similarly, programs providing home visiting services (see Olds et al. 2007; DuMont et al. 2010; Dishion et al. 2008; Chaffin et al. 2012) and parent–child therapy approaches (see Chaffin and Friedrich 2004; Chaffin et al. 2004) hold promise for use with diverse families. At the community level, both Triple P (Prinz et al. 2009) and the Incredible Years (2013) have been used with success with diverse populations.

Although some data suggest that such evidence-based programs are robust enough to be effective with diverse families without adaptation (Damashek et al. 2012; Kataoka et al. 2010; Chaffin et al. 2012), or that culturally tailored interventions may be efficacious but inefficient or unnecessary (Huey et al. 2014), it is not clear that most existing cultural adaptations have been targeted or strong enough to affect meaningful differences in participants' experiences (Falicov 2009). While evidence-based programs may be efficacious or effective with diverse groups, these conclusions have been drawn from a limited number of assessed outcomes, such as reduced child welfare recidivism. Such evaluations do not typically emphasize the experiences of diverse cultural groups or the process of service delivery—thus, measures that represent cultural sensitivity or cultural resonance are rarely a focus of inquiry. This raises questions as to the effectiveness of such programs in the long-term. Specifically, to what extent might culturally diverse families be adopting parenting practices in the short term in an effort to comply with services that do not necessarily resonate with their traditions, beliefs, values, and understandings?

Moreover, the term "culture" has generally been broadly defined (namely with a focus on ethnicity) for the adaptation of programs, calling into question whether the adaptations are indeed culturally based. Of course, it may not be realistic to imagine that all programs can be designed and evaluated for relevance to all cultural groups, nor that there are even a finite number of cultural groups in the US. Despite this challenge moving forward, it is imperative to consider: (1) exactly whose parenting styles and norms are driving intervention development and normalization; (2) to which populations these interventions are available; (3) who is developing and evaluating such programs; and (4) how we are defining "effectiveness" when attempting to understand which maltreatment prevention programs work best and for whom.

Other program improvement efforts have addressed the issue of culture by focusing on professional skill building and organizational capacity. Over the past several decades, much has been written on the need for child welfare agencies and service providers to assess parenting processes and maltreatment risk while delivering services through a "culturally competent" lens. However, perceptions of what constitutes cultural competence have evolved and shifted over time. In a recent review of the literature, a summary of the process for achieving cultural competence included the efficient use of agency resources, specialized training and education of professionals, availability of culturally appropriate services, and matching race and language between the provider and the family (Fluke et al. 2011). Such practice standards for culturally competent interventions for child welfare systems are rooted in the National Standards for Culturally and Linguistically Appropriate Services (CLAS) in Health Care (U.S. Department of Health and Human Services, Office of Minority Health 2015). However, only six states have legislation requiring or strongly recommending cultural competence training among professionals. Moreover, training content and requirements related to cultural competence vary substantially between training programs for professionals engaged with child welfare agencies, creating uneven responses to diverse families in these systems.

Perhaps even more concerning is that it is not clear that cultural *competence* is the ultimate goal for professionals. Alternatively, we might imagine it possible that in a heterogeneous and culturally diverse country like the US, more than one single culturally normative framework for parenting could exist. The concept of cultural *reciprocity* aptly supports this possibility and the truly fluid nature of culture, in which professionals engage in a self-reflective and dialogic process toward identifying both their own and their families' cultural norms in a collaborative exchange to provide effective services (Harry et al. 1999). For instance, a culturally competent heterosexual practitioner may recognize that her background and beliefs about parenting differ from those of a homosexual client, whereas a practitioner engaging in cultural reciprocity may try to understand where such differences come from and recognize how that might influence the way she should approach working with the family. An ultimate goal may involve a continuing commitment to understanding the overlapping influences of culture, context, and social stratification, as well as learning from individual families, better described as cultural humility (Tervalon and Murray-García 1998).

In addition to the importance of supporting practitioners to engage in cultural reciprocity, it is equally important to build a workforce that is culturally diverse. Not only will greater diversity in the child welfare workforce facilitate deeper dialogue and awareness of culture among practitioners who train and work with diverse colleagues, it will also contribute to making culture and diversity a normative part of understanding family processes and individual client goals. The goals of training practitioners to use cultural reciprocity and increasing the diversity of the child welfare workforce should not be considered mutually exclusive or separate goals. Combining these strategies may form the most sustainable approach to using culture as a central organizing construct in understanding, preventing, and intervening to reduce child maltreatment.

Culture, Parenting, and Child Maltreatment at the Individual Level

Individual parents' beliefs and expectations are central to understanding variability in parenting behaviors (Cote and Bornstein 2009; Miller and Harwood 2002; Morelli et al. 1992), including which child behaviors elicit parents' attention and how parents respond to these behaviors (Tamis-LeMonda and Song 2012). Individual parenting practices are also influenced by culturally conditioned forces, including beliefs about character traits in children that are desirable or encouraged, prevailing advice about childrearing, suggestions from family and friends, and direct observations of the parenting behaviors of others (Bornstein and Lansford 2010). Culturally normative parenting in the US, from a European American perspective, focuses on separation and autonomy within a supportive and responsive relationship. In contrast, many other cultures traditionally engage in authoritarian parenting, emphasizing obedience and conformity (Bornstein and Lansford 2010).

Culture-specific patterns of childrearing also adapt and evolve depending on location, suggesting that cultural variation in philosophies, values, and beliefs may mediate differences in childrearing practices depending on the context of physical and social environments (Bornstein and Lansford 2010; Tamis-LeMonda and Kahana-Kalman 2009). To date, there is no clear formula for understanding to what extent different parenting styles and practices are adopted, and in what contexts, by families with diverse cultural backgrounds. One example from existing research suggests that authoritarian parenting behaviors may be linked with behavior problems in European American children, but is unrelated to the behavior of Mexican American children and can have positive associations with school performance among Chinese American children (Bornstein and Lansford 2010). Other literature suggests that the use of physical discipline may be less correlated with children's externalizing problems when the cultural norms and neighborhood quality are considered (Lansford et al. 2004, 2005; Polaha et al. 2004). Furthermore, some parenting practices, such as the use of folk remedies in lieu of Western medical treatments, may become problematic when parents use them outside of their normative cultural context (e.g., after immigrating to the US). Coining, a traditional medical treatment utilized in many Southeast Asian cultures, in which the skin is scraped to release unhealthy elements from injuries and stimulate blood flow and healing, is one of the example of non-Western medical remedies that have been often perceived as physical abuse.

Although parents from diverse cultures in the US generally agree on definitions of child maltreatment, the increasing complexity of diversity in the US and concomitant variability in parenting behaviors—particularly to the degree these behaviors diverge from the norms of the majority group—may elicit differential levels of attention from the child welfare system (Evans-Campbell 2008; Korbin and Spilsbury 1999; Rose and Meezan 1996). Therefore, observable risks for child maltreatment and higher rates of reporting for some groups are not only due to cultural influences. Their interaction with factors related to the process of social stratification and the broader ecological context that form.

In the US, research shows that ethnic minority families face many similar challenges, as well as show considerable differences in their root childrearing practices and beliefs. Such examinations of parenting in different racial or ethnic groups can contribute to overgeneralization and stereotyping. Nevertheless, existing literature focusing on specific ethnic groups may be able to enhance our understanding of parenting behaviors across and within some cultural groups that can contribute to risk for child maltreatment. For instance, among Latino families, studies suggest that relative to English-speaking mothers in the US, those who are Spanish-speaking are more likely to endorse parenting beliefs associated with use of physical punishment and risk for maltreatment (Acevedo 2000). Spanish-speaking mothers are also more likely to use more hostile control and inconsistent discipline (Hill et al. 2003). More detailed analysis of the Mexican American population specifically reveals that, to some extent, differences in acculturation may be associated with the adoption of these and other parenting strategies (Varela et al. 2004).

Immigration-related issues comprise an important set of factors that could potentially be conflated with issues of culture and parenting practices. As noted, cultural emphasis on child behaviors is dependent on a parent's level of acculturation in the US, which is likely to affect the strategies parents use with their children (Chao and Kanatsu 2008; Johnson et al. 2003). In contrast to indications that immigrant parents experience elevated stress relative to nonimmigrant parents, nationally representative data suggest that parents' mental health does not vary systematically by immigrant status (Reardon-Anderson et al. 2002; Takanishi 2004). Nonetheless, immigrant parents are less likely than nonimmigrant parents to know where to seek help for mental health issues when they do need it (Reardon-Anderson et al. 2002). Additionally, legal factors influenced by the socio-political environment affect immigrant parents' behaviors. Immigrant families may be less likely to access needed support services and more often remain socially isolated, due to concerns surrounding legal status and documentation and fear of deportation. This is true even among legal residents and families with children who are US citizens (Borjas 2011; Finno-Velasquez 2013). Finally, the neighborhoods where immigrants tend to live often have fewer and lower quality resources than the neighborhoods where nonimmigrants live (Leventhal and Shuey 2014; Matthews 2009; Matthews and Jang 2007). As immigrants are likely to be less familiar with resources available in the US (Chaudry et al. 2011; Simpkins et al. 2012), these limitations may create barriers for families trying to adjust to mainstream U.S. values, norms, and practices.

Neighborhood circumstances may also contribute to a risk for involvement in the child welfare system for many families—not only immigrants (Belsky 1984; Garbarino et al. 2005; Korbin 2002; Kotchick et al. 2005). Higher poverty rates and lower residential stability rates are associated with higher rates of child maltreatment (Coulton et al. 1995; Drake and Pandey 1996; Ernst 2001; Freisthler et al. 2006; Garbarino et al. 2005), although this relationship appears to be stronger in predominantly European American compared with predominantly African American neighborhoods (Korbin et al. 1998). This fact suggests potential protective mechanisms in place among African American families in poor neighborhoods. Much of the literature on neighborhoods and culture stresses the beneficial role of restrictive and controlling parenting in African American families living in disadvantaged or dangerous neighborhoods (Furstenberg 1993; Lamborn et al. 1996; McLoyd 1990). However, it is unclear under what conditions strict control and discipline may be beneficial for African American children, whether these patterns might hold for other ethnic groups or for immigrant families, and how these parenting strategies may contribute to risk for child maltreatment (Shuey and Leventhal under review). Nevertheless, data from the neighborhood level may be useful for understanding links between culture and child maltreatment when the definition of culture is restricted to a local, contextual level (Korbin 2002).

In summary, to better uncover the role of culture in parenting and risks for maltreatment, any examination of the cultural circumstances of individual families should be considered in relationship to other risks for maltreatment and within a broader cultural and ecological context. In clinical practice, practitioners may be well-served in understanding the cultural values driving the behaviors of an individual family, while remaining mindful of the cultural lens from which decisions and judgments about families are made. The focus of change should not necessarily be on cultural practices or behaviors that diverge from accepted norms, unless such factors are *directly* contributing to maltreatment. Unfortunately, this does not resolve the ongoing challenge of assessment and child welfare decision making: balancing a threshold for standards of safety that are evolving and culturally bounded, while sensitively acknowledging and supporting individuals' culturally situated parenting practices. We consider ways to achieve this balance in our final section.

Strategies for Moving Forward

Significant disadvantages and disproportionate representation in the child welfare system among racial and cultural minority families in the US remain a serious social issue. In response, researchers, policymakers, and practitioners are increasingly including an examination of culture as an integral part in developing child maltreatment prevention and intervention efforts. While the field has attempted to make—and has made—advancements in understanding the disproportionality of minority groups in the child welfare system, these advancements have only served to highlight the complex and multifaceted nature of culture, as well as its interaction with social stratification by race and ethnicity and socioeconomic status (Institute of Medicine and National Research Council 2013). The necessity of capturing and examining the dynamic nature of culture in relation to child maltreatment is clear; thus, to continue efforts to reduce disparities and improve outcomes for all children and families in the U.S., we present four primary recommendations for moving the field forward.

Recalibrating the Conceptualization of Culture

Increasingly, culture is recognized not as a static set of values, norms, and practices that reside solely within the individual but rather as a dynamic concept continuously shaped by the ongoing interactions among individuals, families, professionals, organizations, policies, and societies. Culture is learned, transmitted and adapted by social interactions, conflicts, and power relations (Alegria et al. 2010; Cabassa and Baumann 2013; Castro et al. 2010; Kleinman and Benson 2006). Yet capturing the dynamic nature of culture in tangible forms presents many practical challenges. The constantly evolving nature of culture and risk for child maltreatment and involvement in the child welfare system resulting from many factors at many levels elicits more questions than answers. Some of these questions include: Given that the US continues to be the top receiving country of immigrants from all over the world (Nwosu et al. 2014), what constitutes a culture? What experiences do we examine to understand the role of culture? The key is to continue instilling the notion that a family's culture is a product of experiences that cannot be categorized monolithi-cally with easily visible shared characteristics and features such as racial or ethnic labels (Rogoff 2003). The examination of the role of culture in child maltreatment necessitates a close look at each family's heterogeneous experiences, beliefs, and practices across multiple contexts that are uniquely relevant to each family's func-tioning, with the goal of addressing cultural processes involved in child maltreat-ment prevention and intervention efforts in a more nuanced manner.

Related to this is the need to refine our understanding and use of the phrase "cul-tural competence" in supporting racially and culturally diverse families. Given the longstanding cultural discriminatory practices and policies within child welfare agencies (Fluke et al. 2011; Roberts 2002), cultural competence has been identified as a key strategy for reducing bias in decision making and reducing disparate out-comes for minority groups (Falicov 2009). There is an ongoing call for standardiza-tion of the definition and measurement of cultural competence (Andrulis et al. 2010; Betancourt et al. 2005; Vega 2005); however, our current understanding and execu-tion of cultural competence may be questionable. First, the definition of culture has often been overly broad for the purposes of program adaptations, such that "culturally-informed" modifications may not truly target or be strong enough to effect meaningful differences in participants' experiences (Falicov 2009). Second, cultural competence often implies superiority of dominant professional practices and beliefs and evokes the notion that culture is something in which professionals can become an "expert." It fails to recognize the mutual interaction that goes on between an individual and a family and the environment, including interactions with the child welfare system.

To effectively serve culturally diverse families, practicing cultural reciprocity or humility may be more appropriate. Cultural reciprocity places responsibility on the professional to engage in self-reflection and dialogue to consider their own and families' cultural norms and participate in collaborative exchange to provide effec-tive services (Harry et al. 1999). Cultural humility or attunement can be understood as respect for families' heritage and tools, commitment to understanding the over-lapping influences of culture, context, and social stratification, and learning from individual families about the aspects of culture and context most important to them (Falicov 2009; Tervalon and Murray-García 1998).

Refining Child Maltreatment Research for Diverse Cultural Groups

Continuing efforts are needed to define and measure child maltreatment for diverse racial or ethnic and cultural groups, as well as to better understand differences and similarities in the causes of maltreatment among many types of families. From a research perspective, scholars may help to advance this goal by carefully articulat-ing the definitions and operationalization of maltreatment constructs included in studies, as well as assumptions about the cultural relevance of these constructs for the study population. Although it will not be possible for any single study to com-prehensively address all aspects of culture, we can at least move towards explicitly stating the strengths and limitations of the measures used to capture culture as a research construct. Recent decades have seen more research investigating the meaning and measurement of parenting behaviors, with particular attention to corporal punishment, as well as potential moderators of associations between parenting behaviors and child outcomes (e.g., Bradley et al. 1996; Lansford et al. 2005; Leyendecker et al. 2005; Bornstein and Lansford 2010). However, further work is needed, both within and across cultural groups, to understand how contexts (e.g., neighborhoods, federal family and immigration laws, and local child welfare policies and practices) and family characteristics (e.g., household structure and primary language) interact with parents' culturally bound beliefs and behaviors in the US. The benefit of this work may not be limited to identifying risk factors for child maltreatment, as it can also inform our understanding of the many strengths that diverse parents bring to their roles as caregivers. This understanding will allow prevention efforts to bolster existing family and parental assets.

From a research perspective, the prevalence of corporal punishment in the US offers an important means of understanding differences in how parents perceive and use these behaviors. These differences could be based on societal values and the role of the family as espoused by their cultures and countries of origin. The prevalence of corporal punishment could also help identify potential disparities in how the child welfare system distinguishes discipline from maltreatment. Along these lines, research would benefit from carefully defining child neglect so as to clearly distinguish it from family poverty. Despite the risks poverty creates—both for child development generally and for child neglect specifically—more focused research and clearer definitions of neglect and risks for neglect within culturally diverse groups could contribute substantially to the ability of policymakers and practitioners to address these issues and promote child well-being.

Enhance Intervention Design and Testing with Diverse Cultural Groups

Several strategies exist to intentionally emphasize culture when improving interventions that promote child well-being at multiple levels. At the forefront is a need to diversify the parenting styles and norms that are driving intervention development and normalization. Research is desperately needed to advance interventions that promote child well-being in diverse cultural groups, both in effectiveness studies in controlled settings as well as in the implementation of existing interventions. By design, existing interventions often rely on twentieth century, European American, middle-class values. They may unintentionally impose and reinforce strategies and techniques that are based on values that are grounded in mainstream culturally normative behaviors. In order to avoid misperceptions of positive parenting practices being universal, as well as bias that can arise from such approaches, experts may want to consider more rigorous and targeted testing of existing child welfare interventions with diverse cultural groups. They may also consider development of culturally driven interventions designed for specific groups.

Furthermore, to advance the impact of interventions on culturally diverse groups, more holistic and innovative strategies are needed. Maltreatment prevention interventions could address multiple stressors typically clustered together within a specific racial or ethnic group or community context, including economic and cultural stressors, to focus on reducing numerous risks associated with maltreatment and family stress at the same time. Innovative interventions might also be designed and evaluated for impact at several levels at once—for instance, by modifying the behaviors of individual families, increasing racial and cultural minorities' access to existing services and making services more culturally relevant, and reforming child welfare policy and the workforce to better serve diverse families and communities. This multipronged strategy for maltreatment prevention and intervention could be adapted from similar existing models in health care (Fischer et al. 2007). At a minimum, child welfare system reforms could contain multiple culturally adaptive components, including adequate skilled bilingual providers, language-appropriate educational materials, and specialized case management (Chin et al. 2007). Additionally, some programs have been more successful in reducing maltreatment risks when they included the provision of concrete services in an intervention, integrating components such as financial assistance, clothing, housing, and support for everyday tasks (MacLeod and Nelson 2000). Because access to basic supports are lacking in racially and culturally diverse families and communities (Johnson-Motoyama 2013), they may need assistance with concrete needs to lower their risk for involvement with the child welfare system.

The diversification of interventions goes hand in hand with diversifying who is developing and evaluating such programs. A majority of researchers and interventionists of existing programs are from the same ethnic and demographic circumstances as those studied or those they work with. Likewise, intended audiences of scientific investigation have been restricted socio-demographically (Bornstein and Lansford 2010). Therefore, a crosscutting and intentional commitment to increasing the racial and cultural diversity of leading researchers, teachers, service providers, and policymakers in the field of child maltreatment prevention may be critical to improving interventions and supporting the well-being of an increasingly diverse pool of families.

We also challenge the definition of "effectiveness" when attempting to understand which programs work best and for whom. Although diverse groups may have similar outcomes on common evidence-based program indicators, such as retention and treatment outcomes (Chaffin et al. 2012; Damashek et al. 2012), can we conclude that diverse families have equally positive experiences with the intervention? Are there unintended consequences for family dynamics among program participants whose cultural backgrounds differ from the values inherent to the interventions? Are there ways we might be able to improve the experiences of diverse families in intervention programs? Research could be strengthened by placing greater emphasis on the process and experiences of diverse families throughout the implementation and sustainment of interventions. Such research might document perceptions of cultural relevance or resonance, shared understandings and shared worldviews among program participants and providers, experiences of discrimination or empowerment, and overall client satisfaction with providers and services. Perhaps more importantly, longitudinal data could be utilized to understand whether the effects of parenting interventions on culturally diverse groups hold in the long term and prevent maltreatment. This information, along with more data about families' origins and cultural identities, could be collected and analyzed within the context of implementation trials to better understand the role of culture in responses to intervention. Moreover, even when evidence-based programs may be effective in promoting positive parenting outcomes for families with diverse cultural beliefs and backgrounds, alternatives could exist that work just as well. Such alternatives might not require assimilation and adoption of culturally relative practices that may force suppression of divergent cultural values. Funding institutions should consider prioritizing intervention testing with culture as a central organizing concept. This would allow testing to be aligned with the values and thinking of, at the very least, a large number of racial and cultural groups. The testing could then be adapted for application in a local community's subcultural contexts.

Finally, although existing evidence-based programs may demonstrate effectiveness in diverse settings without introducing laboratory-designed cultural adaptations (Huey et al. 2014), the reality of front line practice is that, during implementation, local practitioners are constantly using clinical and personal judgment to adapt interventions to fit the cultural needs of individual families. Because culture is often not a central focus of implementation studies, research does not always document cultural adaptations, even though they are naturally occurring all the time. The little research that does exist suggests that evidence-based programs can have relevance for clients of diverse cultures when implemented in real-world settings, especially when allowing for flexible cultural adaptation throughout the process to meet the needs of local communities (Finno-Velasquez et al. forthcoming.) If the process of adaptation were more consciously documented and analyzed, it could improve our understanding of the role of culture in parenting and in making interventions function across cultures. Increasing recognition of this issue is evident in researchers calling for clear documentation of when and how cultural adaptations are occurring during implementation, as well as documentation of service outcomes associated with adapted programs for diverse cultural groups, in order to generate knowledge on when and how to adapt existing programs (Cabassa and Baumann 2013). For example, ongoing coaching on implementation, extra efforts to help families understand program goals and purpose, and integrating content that supports families' cultural values, may be useful in helping providers use evidence-based programs in ways that are culturally relevant. Conducting studies that examine implementations within cultural groups, rather than across broad domains defined by socio-demographic features, might also be beneficial for understanding the process aspect of intervention and the strengths and weakness in implementation for different cultural groups.

Conclusion

Throughout this chapter we have argued for increased attention to and better definitional clarity of culture. By using culture as a central organizing concept to understand the history, beliefs, and behaviors shared among communities in the US, as well as in intervention design and implementation, we believe that it will be possible to better serve diverse families and ultimately reduce the existing disproportionality of child maltreatment and child welfare service involvement among minority groups. Moving forward, research should focus on how parents engage in their cultural communities, how culture shapes their parenting beliefs and strategies, how these differences in parenting may affect the meaning and effectiveness of child maltreatment prevention and intervention programs, and how existing strategies and interventions for addressing issues of culture may be improved.

Reflection: Listen to All Voices

Ellen E. Pinderhughes
Tufts University, Medford, MA, USA

Whether as practitioner or researcher, I have participated in the field of child maltreatment for over 40 years. Reflecting on the changes during this period, I am struck by the importance of voices—those that are and are not privileged.

Terminology In the 60s and 70s, terms pervaded the literature reflecting white middle class families as the standard bearer. (I remember being asked why I was bothering to learn about the demographics and cultural backgrounds of families as I prepared to evaluate an agency's services.) The prevailing approaches were founded on a deficit approach to families who were not white, middle class, and headed by two straight parents. In 2014, we hear terms suggesting the importance of empowerment, practitioners as allies, and understanding families' culture and position in the social system.

Disciplinary Relationships Four to five decades ago, the fields charged with addressing child abuse were disconnected and focused on their own power and privilege stratification. Today, interventions and evaluations benefit from interdisciplinary collaborations of scientists/practitioners, quantitative/qualitative experts, embracing social work, psychology, health sciences, education, sociology, anthropology, policy, and other fields. Most recently, community-based collaborations have emerged, shaped in part by voices in the community supporting this approach.

Context Forty years ago, our considerations of contextual influences were unidirectional and in their infancy. We now consider multiple and intersecting layers of context that directly (family, neighborhood, school) and indirectly (workplace, extended families/support networks, and policies) transact with parenting and are relevant to addressing child maltreatment. Perhaps most importantly of all, we now work to incorporate an understanding of culture and culturally related processes into our understanding of child abuse prevention and intervention and its effectiveness.

Who's the Expert? A critical change occurred in the framing of professionals or researchers and clients or research participants. Fifty years ago, guided by values privileging "objectivity" in science and in service delivery, the field viewed professionals and researchers as the expert. The field did not value the perspectives of those we sought to help. The field also did not value the perspectives of professionals of color that differed from mainstream views. Over time, the voices of professionals of color grew in decibel, number, persistence, and insistence, calling for attention to culturally based processes in research, theoretically based reasons for studying differences in parenting and child functioning between cultural groups, and strength-based approaches to studying diverse families. These approaches would require listening to families. Gradually, the voices of mainstream and dominant group allies joined this effort. Voices from multiple fields also have converged to highlight the importance of cultural sensitivity and humility and distinguishing social stratification processes from cultural processes and their effects in defining the target problem, developing interventions and designing evaluations.

Self-inquiry We also learned the importance of understanding the voices (explicit and implicit) we each carry with us as we engage with others (whether colleague, peer, client or participant) who are culturally different. Each of us has values, attitudes, and beliefs that have been shaped by our experiences and our cultural characteristics (e.g., race/ethnicity, gender, SES, sexual/romantic orientation, nationality, religion, etc.). Those experiences shape how we view and interact with others. Understanding our own voices has become increasingly critical to understanding the voices of others. As we become aware of our own voices and our underlying beliefs and values, we become better able to listen and better hear others' voices.

The Tools We Use As a result of these changes, we have a greater appreciation of the complex influences on child abuse, the varied outcomes, and the complexities associated with addressing child abuse effectively. Modeling these complexities has been facilitated by tremendous change in methodological and analytical approaches, along with increased access to large datasets relevant for studying child maltreatment. In combination, these latter advances have enabled more sophisticated and cost-effective studies than was possible when researchers only gathered original data. In keeping with the voices calling for cultural sensitivity, we must interrogate these datasets and the methods and analyses used for the voices within and the voices that shaped them.

In sum, listening to diverse voices has facilitated a more comprehensive and nuanced understanding about child maltreatment, as well as more informed decisions about the design or adaptation of interventions for specific populations and examinations of their effectiveness. As the field of child maltreatment looks ahead to the next fifty years, and we develop even more sophisticated approaches to better understand and address these complexities, let us be sure that the voices of those who can most benefit are at the table.

References

Acevedo, M. C. (2000). The role of acculturation in explaining ethnic differences in the prenatal health-risk behaviors, mental health, and parenting beliefs of Mexican American and European American at-risk women. *Child Abuse & Neglect, 24*(1), 111–127.

Alegria, M., Atkins, M., Farmer, E., Slaton, E., & Stelk, W. (2010). One size does not fit all: Taking diversity, culture and context seriously. *Administration and Policy in Mental Health, 37*(1–2), 48–60.

Andrulis, D. P., Siddiqui, N. J., Purtle, J. P., & Duchon, L. (2010). *Patient Protection and Affordable Care Act of 2010: Advancing health equity for racially and ethnically diverse populations.* Washington, DC: Joint Center for Political and Economic Studies.

Bartholet, E. (2009). The racial disproportionality movement in child welfare: False facts and dangerous directions. *Arizona Law Review, 51*, 871–932.

Belsky, J. (1984). The determinants of parenting: A process model. *Child Development, 55*, 83–96.

Betancourt, J., Green, A., Carrillo, E., & Park, E. (2005). Cultural competence and health care disparities: Key perspectives and trends. *Health Affairs, 24*(2), 499–505.

Borjas, G. J. (2011). Poverty and program participation among immigrant children. *The Future of Children, 21*(1), 247–266.

Bornstein, M. H., & Lansford, J. E. (2010). Parenting. In M. H. Bornstein (Ed.), *The handbook of cross-cultural developmental science* (pp. 259–277). New York: Taylor & Francis.

Bradley, R. H., Corwyn, R. F., & Whiteside-Mansell, L. (1996). Life at home: Same time, different places—An examination of the HOME inventory in different cultures. *Early Development and Parenting, 5*(4), 251–269.

Broman, C. L. (2012). Race differences in receipt of mental health services among young adults. *Psychological Services, 9*(1), 38–48.

Cabassa, L. J., & Baumann, A. A. (2013). A two-way street: Bridging implementation science and cultural adaptations of mental health treatments. *Implementation Science, 8*(90), 1–14. doi:10.1186/1748-5908-8-90.

Castro, F. G., Barrera, M., Jr., & Holleran Steiker, L. K. (2010). Issues and challenges in the design of culturally adapted evidence-based interventions. *Annual Review of Clinical Psychology, 6*, 213–239.

Chaffin, M., & Friedrich, B. (2004). Evidence-based treatments in child abuse and neglect. *Children and Youth Services Review, 26*, 1097–1113. doi:10.1016/j.childyouth.2004.08.008.

Chaffin, M., Silovsky, J. F., Funderburk, B., Valle, L. A., Brestan, E. V., Balachova, T., et al. (2004). Parent–child interaction therapy with physically abusive parents: Efficacy for reducing future abuse reports. *Journal of Consulting and Clinical Psychology, 72*(3), 500–510.

Chaffin, M., Bard, D., Bigfoot, D. S., & Maher, E. J. (2012). Is a structured, manualized, evidence-based treatment protocol culturally competent and equivalently effective among American Indian parents in child welfare? *Child Maltreatment, 17*(3), 242–252.

Chao, R., & Kanatsu, A. (2008). Beyond socioeconomics: Explaining ethnic group differences in parenting through cultural and immigration processes. *Applied Developmental Science, 12*(4), 181–187.

Chaudry, A., Capps, R., Pedroza, J. M., Castaneda, R. M., Santos, R., & Scott, M. M. (2010). *Facing our future: Children in the aftermath of immigration enforcement.* Washington, DC: Urban Institute.

Chaudry, A., Pedroza, J. M., Sandstrom, H., Danziger, A., Grosz, M., & Scott, M. (2011). *Child care choices of low-income working families.* Washington, DC: Urban Institute.

Chin, M. H., Walters, A., Cook, S., & Huang, E. S. (2007). Interventions to reduce racial and ethnic disparities in health care. *Medical Care Research and Review, 54*(5), 7s–28s.

Cote, L. R., & Bornstein, M. H. (2009). Child and mother play in three U.S. cultural groups: Comparisons and associations. *Journal of Family Psychology, 23*(3), 355–363.

Coulton, C. J., Korbin, J. E., Su, M., & Chow, J. (1995). Community level factors and child maltreatment rates. *Child Development, 66*(5), 1262–1276.

Cross, T. L., Bazron, B. J., Dennis, K. W., & Isaacs, M. R. (1989). *Towards a culturally competent system of care: A monograph on effective services for minority children who are severely emotionally disturbed.* Washington, DC: CASSP Technical Assistance Center.

Cyr, C., Michel, G., & Dumais, M. (2013). Child maltreatment as a global phenomenon: From trauma to prevention. *International Journal of Psychology, 48*(2), 141–148.

Damashek, A., Bard, D., & Hecht, D. (2012). Provider cultural competency, client satisfaction, and engagement in home-based programs to treat child abuse and neglect. *Child Maltreatment, 17*(1), 56–66. doi:10.1177/1077559511423570.

Dettlaff, A. J. (2008). Immigrant Latino children and families in child welfare: A framework for conducting a cultural assessment. *Journal of Public Child Welfare, 2*, 451–470.

Dishion, T. J., Shaw, D., Connell, A., Gardner, F., Weaver, C., & Wilson, M. (2008). The family check-up with high-risk indigent families: Preventing problem behavior by increasing parents' positive behavior support in early childhood. *Child Development, 79*(5), 1395–1414.

Drake, B., & Pandey, S. (1996). Understanding the relationship between neighborhood poverty and specific types of child maltreatment. *Child Abuse & Neglect, 20*, 1003–1018.

Drake, B., Lee, S. M., & Jonson-Reed, M. (2009). Race and child maltreatment reporting: Are Blacks overrepresented? *Children and Youth Services Review, 31*, 309–316.

DuMont, K., Kirkland, K., Mitchell-Herzfeld, S., Ehrhard-Dietzel, S., Rodriguez, M. L., Lee, E., et al. (2010). *A randomized trial of Healthy Families New York (HFNY): Does home visiting prevent child maltreatment.* Washington, DC: National Institute. https://www.ncjrs.gov/pdffiles1/nij/grants/232945.pdf

Durrant, J. E. (2008). Physical punishment, culture, and rights: Current issues for professionals. *Journal of Developmental Behavioral Pediatrics, 29*(1), 55–66.

Dykeman, C., Nelson, J. R., & Appleton, V. (1996). Building strong working alliances with American Indian families. In P. L. Ewalt, E. M. Freeman, S. A. Kirk, & D. L. Poole (Eds.), *Multicultural issues in social work* (pp. 336–349). Washington, DC: NASW Press.

Ernst, J. S. (2001). Community-level factors and child maltreatment in a suburban county. *Social Work Research, 25*(3), 133–142.

Evans-Campbell, T. (2008). Perceptions of child neglect among urban American Indian/Alaska Native parents. *Child Welfare, 87*(3), 115–142.

Faircloth, C., Hoffman, D. M., & Layne, L. L. (Eds.). (2013). *Parenting in global perspective: Negotiating ideologies of kinship, self and politics.* New York: Routledge.

Falicov, C. J. (2009). Commentary: On the wisdom and challenges of culturally attuned treatments for Latinos. *Family Process, 48*(2), 292–309.

Finno-Velasquez, M. (2013). The relationship between parent immigration status and concrete support service use among Latinos in child welfare: Findings using the National Survey of Child and Adolescent Well-being (NSCAWII). *Children and Youth Services Review, 35*(12), 2118–2127.

Finno-Velasquez, M., Fettes, D., Aarons, G. A., & Hurlburt, M. S. (2014). Cultural adaptation of an evidence-based home visitation programme: Latino clients' experiences of service delivery during implementation. *Journal of Children's Services, 9*(4), 280–294.

Fischer, T. L., Burnet, D. L., Huang, E. S., Chin, M. H., & Cagney, K. A. (2007). Cultural leverage: Interventions using culture to narrow racial disparities in health care. *Medical Care Research and Review, 64*(5), 243s–282s.

Fluke, J. D., Yuan, Y. T., Hedderson, J., & Curtis, P. A. (2003). Disproportionate representation of race and ethnicity in child maltreatment: Investigation and victimization. *Children and Youth Services Review, 25*, 359–373.

Fluke, J. D., Harden, B. J., & Jenkins, M. (2011). *A research synthesis on child welfare disproportionality and disparities.* Paper presented at the Disparities and Disproportionality in Child Welfare: Analysis of the Research. Annie E. Casey Foundation. Retrieved from http://www.aecf.org/m/resourcedoc/AECF-DisparitiesAndDisproportionalityInChildWelfare-2011.pdf#page=11

Freisthler, B., Merritt, D. H., & LaScala, E. A. (2006). Understanding the ecology of child maltreatment: A review of the literature and directions for future research. *Child Maltreatment, 11*(3), 263–280.

Furstenberg, F. F., Jr. (1993). How families manage risk and opportunity in dangerous neighborhoods. In W. J. Wilson (Ed.), *Sociology and the public agenda* (pp. 231–258). Newbury Park: Sage.

Garbarino, J., & Ebata, A. (1983). The significance of ethnic and cultural differences in child maltreatment. *Journal of Marriage and Family, 45*(4), 773–783.

Garbarino, J., Bradshaw, C. P., & Kostelny, K. (2005). Neighborhood and community influences on parenting. In T. Luster & L. Okagaki (Eds.), *Parenting: An ecological perspective* (2nd ed., pp. 297–318). Mahwah: Lawrence Erlbaum Associates, Inc.

Gershoff, E. T. (2013). Spanking and child development: We know enough now to stop hitting our children. *Child Development Perspectives, 7*(3), 133–137.

Harris, M. S., & Hackett, W. (2008). Decision points in child welfare: An action research model to address disproportionality. *Children and Youth Services Review, 30*, 199–215.

Harris, M. S., & Skyles, A. (2008). Kinship care for African American children: Disproportionate and disadvantageous. *Journal of Family Issues, 29*(8), 1013–1030.

Harry, B., Rueda, R., & Kalyanpur, M. (1999). Cultural reciprocity in sociocultural perspective: Adapting the normalization principle for family collaboration. *Exceptional Children, 66*(1), 123–136.

Hawkins, A. O., Danielson, C. K., de Arellano, M. A., Hanson, R. F., Ruggiero, K. J., Smith, D. W., et al. (2010). Ethnic/racial differences in the prevalence of injurious spanking and other child physical abuse in a National Survey of Adolescents. *Child Maltreatment, 15*(3), 242–249.

Hays, P. A. (2001). *Addressing cultural complexities in practice: A framework for clinicians and counselors*. Washington, DC: American Psychological Association.

Hill, R. B. (2004). Institutional racism in child welfare. *Race and Society, 7*(1), 17–33.

Hill, N. E., Bush, K. R., & Roosa, M. W. (2003). Parenting and family socialization strategies and children's mental health: Low-income Mexican-American and Euro-American mothers and children. *Child Development, 74*(1), 189–204.

Hines, A. M., Lemon, K., Wyatt, P., & Merdinger, J. (2004). Factors related to the disproportionate involvement of children of color in the child welfare system: A review of emerging themes. *Children and Youth Services Review, 26*, 507–527.

Huebner, C. E. (2002). Evaluation of a clinic-based parent education program to reduce the risk of infant and toddler maltreatment. *Public Health Nursing, 19*(5), 377–389.

Huey, S. J., Tilley, J. L., Jones, E. O., & Smith, C. (2014). The contribution of cultural competence to evidence-based care for ethnically diverse populations. *Annual Review of Clinical Psychology, 10*, 305–338.

Immigration Policy Center. (2012). *Falling through the cracks: The impact of immigration enforcement on children caught up in the child welfare system*. Washington, DC: American Immigration Council.

Institute of Medicine & National Research Council. (2013). *New directions in child abuse and neglect research*. Washington, DC: The National Academies Press.

Johnson, D. J., Jaeger, E., Randolph, S. J., Cauce, A. M., Ward, J., & NICHD Early Child Care Research Network. (2003). Studying the effects of early child experiences on the development of children of color in the U.S.: Toward a more inclusive research agenda. *Child Development, 74*(5), 1227–1244.

Johnson-Motoyama, M. (2013). Does a paradox exist in child well-being risks among foreign-born Latinos, US-born Latinos, and Whites?: Findings from 50 California cities. *Child Abuse & Neglect, 38*(6), 1061–1072.

Kataoka, S., Novins, D. K., & DeCarlo Santiago, C. (2010). The practice of evidence-based treatments in ethnic minority youth. *Child and Adolescent Psychiatric Clinics of North America, 19*(4), 775–789. doi:10.1016/j.chc.2010.07.008.

Kleinman, A., & Benson, P. (2006). Anthropology in the clinic: The problem of cultural competency and how to fix it. *PLoS Medicine, 3*(10), e294.

Knott, T., & Donovan, L. (2010). Disproportionate representation of African-American children in foster care: Secondary analysis of the National Child Abuse and Neglect Data System, 2005. *Children and Youth Services Review, 32*, 679–684.

Korbin, J. E. (2002). Culture and child maltreatment: Cultural competence and beyond. *Child Abuse & Neglect, 26*, 637–644.

Korbin, J. E., & Spilsbury, J. C. (1999). Cultural competence and child neglect. In H. Dubowitz (Ed.), *Neglected children: Research, practice, and policy* (pp. 69–88). Thousand Oaks: Sage Publications.

Korbin, J. E., Coulton, C. J., Chard, S., Platt-Houston, C., & Su, M. (1998). Impoverishment and child maltreatment in African American & European American neighborhoods. *Development and Psychopathology, 10*, 215–233.

Kotchick, B. A., Dorsey, S., & Heller, L. (2005). Predictors of parenting among African-American single mothers: Personal and contextual factors. *Journal of Marriage and Family, 67*, 448–460.

Kraizer, S., Witte, S. S., & Fryer, G. E. (1989, September–October). Child sexual abuse prevention programs: What makes them effective in protecting children? *Children Today*, pp. 23–27.

Lamborn, S. D., Dornbusch, S. M., & Steinberg, L. (1996). Ethnicity and community context as moderators of the relations between family decision making and adolescent adjustment. *Child Development, 67*(2), 283–301.

Lansford, J. E., Deater-Deckard, K., Dodge, K. A., Bates, J. E., & Pettit, G. S. (2004). Ethnic differences in the link between physical discipline and later adolescent externalizing behaviors. *Journal of Child Psychology and Psychiatry, 45*(4), 801–812.

Lansford, J. E., Chang, L., Dodge, K. A., Malone, P. S., Oburu, P., Palmerus, K., et al. (2005). Physical discipline and children's adjustment: Cultural normativeness as a moderator. *Child Development, 76*(6), 1234–1246.

Lau, A. S. (2006). Making the case for selective and directed cultural adaptations of evidence-based treatments: Examples from parent training. *Clinical Psychology: Science and Practice, 13*(4), 295–310.

Le, H.-N., Ceballo, R., Chao, R., Hill, N. E., Murry, V. M., & Pinderhughes, E. E. (2008). Excavating culture: Disentangling ethnic differences from contextual influences in parenting. *Applied Developmental Science, 12*(4), 163–175.

Leventhal, T., & Shuey, E. A. (2014). Neighborhood context and immigrant young children's development. *Developmental Psychology, 50*(6), 1771–1787. doi:10.1037/a0036424.

Leyendecker, B., Harwood, R. L., Comparini, L., & Yalcinkaya, A. (2005). Socioeconomic status, ethnicity, and parenting. In T. Luster & L. Okagaki (Eds.), *Parenting: An ecological perspective* (2nd ed., pp. 319–341). Mahwah: Lawrence Erlbaum Associates, Inc.

Lu, Y. E., Landsverk, J., Ellis-Macleod, E., Newton, R., Ganger, W., & Johnson, I. (2004). Race, ethnicity, and case outcomes in child protective services. *Children and Youth Services Review, 26*, 447–461.

Lubell, K. M., Lofton, T., & Singer, H. H. (2008). *Promoting healthy parenting practices across cultural groups: A CDC research brief.* Atlanta: Centers for Disease Control and Prevention, National Center for Injury Prevention and Control.

Lum, D. (1992). *Social work practice and people of color.* Belmont: Brooks/Cole Publishing Company.

MacLeod, J., & Nelson, G. (2000). Programs for the promotion of family wellness and the prevention of child maltreatment: A meta-analytic review. *Child Abuse & Neglect, 24*, 1127–1149. doi:10.1016/S0145-2134(00)00178-2.

Maiter, S., Allagia, R., & Trocme, N. (2004). Perceptions of child maltreatment by parents from the Indian subcontinent: Challenging myths about cultural based abusive parenting practices. *Child Maltreatment, 9*, 309–324.

Matthews, H. (2009). *Ten policies to improve access to quality child care for children in immigrant families.* Washington, DC: Center for Law and Social Policy.

Matthews, H., & Jang, D. (2007). *The challenges of change: Learning from the child care and early education experiences of immigrant families.* Washington, DC: Center for Law and Social Policy.

McCall, L. (2005). The complexity of intersectionality. *Signs, 30*(3), 1771–1800.

McLoyd, V. C. (1990). The impact of economic hardship on Black families and children: Psychological distress, parenting, and socioemotional development. *Child Development, 61*(2), 311–346.

Miller, A., & Harwood, R. L. (2002). The cultural organization of parenting: Change and stability of behavior patterns during feeding and social play across the first year of life. *Parenting: Science and Practice, 2*(3), 241–272.

Morelli, G. A., Rogoff, B., Oppenheim, D., & Goldsmith, D. (1992). Cultural variation in infants' sleeping arrangements: Questions of independence. *Developmental Psychology, 28*(4), 604–613.

Needell, B., Brookhart, M. A., & Lee, S. (2003). Black children and foster care placement in California. *Children and Youth Services Review, 25*, 393–408.

Nwosu, C., Batalova, J., & Auclair, G. (2014, April 28). *Frequently requested statistics on immigrants and immigration in the United States*. Washington, DC: Migration Policy Institute. Retrieved from http://www.migrationpolicy.org/article/frequently-requested-statistics-immigrants-and-immigration-united-states.

Obeng, C. S. (2007). Immigrants families and childcare preferences: Do immigrants' cultures influence their childcare decisions? *Early Childhood Education Journal, 34*(4), 259–264.

Olds, D. L., Kitzman, H., Hanks, C., Cole, R., Anson, E., Sidora-Arcoleo, K., et al. (2007). Effects of nurse home visiting on maternal and child functioning: Age-9 follow-up of a randomized trial. *Pediatrics, 120*(4), e832–e845.

Pierce, R., & Pierce, L. (1996). Moving towards cultural competence in the child welfare system. *Children and Youth Services Review, 18*, 713–731.

Polaha, J., Larzelere, R. E., Shapiro, S. K., & Pettit, G. S. (2004). Physical discipline and child behavior problems: A study of ethnic group differences. *Parenting: Science and Practice, 4*(4), 339–360.

Prinz, R. J., Sanders, M. R., Shapiro, C. J., Whitaker, D. J., & Lutzker, J. R. (2009). Population-based prevention of child maltreatment: The U.S. Triple P system population trial. *Prevention Science, 10*(1), 1–12.

Putnam-Hornstein, E. (2011). Report of maltreatment as a risk factor for injury death: A prospective birth cohort study. *Child Maltreatment, 16*(3), 163–174.

Putnam-Hornstein, E., Needell, B., King, B., & Johnson-Motoyama, M. (2013). Racial and ethnic disparities: A population based examination of risk factors for involvement with child protective services. *Child Abuse & Neglect, 37*(1), 33–46.

Reardon-Anderson, J., Capps, R., & Fix, M. (2002). *The health and well-being of children in immigrant families*. Washington, DC: The Urban Institute.

Roberts, D. (2002). Shattered bonds: The color of child welfare. *Children and Youth Services Review, 24*, 877–880.

Rogoff, B. (2003). *The cultural nature of human development*. New York: Oxford University Press.

Rose, S. J., & Meezan, W. (1996). Variations in perceptions of child neglect. *Child Welfare, 75*(2), 139–160.

Shuey, E. A., & Leventhal, T. (under review). Overlapping contexts: The role of neighborhoods and parenting for child development.

Simpkins, S. D., Delgado, M. Y., Price, C. D., Quach, A., & Starbuck, E. (2012). Socioeconomic status, ethnicity, culture, and immigration: Examining the potential mechanisms underlying Mexican-origin adolescents' organized activity participation. *Developmental Psychology, 49*(4), 706–721.

Small, M., Harding, D. J., & Lamont, M. (2010). Reconsidering culture and poverty. *The Annals of the American Academy of Political and Social Science, 629*, 6–27. doi:10.1177/0002716210362077.

Stevenson, K. M., Cheung, K. M., & Leung, P. (1992). A new approach to training child protective services workers for ethnically sensitive practice. *Child Welfare, 71*(4), 291–305.

Takanishi, R. (2004). Leveling the playing field: Supporting immigrant children from birth to eight. *The Future of Children, 14*(2), 61–79.

Tamis-LeMonda, C. S., & Kahana-Kalman, R. (2009). Mothers' view at the transition to a new baby: Variation across ethnic groups. *Parenting: Science and Practice, 9*(1–2), 36–55. doi:10.1080/15295190802656745.

Tamis-LeMonda, C. S., & Song, L. (2012). Parent-infant communicative interactions in cultural context. In R. M. Lerner, M. A. Easterbrooks, & J. Mistry (Eds.), *Handbook of psychology* (2nd ed., Vol. 6, pp. 143–172). Hoboken: Wiley.

Tervalon, M., & Murray-García, J. (1998). Cultural humility versus cultural competence: A critical distinction in defining physician training outcomes in multicultural education. *Journal of Health Care for the Poor and Underserved, 9*(2), 117–125.

The Incredible Years. (2013). Evaluation. Retrieved January 5, 2014, from http://incredibleyears.com/for-researchers/evaluation/

Tower, C. (1996). *Child abuse and neglect.* Boston: Allyn & Bacon.

U.S. Department of Health and Human Services, Office of Minority Health. (2015). *Think Cultural Health: CLAS Legislation Map.* Available at https://www.thinkculturalhealth.hhs.gov/Content/LegislatingCLAS.asp

Varela, R. E., Vernberg, E. M., Sanchez-Sosa, J. J., Riveros, A., Mitchell, M., & Mashunkashey, J. (2004). Parenting style of Mexican, Mexican American, and Caucasian–Non-Hispanic families: Social context and cultural influences. *Journal of Family Psychology, 18*(4), 651–657.

Vega, W. A. (2005). Higher stakes ahead for cultural competence. *General Hospital Psychiatry, 27*(6), 446–450. doi:10.1016/j.genhosppsych.2005.06.007.

Wagner, M., Spiker, D., & Linn, M. I. (2002). The effectiveness of the Parents as Teachers Program with low-income parents and children. *Topics in Early Childhood Special Education, 22*(2), 67–81.

Wells, S., Merritt, L. M., & Briggs, H. E. (2009). Bias, racism, and evidence-based practice: The case for more focused development of the child welfare evidence base. *Children and Youth Services Review, 33*, 1160–1171.

Megan Finno-Velasquez is a Ph.D. candidate at the University of Southern California School of Social Work. Her research interests center broadly around Latino child and family well-being, maltreatment prevention strategies for immigrant families, and improving service system responses to the needs of for Latino immigrant families at risk of child maltreatment. Her dissertation study focuses on understanding patterns of need and service receipt among Latino immigrant families investigated by child welfare agencies. Prior to entering the doctoral program at USC, Ms. Finno-Velasquez served as the immigration liaison for the New Mexico Children, Youth and Families Department. She is a founding member of the Migration and Child Welfare National Network. She received her MSW from New Mexico Highlands University in 2007 and has a BS in psychology and Spanish from the University of Illinois-Urbana/Champaign.

Elizabeth A. Shuey is a doctoral student in the Eliot-Pearson Department of Child Study and Human Development at Tufts University and a Doris Duke Fellow for the Promotion of Child Well-Being. Her work focuses on promoting child and family well-being by bringing a developmental science perspective to bear on social policy issues. She is currently involved in a range of research projects related to this focus, from the housing circumstances of low-income families to the neighborhood context of young immigrant children's development. Ms. Shuey has served as an intern at the Administration for Children and Families (ACF), Region I and at the Federal Reserve Bank of Boston, and worked at RTI International before returning to school to pursue her doctorate. She holds a Bachelor's degree with high honors in psychology from Oberlin College and a Master's degree in clinical psychology from the University of North Carolina at Greensboro.

Chie Kotake is a doctoral student in the Eliot-Pearson Department of Child Study and Human Development at Tufts University. She graduated with a B.A. in psychology from Smith College, and completed her master's degree in child development at Tufts University in May 2010. Her research experiences include working as a research assistant for numerous projects including a project that examines emotional and behavioral regulation of infants adopted internationally and working on an evaluation of early childhood professional trainings. Her research interest focuses on the role of parenting and parent mental health in the social-emotional development of young children facing adversities. She is also interested in the cultural differences in family practices and their influence on children's development. She holds teaching licensure for infant/toddler and preschool level from the Massachusetts Department of Early Education and Care and worked in various school settings, including community-based and university-based educational day care.

J. Jay Miller is an assistant professor in the College of Social Work at the University of Kentucky. His research interests focus on child welfare, particularly outcomes related to foster care. Jay is involved in several community endeavors and has served as the past president of the Louisville Association of Social Workers, founder of the Jefferson Foster Care Peer Support Program and president of the Foster Care Alumni of America—Kentucky. Jay is a past recipient of the CHFS Paul Grannis Award, was recently recognized as an International Graduate Scholar by the Global Sustainability Conference, and is a 2014 inductee into the College of Health and Human Services Hall of Fame at Western Kentucky University. Jay earned his Ph.D. at the University of Louisville. Last but not least, Jay is a proud foster care alum!

Part III
New Generation of Research:
The Nature of the Response

Chapter 6
From Causes to Outcomes: Determining Prevention Can Work

Paul Lanier, Kathryn Maguire-Jack, Joseph Mienko, and Carlomagno Panlilio

Chapter 6 in Brief

Context

- Effective prevention programs incorporate logic models informed by our understanding of the causes of child maltreatment, a challenging but necessary goal.
- Ecological theories, supported by research, show that the causes of maltreatment are dependent on a dynamic interaction of factors at many levels of a child's ecology.
- The effectiveness of prevention programs is facilitated by study designs that isolate the causal relationship between program participation and outcomes.
- Many alternatives to the randomized-controlled trial are available to researchers.

P. Lanier (✉)
School of Social Work, University of North Carolina at Chapel Hill, Chapel Hill, NC, USA
e-mail: planier@unc.edu

K. Maguire-Jack
College of Social Work, The Ohio State University, Columbus, OH, USA
e-mail: maguirejack.1@osu.edu

J. Mienko
School of Social Work, University of Washington, Seattle, WA, USA
e-mail: mienkoja@uw.edu

C. Panlilio
Department of Human Development and Quantitative Methodology, University of Maryland, College Park, MD, USA
e-mail: panlilio@umd.edu

© Springer International Publishing Switzerland 2015
D. Daro et al. (eds.), *Advances in Child Abuse Prevention Knowledge,*
Child Maltreatment 5, DOI 10.1007/978-3-319-16327-7_6

Strategies for Moving Forward

- Translate research and theory on known risk and protective factors into clearly articulated program logic models.
- To determine the overall utility of prevention efforts, identify, and seek to measure a comprehensive set of immediate as well as distal outcomes.
- Integrate continuous quality improvement strategies into an intervention's operational framework to offer an important empirical tool to strengthen service delivery and, potentially, improve outcomes.

Implications for Research

- Increase the level of research rigor by focusing on inferring causality to improve our knowledge regarding effective programs.
- When possible use random assignment to different treatment conditions to fully understand program impacts.
- In addition to using regression-based analyses, explore a range of strong alternative designs for inferring causality including propensity score analysis, instrumental variables, regression discontinuity, and directed acyclic graphs.

Introduction

As priorities for setting policy continue to emphasize the importance of evidence and accountability, understanding whether maltreatment prevention programs are successfully targeting and changing the causal mechanisms at work will be essential to programs seeking funding and support. To be successful in practice and to gain justification for further dissemination, maltreatment prevention interventions must accomplish two goals related to program design and evaluation: develop and implement an intervention logic model informed by theory that targets known causes of child maltreatment and demonstrate evidence of effectiveness with rigorous methodological designs that isolate the causal effects of the program. Our ability to accomplish these two challenging tasks is directly related to our success in preventing child maltreatment.

Isolating and measuring cause and effect is not a new problem for social science and is certainly not limited to maltreatment research. Our modern thinking regarding causality can be traced to the enlightenment and early thinkers such as David Hume (1748). Hume defines a causal relationship between two objects as, "if the first object had not been the second never had existed." It is not enough for us to simply draw an association between a first object and a second object (e.g., an association between participation in a home visiting program and reduced risk for future maltreatment). In order to establish a causal relationship, we need to determine that the second object would not have existed *without* the first object.

Many programs intended to prevent maltreatment were created to address assumed causes of maltreatment without relying on sound theoretical foundations, rigorous research, or program evaluation (Barth et al. 2005; Slack et al. 2009). Further, programs received funding and support with little accountability as to whether they were actually producing the change they were targeting. More recently, programs that have demonstrated effectiveness for other outcomes (e.g., child behavior problems) are being implemented as maltreatment prevention programs. The causal assumptions undergirding the adaptation of these programs, however, must be scrutinized and evaluated for maltreatment prevention as well.

Despite this history, the evidence base for child maltreatment prevention services has come a long way in recent years. Although the effectiveness of many programs is still unknown, there has been a proliferation of high-quality evaluations to understand whether specific programs are successful in reducing behaviors associated with child maltreatment. (For example, Nurse Family Partnership, Olds 2006; Triple P Positive Parenting Program, Prinz et al. 2009; and several others.) We are beginning to see a noticeable shift from an ideology-based field to one that is much more evidence-based (Institute of Medicine and National Research Council 2012). Driven in part by the changing policy environment, many programs have become more deliberate both in terms of creating programs based in theory and including a plan for evaluation.

This chapter focuses on the role of causality in child maltreatment prevention. We organize the discussion around the two major types of causal inquiry that scholars in diverse fields have applied to many domains of scientific inquiry (Holland 1986). As illustrated in Fig. 6.1, the first approach explores "causes of known effects." For maltreatment prevention, this pertains to understanding the etiology of maltreatment—explaining the causes of the human behavior of child abuse and neglect from an epidemiological perspective. We observe a maltreated child or population of maltreated children and attempt to determine the source. The second inquiry encompasses "effects of known causes," which involves creating a treatment or intervention, using it to manipulate the family context, and then attempting to isolate the causal effect of maltreatment.

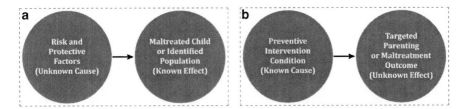

Fig. 6.1 Two approaches to causal inquiry related to designing and testing maltreatment prevention interventions: Determining the causes of known effects (**a**) and determining the effects of known causes (**b**)

These two areas of scientific inquiry must overlap in the context of effective maltreatment prevention in order to move from understanding causes to ensuring positive outcomes. The interventions we deploy are based on our understanding of the causal relationships we think exist. We begin the chapter with a discussion of how theories of maltreatment etiology inform logic models for existing prevention programs. We then move to a summary of exciting statistical methods that bring us closer to inferring causality in observational studies. We end with reflections on how these methods could affect the future of the maltreatment prevention field and discuss discussion on how we can continue to move the field forward.

The Value of Theory

Our efforts to end maltreatment begin with a belief that if we better understand child abuse and neglect, our efforts to halt the occurrence of child maltreatment will be more effective. Using the frame of prevention science, well-specified maltreatment prevention efforts begin with identifying the risk factors that are precursors of abuse (Coie et al. 1993; Kellam and Langevin 2003). Isolating the etiologic causes of maltreatment informs the development of theories that can be tested and refined. Theories validated by research can then be applied to program logic models and tested with rigorous experimental designs.

While a large number of maltreatment prevention programs exist the effectiveness of many is either unknown or not supported (MacMillan et al. 2009), due in part to a lack of synergy between causal theory development and intervention research. Research has uncovered a complex, yet increasingly valid, picture of the causal reality of maltreatment—one that considers overlapping layers of influence. Overly simple logic models and tests of program effectiveness will not suffice. As the rigor of methodology has increased, so too has our ability to isolate program effects and test whether an intervention has truly led to decreased risk for maltreatment. The application of the randomized controlled trial to maltreatment prevention has led this charge. Well-intentioned practitioners and policymakers now have higher confidence in their claims because of this move towards empiricism and evidence-based practice.

Developing a science of maltreatment prevention is a complex and iterative process. The public health model identifies four stages that are directly pertinent to conceptualizing maltreatment prevention: problem definition and surveillance, identifying risk and protective factors, developing and testing interventions, and widespread dissemination of effective models (Coie et al. 1993). The first principle of prevention science is that "prevention trials address fundamental causal processes" (Coie et al. 1993, p. 1014). Specifically, we must attempt to isolate the "causes of known effects" in order to interrupt them. Thus, this seemingly simple process has the impossible methodological and theoretical task of determining true cause and effect.

With regard to maltreatment prevention, the Centers for Disease Control and Prevention have identified a goal of promoting a social context "in which prevention and intervention services are evidence-based, effective, widely available, and socially valued" (Hammond 2003, p. 83). We will assume for this discussion that uniform definitions of maltreatment exist and a robust surveillance system is able to reliably identify true cases of maltreatment. The next task is to identify the risk and protective factors that impact the likelihood of maltreatment. Theory helps us understand where to look for these factors. The theoretical framework for understanding child maltreatment has not changed much in the past two decades. What has changed dramatically is the rate at which interventions have been infused with theory, the rigor with which hypothesized effects have been tested, and the extent to which evidence has begun to penetrate practice. While much work is needed, the gap between what we know can be done to help families and what actually occurs has become smaller.

Theory on Maltreatment Etiology

Decades of research and theorizing on the etiology of maltreatment has yielded a multifaceted and dynamic model of human behavior that depends largely on the unique context of an individual family impacted by broader societal influences (Tzeng et al. 1991). While a restrained and straightforward model would be more satisfying to those developing prevention strategies, complicated multilevel models are likely most valid. The answer "it depends" is not very appealing when attempting to design a universal prevention model that can be taken to scale. It has become apparent that collective multidisciplinary efforts embedded in a nimble and comprehensive system of care must deliver the right support to the right families at the right time. One-size-fits-all, silver-bullet approaches likely do not exist in this field (Greeley 2009).

The evolution of modern theory on maltreatment etiology was sparked when "battered child syndrome" was first introduced by Kempe and colleagues (1962). This new medical classification was identified primarily by patterns of radiological skeletal imaging depicting injuries to children. Although this "discovery" of child abuse generated much social attention and policy action, it did not provide a clear answer to help understand why or how abuse could happen. Early attempts to develop theories on the causes of maltreatment represented the complexity of the issue and had varied disciplinary perspectives. Some focused on profiling maltreating caregivers to identify specific psychopathological dysfunctions that lead to abuse and neglect (National Research Council 1993; Steele and Pollack 1974). Others considered community-level pressures and posited sociological perspectives incorporating the social, political, and cultural environment (Gil 1970; Garbarino 1977). Reviews of theory have acknowledged this division between family and social factors (Daro 1988). Eventually, theories expanded to reflect the transactional nature of risk and protective factors at familial and environmental levels (Belsky

1980; Bronfenbrenner 1979; Bruskas 2008; National Research Council 1993; Sidebotham 2001; Widom 2000; Zielinski and Bradshaw 2006).

Ecological Framework

The ecological perspective of child development was developed to describe the broad experience of human development but has been specifically applied to understanding the causes of maltreatment and its impacts on the developing child (Bronfenbrenner 1977, 1979; Belsky 1980; Cicchetti and Lynch 1993; Lynch and Cicchetti 1998). In the model displayed in Fig. 6.2, the individual exists within a range of social systems that go from the most proximate environments for a child (her family) to the general norms and values that govern the society in which she lives. Since no single factor or level can adequately explain all causes of maltreatment, understanding the problem requires an examination of each level. Further, Cicchetti and Rizley's (1981) transactional model posited that factors at each level dynamically interact over time, further increasing and decreasing the potential for maltreatment.

Belsky (1980) provided the first ecological integration of the parent and child characteristics and environmental factors thought to cause maltreatment. More recent research continues to lend support for this ecological framework. To further explicate the causal theory indicated by the ecological framework, we will provide examples from three factors originally posited by Belsky (1980) to contribute to maltreatment and examine the way in which these factors are understood today. As indicated in Fig. 6.2, multiple levels of ecology have been identified as impacting individual actions, conditions, and outcomes. We describe examples of recent research that support this theory, with a focus on studies that demonstrate the importance of including interactions across multiple levels of a child's ecology.

A caregiver's own childhood history, particularly exposure to maltreatment, is consistently correlated with an intergenerational transmission of maltreating behav-

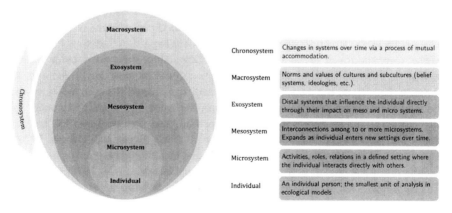

Fig. 6.2 Levels of an ecological system

ior (see, for example, Widom 1989). The simplest inductive formulation of this observation is that exposure to abuse or neglect as a child *causes* a parent to abuse or neglect his or her own child. However, this relationship is not deterministic. Not all individuals who were maltreated as children grow up to maltreat their own children. Subsequent research has found support for an interactional influence of the individual's genotype in this causal pathway. When a specific gene is present in a maltreatment victim, they are less likely to become violent and have antisocial problems as adults (Caspi et al. 2002; Widom and Brzustowicz 2006). Understanding the interaction of genotype and environmental influences is a largely undeveloped area of research in this field.

Our understanding of the causal factors at the family level, or microsystem, has also evolved over recent years. Belsky (1980) cites observational studies indicating disproportionate representation of infants born premature or low birth weight among samples of maltreated children. Recent epidemiological research using population-based birth cohorts and official reports of maltreatment have found that children born low birth weight are more likely to later be maltreated (Parrish et al. 2011; Putnam-Hornstein and Needell 2011; Wu et al. 2004). However, the research indicates that this pattern reflects a complex interplay between the caregiver and the infant, as well as the supports available to the family. Studies have found that risk for maltreatment among low birth weight infants is largely driven by parental mental health symptoms and not by infant factors such as disability (Strathearn et al. 2001; Zelkowitz et al. 2007). Based on this research, those developing interventions targeting expectant parents at risk for maltreatment might choose to focus on providing mental health services for families with low birth weight infants.

Our understanding of causal processes diminishes as we move away from the family level. At the societal or macrosystem level, the "cultural fabric" dictates social norms and defines social constructions of children and parenting (Belsky 1980). While direct evidence of the causal influence of society is often difficult to measure, its impact is widely acknowledged. One example is the social acceptance of corporal punishment as a suitable form of discipline. In many states, corporal punishment is still legally and commonly practiced in public schools (Sacks 2008). If parents are grappling with selecting an effective method of discipline for their child, it may make sense to model their strategies after a practice sanctioned and demonstrated by educators and administrators at their child's school. A review of studies examining the effect of policies banning corporal punishment in other countries found a decline in support for and use of corporal punishment after the policy change (Zolotor and Puzia 2010).

These are just some examples of the support for the ecological framework to explain the etiology of maltreatment. It is unlikely that one single program or intervention could be developed to address all risk factors experienced by a family at all levels of ecology. Therefore, programs embedded within systems of care serving defined child populations may be able to identify areas of overlap and need for services to provide a comprehensive prevention service continuum. There are interventions that engage with a defined service population that can begin to address a wide array of risk factors using these advances in theory.

Using Theory to Move Forward

Many model developers are beginning to use theory more explicitly in describing the rationale for interventions. There are many examples of models that explicitly integrate causal theory to varying extents. While a comprehensive review of this process is beyond the scope of this chapter, we provide one example. Developers of the Nurse-Family Partnership (NFP), a well-studied home visiting program with a primary goal of preventing maltreatment, describe their model as "research-based and theory-driven" (Olds 2006, p. 9). Along with ecological and attachment theory, self-efficacy theory informed the development of NFP and is a useful frame for interventions that seek to improve parenting skills among caregivers who may lack motivation to change or perceive the barriers to change as being too great. Providing information about child developmental stages to parents who have low self-efficacy is likely insufficient. Many caregivers did not have examples of positive parenting or a stable family environment as children. As caregivers, they may have limited social support and few models of effective and nurturing parents. Self-efficacy theory was integrated into this program by including components that focus on improving maternal confidence through setting short-term, achievable goals towards attainment of long-term change (Olds et al. 1997). NFP and other evidence-based models have clearly articulated logic models that use theory to inform the specific inputs prescribed by the intervention.

Over the past decade, with the integration of theory with methodology from public health and prevention science, the rigor of intervention research in behavioral and social sciences has yielded a massive increase in available evidence. Armed with this new knowledge—which is often accompanied by promising cost-benefit analyses—policymakers now demand public dollars be spent on interventions that are "evidence-based." The next section will discuss how to design research studies that can assess the causal impact of such programs. We shift to causal inferences regarding "effects of known causes" to better understand whether our interventions were truly effective.

Methods to Infer Causality in Observational Studies

Much of the current language and theory that has developed in the two centuries since Hume articulated the problem of causality is based on the work of Neyman (1990 version) and their approach to experimental crop trials. When comparing several different varieties of crops in multiple plots of land, they noted a crucial limitation of observational research: we only ever observe the yield of one particular variety on one particular plot. Expanding on this work, Rubin (1974) observed that the same problem also existed in any setting of causal analysis: it is impossible for the same family to be in both the treatment and control conditions of a maltreatment prevention study at the same time. After the intervention, we observe whether or not the parent engaged in child maltreatment (i.e., the outcome). This phenomenon is known as the fundamental problem of causal inference (Holland 1986); we are only able to observe a single outcome for a given subject.

Average Causal Effect and Random Assignment

Rubin (1974) suggests that our limited observations do not prevent us from making statements about the causal relationship between an intervention and an outcome. In most cases, we cannot assess the effect of an intervention on a particular subject. We can, however, assess an average causal effect for a larger population (e.g., families at risk for child maltreatment). As long as all parents have an equal chance of entering into the treatment or control condition, we can calculate the average causal effect by comparing the difference between treatment and control groups on the given outcome (e.g., mean parenting change scores or rates of later maltreatment reports).

A key factor for inferring causality is the notion that all parents have an equal chance of entering into the treatment or control condition. In an ideal situation, this takes place by randomly assigning a properly drawn sample from the population into a treatment or control group. If the randomization is successful, the researcher can assume that the outcomes in the treatment group are approximately what would be seen if all members of the population received an intervention.

However, randomized experiments are not always practical or feasible. The next section provides some solutions for how to infer causality in the absence of a randomized experiment. It is important to note that these approaches could (in principle) be used to evaluate etiological frameworks (causes of known effects) *in addition to* evaluating interventions (effects of known causes). In other words, there are many etiological conditions (such as poverty) to which we could never ethically (or practically) randomly assign people. We can, however, make use of extensions of the Neyman-Rubin framework to assess both our etiological assumptions and interventions made given an assumed etiological context.

Thinking Causally

As a preliminary step, it is worth noting some recent advances in causal thinking that can help inform methodological approaches. While a detailed treatment is beyond the scope of this chapter, the use of directed acyclic graphs (DAGs) is discussed here briefly as a potential means of properly scoping statistical problems prior to engaging in statistical analyses.[1] These models are based on the theory of

---

[1] The reader is directed to Pearl (1988, 2009) for a more formal and complete treatment of DAGs and d-separation.

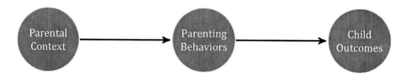

Fig. 6.3 Simple DAG

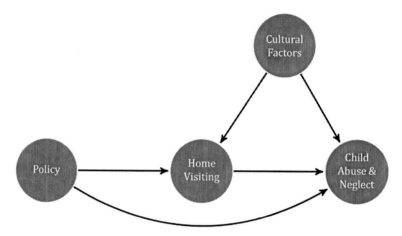

Fig. 6.4 Complex DAG

inferred causation that suggests that the task of causal modeling is really involved with "finding a satisfactory *explanation* to a given set of observations" (Pearl and Verma 1995, p. 789). A DAG is a causal model that includes a set of points connected by unidirectional arrows (often referred to as "edges"). The models identify potential confounding variables, establish temporal ordering, and then use observed data and probability theory to identify the best causal explanation. While the points are frequently given variable names (e.g., X, Y, or Z), we label them with plain text here. Figure 6.3 provides an example of a DAG using a home visiting program. The direction of a potential "effect" (i.e., positive or negative) represented along a given edge is irrelevant—the direction could be positive or negative. A DAG and mathematical operations on DAGs illustrate the causal relationship between two random variables independent of the direction of that relationship.

Figure 6.4 depicts a slightly more complex DAG, which shows a potential confounding variable (i.e., cultural factors) and a possible connection between a policy designed to promote home visiting (i.e., policy) and the outcome of interest (i.e., child abuse and neglect). What remains is to decide how to handle these variables in analysis. The simple act of mapping causal factors in a DAG is useful in conceptualizing the relationships between variables under study. However, a DAG can also be reduced to a mathematical and probabilistic representation, which can, in turn, be used to better determine what factors should be addressed in a given analysis. In other words, a DAG can serve as *both* a visual and a mathematical representation of theory.

One of the more common approaches of analyzing a DAG is known as assessing a graph for directional or "d-separation" (Pearl 1988). The basics of the process involve checking whether one or more points on the DAG block all available paths between two variables. If all paths are determined to be blocked, they are said to be d-separated (see Pearl 1988, 2009). Depending on the research question under consideration, such analysis can help prioritize variables for inclusion in a given analysis. In addition to providing a method through which causal models can be assessed, the theory related to DAGs also provides the basis for many of the modern approaches to estimating causal effects in the context of an observational study.

Methods to Handle the Fundamental Problem of Causal Inference

Structural Equation Modeling (SEM) Is Never Enough

Structural equation modeling (SEM) encompasses a diverse set of statistical procedures but typically includes the simultaneous estimation of several multivariate regression models. Because SEM, particularly path analysis, is used to test theoretical causal relationships, it is often equated with an implied causal analysis. The simple act of mapping proposed relationships between manifest or latent variables in an SEM analysis does not allow a researcher to infer a causal relationship between the variables. Although it was never intended to do so, as noted by Bollen and Pearl (2013), there is a pervasive myth throughout the social science community that the use of a structural model can somehow allow a researcher to establish causation through associations alone. Bollen and Pearl reviewed nearly a century of literature on SEM and demonstrated that, despite the clear intentions of the initial developers of path analysis and latent variable approaches (see Wright 1921), social scientists continue to imply or even explicitly state that SEMs provide researchers with an ability to determine causal relationships between variables.

Structural models provide researchers with a valuable tool with which they can isolate the effects of individual variables on other variables in a complex model while simultaneously controlling for measurement error in latent variables. They do not, however, provide researchers with a solution to inferring causality where random assignment has not been employed. Other approaches, which can be used in conjunction with SEM, can help get researchers closer to simulating the experimental condition and are discussed in more detail below.

Creating Control Groups in the Absence of Randomized Trials

Instrumental Variable Models

While some methods focus on identifying comparable groups, others focus on trying to mimic assignment to treatment and control conditions. One such approach is referred to as the instrumental variable approach.[2] The term "instrumental" comes from the goal of the approach in finding an assignment mechanism (i.e., an instrument) to treatment and control conditions within observational data. This approach requires that the instrument randomly assign participants to condition of treatment and the instrument to be unrelated to the outcome of interest.

For example, imagine a jurisdiction with a robust differential response system. In this system, intake workers on a child abuse hotline could make decisions about whether or not to refer low-risk cases alleging child maltreatment to a home visiting program designed to prevent child maltreatment. Intake workers are likely to vary substantially in their propensity to refer clients the home visiting program; some intake workers will be more likely to refer and some will be less likely to refer. Since cases are effectively randomly assigned to intake workers and one can reasonably assume that there is no correlation between the intake worker and future incidents of child maltreatment, a reasonable instrumental variable model focused on the home visiting program might look something like the depiction in Fig. 6.5 below.[3]

This basic logic has been previously applied to a rigorous study of the foster care system (Doyle 2011). Doyle attempted to examine the causal effects of foster care on future outcomes (such as medical service usage) and utilized investigator assignment as the instrumental variable. Doyle observed that investigators can be gener-

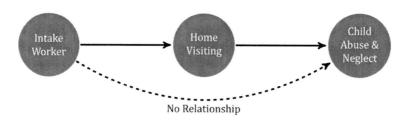

No Relationship

Fig. 6.5 Hypothetical instrumental variable DAG

---

[2] We direct the reader to Heckman (1997) for a discussion of the use of instrumental variables in program evaluation and to Hogan and Lancaster (2004) for application in longitudinal studies of public health outcomes.

[3] As with all DAGs, the depiction represents relationships between variables. These variables can take on many potential values. In the case of home visiting, a child can be assigned to the home visiting program (i.e., Home Visiting = 1) or not (i.e., Home Visiting = 0). Both conditions are implicit in the single vertex.

ally classified into two categories: strict and lenient. Strict workers have an above average placement rate amongst workers in their unit and lenient workers have a below average placement rate. As assignment to a given worker is a largely random process, the assignment can be used to mimic random assignment to foster care (at least for marginal cases—those cases in which worker assignment mattered).

Propensity Score Matching

Estimation of causal effects from nonexperimental designs, even those using matching or statistical controlling, can be biased due to sample selection (Guo et al. 2006). One statistical approach that has potential in effectiveness research using nonrandom groups is propensity score matching (PSM).[4] PSM is appropriate in situations where a comparison group has been identified but concerns about sample selection bias remain. There must be sufficient information about the treatment and comparison groups to create the propensity score and assess the balance of groups. The propensity score is estimated by modeling the probability of being treated "as a function of all relevant observed covariates—that is, observed pretreatment measurements possibly related to posttreatment outcomes" (Rubin 2010, p. 7). In the example of a randomized study in which each subject has a 50/50 chance of being selected into the treatment or control group, the propensity score for all subjects, treatment and control, is one-half (0.5). In an observational study with individuals who self-select into treatment, other factors will influence the chances of being in the treatment or comparison group. For example, if the treatment is provided in an office setting, individuals with access to transportation may be more likely to self-select into the treatment condition. But, if groups are randomized, access to transportation would not influence treatment assignment.

The PSM procedures use this propensity score to balance the treatment and comparison groups by creating ideal matches on the propensity score. Decision algorithms are used to complete this matching process (Coca-Perraillon 2007; Thoemmes and Kim 2011). The adequacy of the matching procedure can be assessed by comparing the differences on observed variables between the conditions before and after matching. There are a variety of PSM strategies and other analytic approaches using the propensity score, including stratification, weighting, and regression adjustment (D'Agostino 1998; Myers and Louis 2010; Rosenbaum and Rubin 1983). These techniques all seek to remove the effect of bias and isolate a true causal effect.

Instrumental variable and propensity score approaches are examples of two analytic techniques that can be used to assess causality in intervention studies. The next section provides additional considerations for designing rigorous studies to advance our understanding of what works.

---

[4] Propensity score matching is just one type of propensity score analysis. Guo and Fraser's (2010) text provides a useful review of the need for propensity score methods in observational studies and provides examples of software analysis code and output.

Moving Forward

In moving the prevention field forward, it is important to develop a roadmap with clear indicators of causes and their relationships to intermediate and long-term outcomes, as well as a means to evaluate each of these indicators. Developing a logic model can help achieve this by setting the stage for designing, implementing, and evaluating programs aimed at preventing maltreatment.

Logic Model

The evaluation of program effectiveness is well served by beginning with a clear understanding of the conceptual framework utilized in its design. The creation of a logic model provides a theoretical causal mechanism, which serves as a "roadmap" in designing interventions. This mechanism, along with key program components, would shift an outcome's trajectory and inform methodologies to evaluate its efficacy and effectiveness. For example, the ecological framework highlights the importance of *proximal processes* as the key mechanism that drives human growth and development (Bronfenbrenner and Morris 2006). These processes occur between the child and his or her immediate and distal environments. Parent–child interaction is one example of this process, which serves as the mechanism for change that can be targeted by interventions such as Parent–child Interaction Therapy and Attachment and Biobehavioral Catch-up.

Application of this roadmap in the area of maltreatment prevention, however, requires understanding complex dynamic causes leading to maltreatment behaviors and adverse child outcomes. Programs and intervention components should be able to take the dynamic interplay of these complexities into account, such as with the examples discussed in the prior section on theory. In the creation of a logic model to inform program development or evaluate program effectiveness, the selected framework should allow for the inclusion of causal inputs from an ecological perspective that takes into account individual-level and contextual factors. Contextual factors in this case would include key program components that might have an influence on the theoretical change mechanisms within the selected framework. An important component for later evaluation is monitoring processes and outcomes to ensure fidelity in the delivery of an intervention or program that targets specific family processes.

Adopting attachment-based models such as Parent–child Interaction Therapy (Herschell et al. 2002) or Attachment and Biobehavioral Catch-up (Dozier et al. 2006) allows for the inclusion of evidence-based interventions within an ecological framework. These interventions may intervene on *proximal processes* between parent and child to affect positive outcomes, such as decreased incidence of maltreatment. Inclusion of program factors in addition to family-level factors could allow for the partitioning of variances accounted for in the outcomes. That is, examining the outcomes and attributing change, or lack thereof, to the proposed causal inputs related to either program components or family-level factors.

The etiology of maltreatment is seldom a simple linear relationship between an explanatory factor and the resulting incidence of maltreatment. Additional risk and protective factors should be considered for inclusion in a logic model to examine moderating and mediating factors that may influence the causal chain associated with the outcomes of interest. In designing studies, a reasonably comprehensive set of covariates should be selected for measurement to allow for the inclusion of other necessary resources in the causal input of the program. For example, looking at food security issues as a risk factor in increasing the incidence or prevalence of neglect could prompt the inclusion of community partners that might mitigate this risk (Carter and Myers 2007).

With a list of some potential items to include in our logic model, we can now move forward into the next steps, program design, implementation, and evaluation. More specifically, we offer suggestions on how to develop stronger prevention programs and improve upon the quality of existing programs. The scope of this section focuses on the relationship between family and program causal inputs on short- and long-term child and family outcomes.[5]

Design

Challenges such as cost, resource allocation, attrition, and prohibition of random assignment may impact program design. These challenges may alter the evaluation of causal effects on outcomes of interest. Although random assignment is the ideal strategy to determine a program's average causal effects, randomized control studies are not often available and implementation may be cost prohibitive. Thus, alternative nonexperimental research designs, including those we have introduced (PSM and instrumental variables) and others (such as regression discontinuity and longitudinal prospective designs), should be considered in the context of the research questions and feasibility constraints.

Central to these alternative program designs is the importance of key constructs and measures. It is imperative that the measures included in the program or study have sound psychometric properties. That is, accuracy, sensitivity, validity, and reliability properties have been established and have followed the process of inquiry outlined in test theory. These include clear operationalization of the construct of interest, development of appropriate measures, testing of the instruments for accuracy and sensitivity, collection of experimental data to confirm psychometric properties, and statistical summarization (Crocker and Algina 1986). Measurement properties are important in the nonexperimental models (e.g., regression discontinuity and instrumental variables) mentioned above because of the nature in which instrumental variables will be used for participant assignment. Accuracy of the measure(s) used will allow for improvements in unbiased estimates on the intended outcomes. Additionally, in considering longitudinal research designs, stability of measures over time should be taken into account.

---

[5] For additional information on the design and implementation of an evaluation system for program components, see McCabe et al. 2012.

One way to improve upon current measures is the inclusion of physiological measures to complement behavioral self-report and observational measures. Physiological measures offer researchers a way to evaluate the reliability and validity of currently employed behavioral measures. They also offer a new and exciting way to examine causal effects on outcomes, and may result in fewer measurement errors. These physiological measures have been devised in part due to recent advances in neuroscience. One example of an intervention that employs physiological measures is the Attachment and Biobehavioral Catch-up intervention, which targets emotion regulatory capabilities of young children in foster care. Outcome measures on these regulatory processes are collected in the form of parent reports as well as saliva cortisol. Dozier et al. (2009) stated that dysregulation can occur at the behavioral, emotional, and neuroendocrine levels. (Saliva cortisol is one way to measure neuroendocrine levels.) Emotional dysregulation may not be directly observed, but can be inferred in the measurement of both behavioral and neuroendocrine levels. In doing so, estimation of the direct and indirect effects of the intervention on child outcomes can be more accurately assessed.

Cost and attrition rates bring about problems, not only in program design but in evaluating effectiveness as well, particularly in longitudinal designs. One option for addressing missing data that result from attrition or limitations due to cost is to adopt planned missing data designs. These designs allow for the collection of missing data through randomly assigning participants to have missing items, missing measurement occasions, or missing measures. These correspond to the different types of designs such as multiform design, wave missing design, and two-method measurement design (Little and Rhemtulla 2013). Modern analytic methods allow for the analysis of missing data (e.g., multiple imputation and full information maximum likelihood).[6]

For example, a two-method measurement design allows for the use of two measures: one that is cheap and easy to administer but with potentially low validity and a second, more expensive, higher quality measure. In this design scenario, the cheaper measure is administered to the entire sample while the more expensive, higher quality measure is administered to a random subsample of those participants.[7] In the Attachment and Biobehavioral Catch-up intervention above, collection of salivary cortisol may prove to be too expensive and time consuming to administer to the entire sample. Therefore, a two-method measurement design could be implemented, with all the participants completing the parent-report measure on regulatory capabilities and a random subset of the sample being assigned to collection of cortisol. In a study by Hogue et al. (2013), the authors employed six

---

[6] For more information on missing data see Enders (2010). For the strategies mentioned, data that are missing have to assume missing at random (MAR) or missing completely at random (MCAR) types, which means that there is little to no correlation between the variable that caused the missingness and the variable containing the missingness. By incorporating planned missing data designs, MAR and MCAR assumptions can be under the researchers' control (Graham et al. 2006).

[7] For further information on two-method design issues such as power, sample size considerations, and effect sizes, please see Graham et al. (2006) and Little and Rhemtulla (2013).

planned missing data designs in salivary cortisol research that were analyzed using growth curve modeling. They found that these designs provided similar results to complete case analysis but with lower associated costs.

Implementation

The translation of prevention research has its own set of challenges as interventions progress from rigorously controlled efficacy studies to testing programs in the "real world" with broader populations using effectiveness research. The Society for Prevention Research set forth a set of standards to identify prevention programs that could be considered efficacious and effective (Standards of Evidence Committee 2004). Efficacy studies are conducted under highly controlled conditions and are a direct test of internal validity. Effectiveness studies test interventions under real-world conditions and therefore increase external validity. The use of interventions deemed efficacious by predetermined standards is important in ensuring the success of a prevention program, especially in the area of maltreatment prevention and promotion of child well-being. However, issues of generalizability (external validity) may arise when attempting to implement interventions from a randomized trial or basic science context to a broader, population-based target (i.e., program effectiveness).

This particular task is one of the responsibilities of the Office of Behavioral and Social Sciences Research at the National Institutes of Health. Under its dissemination and implementation activities, this office performs "translational research" in order to "address gaps between scientific discovery and program delivery."[8] It contains resources to guide program development and evaluation efforts in scaling up evidence-based interventions for community delivery. Additional statistical considerations can be employed in assessing the generalizability of randomized trial efficacy results to the general population. For example, Stuart et al. (2011) proposed that propensity scores could be used as a means to assess the homogeneity between trial samples and target populations of interest. This issue, as it relates to scaling up, will be discussed in the next section.

Evaluation

Agencies that implement maltreatment prevention programs and policies should consider whether the selected strategies are impacting the causal outcomes defined in the program logic model. Ultimately, the effectiveness of a prevention program will be important to assess in evaluating whether proposed causal mechanisms have been addressed in order to prevent first reports of maltreatment (when working with

---

[8] http://obssr.od.nih.gov/scientific_areas/translation/index.aspx?p=104

at-risk families) or to prevent further maltreatment (when working with families that have been reported to child welfare agencies). While it is important for programs to evaluate their success by examining future outcomes such as official maltreatment reports, programs can also monitor intermediate outcomes on an ongoing basis. Engaging in evaluation activities before the conclusion of a program allows dynamic adjustments to be made to meet potential needs of program staff, stakeholders, and participants in a timely manner.

McCabe et al. (2012) proposed that incorporating a continuous quality improvement process is a central component in evaluating program effectiveness. The authors defined continuous quality improvement as a systematic approach that applies scientific methods in defining processes and outcomes that allow testing of changes aimed at improving a program. Specifically, there are five principles that govern a continuous quality improvement approach. These include a focus on the process or system as causes for intervention effects rather than at the participant level; troubleshooting approaches based on the application of statistical methods; use of cross-functional employee teams within a program; identification of problems and opportunities that are employee-driven; and focus on internal and external stakeholders. By incorporating a continuous quality improvement process, fidelity monitoring at the program level can occur, ensuring that evidence-based interventions are implemented appropriately (see Chap. 8 in this volume). Intermediate and distal outcomes can then be evaluated based on the program-level causal inputs.

At the participant level, intervention and program effects are difficult to detect if attrition and noncompliance rates are high. Unlike laboratory-based, randomized control studies, the rates of noncompliance for large scale, community-based programs are difficult to manage. A study using Monte Carlo simulations examined the effects of noncompliance and other factors on statistical power to estimate intervention effects (Jo 2002). Additionally, the author of the study discussed intent-to-treat analysis and complier average causal effect estimation as options for estimating treatment effects.

Intent-to-treat analysis is a standard method employed in estimating treatment effects by comparing average outcomes of the treatment and control groups, regardless of whether or not individuals in the treatment group received the intervention. Thus, causal effects provided by this method reflect treatment assignment rather than treatment received. Complier average causal effect, on the other hand, compares average outcomes between treatment and control conditions, but only for compliers. Compared with intent-to-treat, the estimates of causal effects using complier average causal effect estimation reflect both treatment assignment and treatment received. Selection of either method depends on the purpose of the intervention. Intent-to-treat is best suited when interested in the overall intervention effects for the entire sample. The use of complier average causal effect is best suited for estimating intervention effects for those participants who comply with treatment.

Evaluation of the causal inputs at the program level and participant level are critical to ensuring that effectiveness and efficacy are both attained in the prevention of initial or ongoing maltreatment experiences. This is particularly important when evaluating programs that scale up evidence-based interventions. This point was echoed in a paper by Chamberlain et al. (2012), where collaborative models for scaling up evidence-based interventions were presented and challenges and successes were discussed. For example, factors similar to continuous quality improvement principles were presented as important in attaining community and research partnership goals of implementation and sustainability for community and research partners.

Conclusion

The field has come a long way in examining the etiology of maltreatment and the nature of its complexity, which expands beyond individual-level factors to broader macrolevel influences. Using theory to guide us, we can apply research designs and methods that could confirm or disprove these hypothetical causes of maltreatment. Understanding these hypothetical causes is important in designing prevention programs that are shown to be efficacious and effective in order to prevent maltreatment behaviors and promote well-being.

Reflection: Nature of Evidence and How We Use It

Lisbeth Schorr
Center for the Study of Social Policy, Washington, DC, USA

Enormous changes have occurred in the last 50 years in how we define evidence and apply it to public policy. My own direct experience with how these changes have played out began when I joined the War on Poverty at its inception. Dozens of initiatives were inaugurated based on high hopes, innovative ideas, and evidence of varying strengths. Efforts to be more systematic focused on recruiting several of Robert McNamara's "whiz kids" from the Pentagon to calculate cost-effectiveness ratios. (Their only unambiguous contribution in the early stages was finding that the cost-effectiveness of a proposed family planning program came in at 17 to 1, allowing the Office of Economic Opportunity to establish the first federal line item funding for contraceptive services. Reflecting the climate of the time, these would be provided only to married women over 21!)

The importance of establishing clear, quantifiable evidence of what works has grown throughout my career. But the current narrow view that randomized control trials and similar experiments are the only credible information to inform decisions about what is worth funding has overshot the mark and undermined many efforts to improve outcomes. You cannot unravel the "why" and "how" if all your knowledge comes from studies that hold an intervention constant and isolated, as though it were operating in a laboratory setting. This emphasis on proving that a defined model "works" has obscured how different contexts—the institutional system, the funding streams, and the participants and their community—influence and shape an intervention's potential to be effective. Insisting that "proven" models be implemented with fidelity discourages local agencies and funders from reaching new populations, addressing emerging issues, and acting on lessons learned.

To make significant progress, we must determine the essential elements of our efforts and then carefully document, on a day to day basis, how our actions impact our ability to achieve outcomes. We need to "steer as we go" and accept the fact that there is no straight line between cause and effect—we need to tolerate some messiness. Failure to be comfortable with "messy" results pushes us away from the type of complex interventions that are needed to successfully reduce child maltreatment and confront other complex problems, like race-, class- and income-based gaps in well-being and achievement.

The key to improvement is not solely a function of creating better program models. Learning about how and why and how well an intervention works, and explicitly taking account of the importance of context, is a different type of learning. This approach takes us beyond yes/no judgments of a defined model and allows us to rank programs not in terms of the elegance with which they have been evaluated, but rather by our understanding of the strategy's potential to improve defined outcomes. It would allow us to make judgments beyond individual programs to identify *strategies*, including the interactions among multiple programs and reforms of systems and policies, that could achieve transformative outcomes.

We have come a long way since the War on Poverty. We no longer rely on justifications or anecdotes that the program worked for *someone, somewhere* as a basis for allocating resources. Gathering, analyzing, and applying a broader range of evidence is particularly important when it comes to initiatives aimed at prevention, where the need to understand context is critical. Building a deeper and wider knowledge base will require the ability to understand the critical elements of diverse interventions that focus on similar outcomes. At present, there are not many vehicles that allow program developers or funders to do that type of cross-strategy learning. In order to develop a broader, deeper understanding of how we might improve outcomes, we need learning communities and learning networks that can build on one another's experience and learn together from research to build a knowledge base and evidence pool sufficiently sturdy to lead to meaningful improvements at scale in the outcomes we most care about.

References

Barth, R., Landsverk, J., Chamberlain, P., Reid, J., Rolls, J., Hurlburt, M., et al. (2005). Parent-training programs in child welfare services: Planning for a more evidence-based approach to serving biological parents. *Research on Social Work Practice, 15*(5), 353–371.
Belsky, J. (1980). Child maltreatment: An ecological integration. *American Psychologist, 35*(4), 320–335. doi:10.1037//0003-066X.35.4.320.

Bollen, K. A., & Pearl, J. (2013). Eight myths about causality and structural equation models. In S. L. Morgan (Ed.), *Handbook of causal analysis for social research* (pp. 301–328). New York: Springer.

Bronfenbrenner, U. (1977). Toward an experimental ecology of human development. *American Psychologist, 32*(7), 513–531.

Bronfenbrenner, U. (1979). *The ecology of human development*. Cambridge, MA: Harvard University Press.

Bronfenbrenner, U., & Morris, P. A. (2006). The bioecological model of human development. In W. Damon & R. M. Lerner (Eds.), *Handbook of child psychology* (Theoretical models of human development 6th ed., Vol. 1, pp. 793–828). New York: Wiley.

Bruskas, D. (2008). Children in foster care: A vulnerable population at risk. *Journal of Child and Adolescent Psychiatric Nursing, 21*(2), 70–77.

Carter, V., & Myers, M. (2007). Exploring the risks of substantiated physical neglect related to poverty and parental characteristics: A national sample. *Children and Youth Services Review, 29*, 110–121.

Caspi, A., McClay, J., Moffitt, T., Mill, J., Martin, J., Craig, I., et al. (2002). Role of genotype in the cycle of violence in maltreated children. *Science, 297*(5582), 851–854.

Chamberlain, P., Roberts, R., Jones, H., Marsenich, L., Sosna, T., & Price, J. (2012). Three collaborative models for scaling up evidence-based practices. *Administration and Policy in Mental Health, 39*, 278–290.

Cicchetti, D., & Lynch, M. (1993). Toward an ecological/transactional model of community violence and child maltreatment: Consequences for children's development. *Psychiatry, 56*, 96–188.

Cicchetti, D., & Rizley, R. (1981). Developmental perspectives on the etiology, intergenerational transmission, and sequelae of child maltreatment. *New Directions for Child and Adolescent Development, 1981*(11), 31–55.

Coca-Perraillon, M. (2007). Local and global optimal propensity score matching. *SAS Global Forum*. Paper 185–2007.

Coie, J. D., Watt, N. F., West, S. G., Hawkins, J. D., Asarnow, J. R., Markman, H. J., et al. (1993). The science of prevention: A conceptual framework and some directions for a national research program. *American Psychologist, 48*(10), 1013–1022.

Crocker, L., & Algina, J. (1986). *Introduction to classical and modern test theory*. Philadelphia, PA: Harcourt Brace Jovanovich College Publishers.

D'Agostino, R. (1998). Tutorial in biostatistics: Propensity score methods for bias reduction in the comparison of a treatment to a non-randomized control group. *Statistics in Medicine, 17*, 2265–2281.

Daro, D. (1988). *Confronting child abuse: Research for effective program design*. New York: Free Press.

Doyle, J. J., Jr. (2011). Causal effects of foster care: An instrumental-variables approach. *Children and Youth Services Review, 35*(7), 1143–1151.

Dozier, M., Peloso, E., Lindhiem, O., Gordon, M. K., Manni, M., Sepulveda, S., et al. (2006). Developing evidence-based interventions for foster children: An example of a randomized clinical trial with infants and toddlers. *Journal of Social Issues, 62*(4), 767–785.

Dozier, M., Lindhiem, O., Lewis, E., Bick, J., Bernard, K., & Peloso, E. (2009). Effects of a foster parent training program on young children's attachment behaviors: Preliminary evidence from a randomized clinical trial. *Child and Adolescent Social Work Journal, 26*, 321–332.

Enders, C. K. (2010). *Applied missing data analysis*. New York: Guilford Press.

Garbarino, J. (1977). The human ecology of child maltreatment: A conceptual model for research. *Journal of Marriage and Family, 39*(4), 721–735.

Gil, D. (1970). *Violence against children: Physical child abuse in the United States*. Cambridge, MA: Harvard University Press.

Graham, J. W., Taylor, B. J., Cumsille, P. E., & Olchowski, A. E. (2006). Planned missing data designs in psychological research. *Psychological Methods, 11*, 323–343.

Greeley, C. S. (2009). The future of child maltreatment prevention. *Pediatrics, 123*(3), 904–905.

Guo, S., & Fraser, M. W. (2010). *Propensity score analysis: Statistical methods and applications.* Thousand Oaks: Sage.

Guo, S., Barth, R., & Gibbons, C. (2006). Propensity score matching strategies for evaluating substance abuse services for child welfare clients. *Children and Youth Services Review, 28*(4), 357–383.

Hammond, W. R. (2003). Public health and child maltreatment prevention: The role of the Centers for Disease Control and Prevention. *Child Maltreatment, 8*(2), 81–83.

Heckman, J. (1997). Instrumental variables: A study of implicit behavioral assumptions used in making program evaluations. *Journal of Human Resources, 32*(3), 441–462.

Herschell, A. D., Calzada, E. J., Eyberg, S. M., & McNeil, C. B. (2002). Parent–child interaction therapy: New directions in research. *Cognitive and Behavioral Practice, 9,* 9–15.

Hogan, J. W., & Lancaster, T. (2004). Instrumental variables and inverse probability weighting for causal inference from longitudinal observational studies. *Statistical Methods in Medical Research, 13,* 17–48.

Hogue, C. M., Porprasertmanit, S., Fry, M. D., Rhemtulla, M., & Little, T. (2013). Planned missing data designs for spline growth models in salivary cortisol research. *Measurement in Physical Education and Exercise Science, 17,* 310–325.

Holland, P. W. (1986). Statistics and causal inference. *Journal of the American Statistical Association, 81*(396), 945–960.

Hume, D. (1748). *Philosophical Essays concerning Human Understanding.* London: A. Millar.

Institute of Medicine & National Research Council. (2012). *Child maltreatment research, policy, and practice for the next decade: Workshop summary.* Washington, DC: The National Academies Press.

Jo, B. (2002). Statistical power in randomized intervention studies with noncompliance. *Psychological Methods, 7,* 178–193.

Kellam, S. G., & Langevin, D. J. (2003). A framework for understanding "evidence" in prevention research and programs. *Prevention Science, 4*(3), 137–153.

Kempe, C. H., Silverman, F. N., Steele, B. F., Droegemueller, W., & Silver, H. K. (1962). The battered-child syndrome. *The Journal of the American Medical Association, 181*(1), 17–24.

Little, T. D., & Rhemtulla, M. (2013). Planned missing data designs for developmental researchers. *Child Development Perspectives, 7,* 199–204.

Lynch, M., & Cicchetti, D. (1998). An ecological-transactional analysis of children and contexts: The longitudinal interplay among child maltreatment, community violence, and children's symptomatology. *Development and Psychopathology, 10*(2), 235–257.

MacMillan, H., Wathen, C., Barlow, J., Fergusson, D., Leventhal, J., & Taussig, H. (2009). Interventions to prevent child maltreatment and associated impairment. *Lancet, 373*(9659), 250–266.

McCabe, B. K., Potash, D., Omohundro, E., & Taylor, C. R. (2012). Design and implementation of an integrated, continuous evaluation, and quality improvement system for a state-based home-visiting program. *Maternal and Child Health Journal, 16,* 1385–1400.

Myers, J. A., & Louis, T. (2010, January). *Regression adjustment and stratification by propensity score in treatment effect estimation* (Working Paper 203). Baltimore: Johns Hopkins University, Department of Biostatistics.

National Research Council. (1993). *Understanding child abuse and neglect.* Washington, DC: National Academy Press.

Neyman, J. (1990). On the application of probability theory to agricultural experiments: Essay on principles. Section 9 (Splawa-Neyman, J., Dabrowska, D. M., & Speed, T. P., Trans.). *Statistical Science, 5,* 465–480.

Olds, D. (2006). The nurse-family partnership: An evidence-based preventive intervention. *Infant Mental Health Journal, 27*(1), 5–25.

Olds, D., Kitzman, H., Cole, R., & Robinson, J. (1997). Theoretical foundations of a program of home visitation for pregnant women and parents of young children. *Journal of Community Psychology, 25*(1), 9–25.

Parrish, J. W., Young, M. B., Perham-Hester, K. A., & Gessner, B. D. (2011). Identifying risk factors for child maltreatment in Alaska: A population-based approach. *American Journal of Preventive Medicine, 40*(6), 666–673.

Pearl, J. (1988). *Probabilistic reasoning in intelligent systems*. San Mateo: Morgan Kaufman.

Pearl, J. (2009). *Causality: Models, reasoning and inference*. Cambridge, MA: MIT Press.

Pearl, J., & Verma, T. S. (1995). A theory of inferred causation. *Studies in Logic and the Foundations of Mathematics, 134*, 789–811.

Prinz, R., Sanders, M., Shapiro, C., Whitaker, D., & Lutzker, J. (2009). Population-based prevention of child maltreatment: The U.S. triple P system population trial. *Prevention Science, 10*(1), 1–12.

Putnam-Hornstein, E., & Needell, B. (2011). Predictors of child protective service contact between birth and age five: An examination of California's 2002 birth cohort. *Children and Youth Services Review, 33*(8), 1337–1344.

Rosenbaum, P. R., & Rubin, D. R. (1983). The central role of the propensity score in observational studies for causal effects. *Biometrika, 70*(1), 41–55.

Rubin, D. B. (1974). Estimating causal effects of treatments in randomized and nonrandomized studies. *Journal of Educational Psychology, 66*(5), 688–701.

Rubin, D. B. (2010). Propensity score methods. *American Journal of Ophthalmology, 149*(1), 7–9.

Sacks, D. P. (2008). State actors beating children: A call for judicial relief. *University of California Davis Law Review, 42*, 1165–1230.

Sidebotham, P. (2001). An ecological approach to child abuse: A creative use of scientific models in research and practice. *Child Abuse Review, 10*(2), 97–112. doi:10.1002/car.643.

Slack, K. S., Maguire-Jack, K., & Gjertson, L. M. (Eds.) (2009). *Child maltreatment prevention: Toward an evidence-based approach*. Madison: Institute for Research on Poverty. http://www.irp.wisc.edu/research/WisconsinPoverty/pdfs/ChildMaltreatment-Final.pdf

Standards of Evidence Committee. (2004). *Standards of evidence: Criteria for efficacy, effectiveness, and dissemination*. Fairfax: Society for Prevention Research.

Steele, B. F., & Pollack, G. (1974). A psychiatric study of parents who abuse their children and infants. In C. H. Kempe (Ed.), *The battered child* (pp. 89–133). Chicago: University of Chicago Press.

Strathearn, L., Gray, P., O'Callaghan, M., & Wood, D. (2001). Childhood neglect and cognitive development in extremely low birth weight infants: A prospective study. *Pediatrics, 108*, 142–151.

Stuart, E. A., Cole, S. R., Bradshaw, C. P., & Leaf, P. J. (2011). The use of propensity scores to assess the generalizability of results from randomized trials. *Journal of the Royal Statistical Society, 174*, 369–386.

Thoemmes, F. J., & Kim, E. S. (2011). A systematic review of propensity score methods in the social sciences. *Multivariate Behavioral Research, 46*(1), 90–118.

Tzeng, O. C., Jackson, J. W., & Karlson, H. C. (1991). *Theories of child abuse and neglect. Differential perspectives, summaries, and evaluations*. Westport: Praeger.

Widom, C. (1989). The cycle of violence. *Science, 244*(4901), 160–166.

Widom, C. (2000). Understanding the consequences of childhood victimization. In R. Reece (Ed.), *Treatment of child abuse: Common ground for mental health, medical, and legal practitioners* (pp. 339–361). Baltimore/London: Johns Hopkins University Press.

Widom, C., & Brzustowicz, L. (2006). MAOA and the "cycle of violence": Childhood abuse and neglect, MAOA genotype, and risk for violent and antisocial behavior. *Biological Psychiatry, 60*, 684–689.

Wright, S. S. (1921). Correlation and causation. *Journal of Agricultural Research, 20*, 557–585.

Wu, S. S., Ma, C. X., Carter, R. L., Ariet, M., Feaver, E. A., Resnick, M. B., & Roth, J. (2004). Risk factors for infant maltreatment: A population-based study. *Child Abuse & Neglect, 28*(12), 1253–1264.

Zelkowitz, P., Bardin, C., & Papageorgiou, A. (2007). Anxiety affects the relationship between parents and their very low birth weight infants. *Infant Mental Health Journal, 28*(3), 296–313.

Zielinski, D., & Bradshaw, C. (2006). Ecological influences on the sequalae of child maltreatment: A review of the literature. *Child Maltreatment, 11*(1), 49–62.

Zolotor, A. J., & Puzia, M. E. (2010). Bans against corporal punishment: A systematic review of the laws, changes in attitudes and behaviours. *Child Abuse Review, 19*(4), 229–247.

Paul Lanier is an assistant professor at the University of North Carolina at Chapel Hill School of Social Work. He received his doctorate from the Brown School at Washington University in St. Louis. The goal of Dr. Lanier's research is to prevent child maltreatment and promote child well-being among vulnerable populations. His work focuses on early childhood interventions designed to enhance healthy parent-child relationships and prepare caregivers to meet their child's developmental needs. He is also interested in health and mental health outcomes of maltreated children. Dr. Lanier's research agenda seeks to inform both policy and practice by testing innovative interventions and improving the availability of evidence-based service strategies.

Kathryn Maguire-Jack is an assistant professor at The Ohio State University, College of Social Work. She has a B.A. in Social Welfare and Political Science, MPA, MSW, and Ph.D. from the University of Wisconsin—Madison. Dr. Maguire-Jack has experience as a fiscal analyst, working on the Wisconsin state budget at the Wisconsin Legislative Fiscal Bureau and as a program and policy analyst at the Wisconsin Children's Trust Fund. Her research interests include child maltreatment prevention, risk and protective factors for maltreatment, neighborhood research, and program evaluation.

Joseph Mienko is a research scientist and Ph.D. candidate at the University of Washington School of Social Work where he has led the design and development of the Washington State Child Well-Being Data Portal—a joint project between the University of Washington, Children's Administration, and the private philanthropic community. Mr. Mienko has over 9 years of experience working with the child welfare system and has also served as an intelligence analyst with the US Army. Mr. Mienko's doctoral studies have focused on public policy, management, and social statistics. His primary research interests include the application of epidemiological and econometric techniques to child welfare data. He is also interested in research related to assessment and intervention in cases of child neglect.

Carlomagno Panlilio is a doctoral candidate in the Department of Human Development & Quantitative Methodology at the University of Maryland, College Park. His area of specialization is in developmental science and he holds a certificate in Education Measurement, Statistics, & Evaluation. Mr. Panlilio's research focuses on longitudinal analyses of early childhood school readiness domains for children with a history of maltreatment. More specifically, the role that emotion regulation, cognitive functioning, language, and context play on influencing later academic outcomes. He has a B.A. in psychology from the California State University at Long Beach and his Master of Science in Family Studies from the University of Maryland, College Park. Mr. Panlilio has also been in clinical practice as a licensed clinical marriage and family therapist since 2005 and continues to work in private practice. He has also worked as a family therapist in community agencies serving foster families, as well as children and families involved with Child Protective Services.

Chapter 7
Evidence-Based Programs in "Real World" Settings: Finding the Best Fit

Byron J. Powell, Emily A. Bosk, Jessica S. Wilen, Christina M. Danko, Amanda Van Scoyoc, and Aaron Banman

Chapter 7 in Brief

Context

- Children's social service systems are under increasing pressure to adopt "evidence-based" programs and practices (EBPPs), of which there are an increasing number.
- Concerns about the quality of prevention and treatment programs persist.
- When proven programs are adopted, implementation problems can limit their impact.
- Implementation research can serve to generate a better understanding of how to improve the quality of intervention and prevention programs.

This work was supported in part by the Doris Duke Charitable Foundation Fellowship for the Promotion of Child Well-Being, which was awarded to all authors; the Fahs-Beck Fund for Research and Experimentation to BJP and EAB; a National Science Foundation Dissertation Research Improvement Grant to EAB; and a Ruth L. Kirschstein National Research Service Award from the National Institute of Mental Health to BJP (F31MH098378).

B.J. Powell (✉)
Center for Mental Health Policy and Services Research, Department of Psychiatry,
Perelman School of Medicine, University of Pennsylvania, Philadelphia, PA, USA
e-mail: byronp@upenn.edu

E.A. Bosk
University of Michigan, Ann Arbor, MI, USA
e-mail: bosk@umich.edu

J.S. Wilen
Washington University in St. Louis, St. Louis, MO, USA
e-mail: jwilen@wustl.edu

C.M. Danko
Mt. Washington Pediatric Hospital, Baltimore, MD, USA
e-mail: cdanko@mwph.org

© Springer International Publishing Switzerland 2015
D. Daro et al. (eds.), *Advances in Child Abuse Prevention Knowledge*,
Child Maltreatment 5, DOI 10.1007/978-3-319-16327-7_7

Strategies for Moving Forward

- Continue to develop and utilize rigorous methods to synthesize the evidence supporting the effectiveness of different programs and practices.
- Consider the "fit" between intervention characteristics, the target population, and setting, and adapt interventions and implementation strategies in thoughtful and systematic ways.
- Test a wide range of implementation strategies, particularly those that are multi-faceted and multi-level.
- Develop "learning organizations" that are capable of innovation, "exnovation," and continuous quality improvement
- Account for contextual influences such as organizational structure, culture, and climate.

Implications for Research

- Partner with a diverse set of stakeholders and utilize a range of methodologies including mixed methods and systems science approaches.
- Integrate theories and conceptual models in the design, conduct, and interpretation of implementation research.
- Improve the measurement of implementation-related constructs.
- Conduct more studies that prospectively test the sustainability of proven programs.
- Develop better methods of selecting implementation strategies that are responsive to the settings, stakeholders, and unique barriers associated with implementation efforts.

Introduction

Organizations and systems that serve children, youth, and families are under increasing pressure to demonstrate that the services they provide are "evidence-based," and that they are achieving desired outcomes related to safety, permanence, and well-being. Fortunately, there are an increasing number of evidence-based programs and

A. Van Scoyoc
University of Oregon, Eugene, OR, USA
e-mail: avanscoy@uoregon.edu

A. Banman
University of Chicago, Chicago, IL, USA
e-mail: abanman@uchicago.edu

practices (EBPPs) related to the prevention and treatment of child abuse and neglect. Prevention programs have largely utilized home visiting models such as Nurse Family Partnership and Parents as Teachers (Institute of Medicine and National Research Council 2013). Treatment programs have targeted the sequelae of trauma or abuse (e.g., Trauma-Focused Cognitive Behavior Therapy) and addressed problematic parenting and behavior problems in children (e.g., Parent–child Interaction Therapy, Triple P, The Incredible Years, PMTO; see Institute of Medicine and National Research Council 2013).

Despite these advances in the prevention and treatment of child maltreatment, rigorously tested interventions remain underutilized in children's social service settings (Garland et al. 2010; Kohl et al. 2009; Raghavan et al. 2010; Zima et al. 2005). When such programs are adopted, implementation problems often diminish their effect (Durlak and DuPre 2008). Indeed, myriad barriers to implementing EBPPs have been identified at the client, provider, team, organizational, system, and policy levels (e.g., Flottorp et al. 2013; Raghavan 2007; Shapiro et al. 2012). It is increasingly clear that EBPPs must be coupled with evidence-based approaches to implementation if they are to achieve the promise of improving the quality of care in the "real world." Accordingly, the National Institutes of Health (2013), the Institute of Medicine (2007, 2009a, b, 2013), and private foundations such as the Doris Duke Charitable Foundation (2010) have prioritized the advancement of implementation science, which is defined as the "...scientific study of methods to promote the systematic uptake of research findings and other evidence-based practices into routine practice..." (Eccles and Mittman 2006, p. 1). Implementation science also includes the study of influences on professional and organizational behavior; thus, much of the broader literature on organizations and organizational change is relevant (Aarons et al. 2012d; Eccles and Mittman 2006).

In this chapter, we review the extant research and discuss ways in which implementation science can contribute to the promotion of child well-being. Given the scope of this topic, our aim is not to provide an exhaustive review, but to offer some examples of innovative approaches to implementation science and practice.[1] The chapter utilizes a conceptual model of implementation in public health developed by Aarons and colleagues (2011), which specifies four phases of implementation: exploration, adoption decision and preparation, active implementation, and sustainment. We discuss some of the factors that stakeholders must consider during the early phases of implementation (i.e., exploration and adoption decision and preparation) and later phases of implementation (i.e., active implementation and sustainment). We then discuss contextual factors that can influence implementation processes, and conclude by presenting some areas that will likely be critical to advancing the science and practice of implementing EBPPs.

---

[1] For broader overviews of implementation research, readers may be interested in several recently published books (Beidas and Kendall 2014, Brownson et al. 2012, Grol et al. 2013, Palinkas and Soydan 2012, Straus et al. 2013). We also point readers to overviews of theories and conceptual frameworks related to implementation science (Grol et al. 2007, Tabak et al. 2012), which may be helpful in facilitating a deeper understanding of some of the key constructs that we discuss in this chapter.

The Current State of Implementation Research

Early Phases of Implementation: Exploration and Adoption Decision and Preparation

Social service systems and organizations faced with the task of implementing effective prevention and treatment programs must choose from a variety of potential programmatic options. Unfortunately, the evidence for the effectiveness and feasibility of various programs is often not clear-cut. In many cases, systems and organizations do not have the option of selecting any intervention, as federal or state funders may require them to implement a specific practice or select from a few options (Pipkin et al. 2013). Even if the choice of intervention is not an option, it remains important for these organizations to engage in thoughtful and systematic implementation planning, execution, and evaluation (Pipkin et al. 2013). There are several challenges related to the initial phases of implementation, including (but not limited to) the assessment of evidence, the consideration of the "fit" of particular EBPPs, and the adaptation of EBPPs to local settings when necessary.

Assessing the Evidence

Assessing the evidence is not an easy task. However, an awareness of the hierarchy of evidence, available systematic reviews and meta-analyses, and evidence-based clearinghouses can facilitate the exploration of programs and practices. The hierarchy of evidence is one of the foundational elements of evidence-based practice (Gibbs 2003; Sackett et al. 1996). It is defined as "the relative weight carried by the different types of primary study when making decisions" about interventions (Greenhalgh 1997, p. 246). The hierarchy of evidence lists (from strongest to weakest) meta-analyses and systematic reviews of multiple randomized controlled trials (RCT), RCTs, cohort studies, case control studies, case series studies, cross sectional studies and case reports, and expert opinion (Fraser et al. 2009). The American Psychological Association has deemed that specific thresholds must be met before an intervention is deemed "evidence-based," "empirically-supported," or (in our terms) an EBPP (Chambless et al. 1998; Roth and Fonagy 2005; Weissman et al. 2006). Chambless and colleagues (1998) note that to be considered "well established," an intervention must prove to be superior to placebos or to another treatment in at least two between-group design experiments *or* have demonstrated efficacy in a large series of single case design experiments. They also state that experiments should have been conducted with treatment manuals, the characteristics of the samples must have been clearly specified, and the effects must have been demonstrated by at least two different investigators or investigative teams (Chambless et al. 1998, p. 4). This approach can be problematic because it does not take into account for whom (i.e., which subgroups) and under what circumstances these treatments are most effective. Additionally, as long as the intervention meets the threshold of having two trials that demonstrate effectiveness, it does not take into account the number of studies that find null or negative effects. This could potentially overstate an intervention's effectiveness.

While the hierarchy of evidence has obtained wide support, there is no shortage of scholars who critique it. Some claim that RCTs are particularly problematic for evaluating complex psychosocial interventions given that they typically exclude potential participants that have comorbid health, mental health, or substance abuse problems. This critique is made despite the fact that patients struggling with these issues are commonly seen in routine settings of care (Fonagy and Target 2001; Westen et al. 2004). Others have noted that findings from designs that are generally considered "less rigorous" can yield remarkably similar results (Concato 2004), or have argued the importance of using a variety of approaches (including qualitative and mixed methods approaches) for determining what works and what will be feasible to implement in real world practice (Bloom et al. 2006; Norcross et al. 2006; Palinkas et al. 2011b). Though these critiques are important to consider, the established hierarchy of evidence remains an important standard. The research designs at the top of the hierarchy provide the highest level of internal validity and hold the potential (through effectiveness and implementation research) to yield results with high levels of external validity as well.

Despite the importance of understanding the hierarchy of evidence, it is unlikely that stakeholders will access and assess reports of primary research findings when considering programs and practices. Rather, implementation stakeholders are more likely to depend upon summaries of the existing research (Harris et al. 2009). Systematic reviews and meta-analyses can be very helpful in summarizing a large body of research. They can be found in a number of sources, most notably the Cochrane (cochrane.org) and Campbell (campbellcollaboration.org) Collaborations. Meta-analyses of randomized clinical trials, considered the "highest" form of evidence, have become even more useful through the use of "network meta-analyses" or "multiple treatment comparisons." These methods allow for multiple interventions to be compared simultaneously (provided they have a common comparator such as a no-treatment control group) even if they have never been tested head-to-head in an RCT (Caldwell et al. 2005; Grant and Calderbank-Batista 2013). Network meta-analyses have more often been used to compare the effects of biomedical interventions; however, they hold promise for comparing psychosocial and educational interventions as well (Grant and Calderbank-Batista 2013). Figure 7.1 presents an example of a network analysis and its potential utility in comparing interventions.

In addition to primary studies and systematic reviews, stakeholders may rely upon research summaries in high profile reports (Harris et al. 2009), such as the Institute of Medicine's reports on preventing mental, emotional, and behavioral disorders and research on child abuse and neglect (Institute of Medicine and National Research Council 2013; Institute of Medicine 2009b). Increasingly, stakeholders also have the opportunity to turn to several evidence-based practice clearinghouses

There are a number of completed randomized controlled trials evaluating different psychosocial treatments available for adult survivors of childhood sexual abuse. However, there is limited information about the comparative effectiveness of these interventions, which limits decisionmakers' ability to select appropriate treatments. A comprehensive systematic review (described more fully in a published protocol, Wilen et al. 2012) sought to provide more complete information about the comparative effectiveness of diverse treatments.

A network meta-analysis of 15 direct comparisons of 568 individuals found that trauma-focused treatments (such as Cognitive Behavioral Therapies, Eye Movement Desensitization and Reprocessing, and psychodynamic therapies) trended in the direction of being more effective than present-centered treatments (such as humanisticand supportive therapies and psychoeducation) at reducing Posttraumatic Stress Disorder symptoms in this population (Wilen 2014). The literature in this area is sparse, which compromised the analyses' power and generalizability, and ultimately limited the clinical usefulness of the review findings. However, this review clarified current holes in the literature and provides a roadmap for future research. Additionally, it demonstrates how network meta-analyses can improve upon traditional meta-analytic approaches by increasing the number of useful comparisons that can be drawn. It also highlights the potential for applying this innovative approach to other prevention and treatment interventions.

Fig. 7.1 A systematic review and meta-analysis of psychosocial interventions for adults who were abused as children

(Soydan et al. 2010), which vet a wide range of mental health treatments, rank them according to their evidentiary support, and provide additional information that may be pertinent to implementing them in real world care (e.g., the populations with which the intervention has been tested, whether there are training manuals, implementation guides, fidelity measures).

The California Evidence-Based Clearinghouse for Child Welfare (2014) is most germane to the prevention of child maltreatment, and (as of June 2014) includes 28 interventions that are deemed "well-supported by research evidence," 41 interventions that are "supported by research evidence," and 97 with "promising research evidence." A limitation of this approach is that the ratings are not based upon formal systematic reviews or meta-analyses, and in some cases are based on a sample of the available research. Programs are classified on the basis of "voting counting," a method some have classified as unreliable (Bushman and Wang 2009). While evidence-based clearinghouses are useful for gathering information about potential interventions, the most robust syntheses of an intervention's evaluation findings are found in rigorously conducted, up-to-date systematic reviews and meta-analyses.

Issues of "Fit" and Adaptation

Stakeholders may also consider whether a given EBPP is a good "fit" within their system or organization, as the characteristics of an intervention may impact rates of adoption and sustainment (for a relatively comprehensive list of these characteristics, see Grol et al. 2007). As noted by Fraser and colleagues (2009), Rogers' (2003) diffusion of innovation theory suggests that interventions will be more likely to be adopted if they are: superior to treatment as usual, compatible with agency practice, no more complex than existing services, easy to try and reject if the effort is not successful, and likely to produce tangible results recognizable by authorities. More recently, Scheirer (2013) has proposed a helpful framework of six different intervention types that vary in complexity and scope, from interventions implemented by individual providers to those requiring coordination across staff and community agencies to those embracing broad-scale system change. Each of these different intervention types carries unique considerations with regard to the strategies that will be needed to implement and sustain them.

Given the importance of fit between the intervention and the context in which it is being implemented, some EBPPs may need to be adapted to enhance fit (Bernal and Domenech Rodriguez 2012; Cabassa and Baumann 2013). A number of different types of adaptations or modifications may occur in either ad hoc or planned fashion. Adaptations can occur at the contextual level, including changes in *format* (e.g., adapting an individual intervention for a group format), *setting* (e.g., adapting an office-based intervention for in-home delivery), *personnel* (e.g., an intervention designed to be delivered by a masters-level clinician that is adapted to be delivered by lay-providers), and *population* (e.g., cultural adaptations) (Wiltsey Stirman et al. 2013b). Wiltsey Stirman and colleagues (2013b) also identify twelve different ways in which the content of interventions can be adapted, such as adding or removing elements, shortening or lengthening the pacing or timing of the intervention, substituting elements, reordering the elements, repeating some elements, or departing from the intervention entirely (i.e., drift). A fundamental challenge during implementation is ensuring that adaptations are executed thoughtfully and that the core elements that contribute to an intervention's effectiveness are not compromised. Figure 7.2 provides an example of how this adaptation process has been applied in the replication of one EBPP (Aarons et al. 2012c).

Later Phases of Implementation: Active Implementation and Sustainment

A number of strategies that can potentially facilitate the implementation and sustainment of EBPPs have been identified (for overviews, see Grimshaw et al. 2012; Grol et al. 2013; Powell et al. 2012; Straus et al. 2013). While evidence to support the use of specific strategies is mounting (Grimshaw et al. 2012), evidence for

Maintaining fidelity to EBPPs is very important (see Chap. 8 of this volume). However, adaptations may be necessary if the intervention proves to be a poor fit with a given setting or population. In fact, there is evidence to suggest that, for better or worse, these adaptations are made routinely (Wiltsey Stirman et al. 2013a). The Dynamic Adaptation Process (DAP) is being developed in order to make the inevitable adaptations to EBPPs more thoughtful and planned rather than haphazard and reactionary (Aarons et al. 2012c). In this way, the developers hope that adaptations are undertaken in a way that allows for the EBPP to be delivered with fidelity in contexts where it otherwise might not fit appropriately.

The DAP is being tested in an effort to implement SafeCare©, a well-known EBPP used to prevent child neglect (Lutzker et al. 1998). The DAP is a four-phased model (the phases are exploration, preparation, implementation, and sustainment; see Aarons et al. 2011) that . . . takes into account the multilevel context of services delivery, engages multiple stakeholders, and provides appropriate expertise and feedback during implementation to guide, monitor, and address system, organization, and model adaptations while maintaining fidelity to the core elements of an [EBPP] (Aarons et al. 2012c, p. 3). Central to the model is the use of an Implementation Resource Team comprised of experts in SafeCare and implementation science as well as members of the county and organizations involved in the implementation process. The Implementation Resource Team meets monthly via conference call and continuously guides the adaptation process by monitoring data and providing ongoing support. The exploration phase involves assessing system-, organizational-, provider-, and client-level factors that may influence the implementation and sustainment of SafeCare. During the preparation phase, the tTeam reviews the data gathered during the exploration phase and determines what adaptations may be necessary and how they might be accomplished.

Provider training and adaptation support commences in the implementation phase, which includes a discussion of adaptation (e.g., why one might adapt, what one may and may not adapt, and when and how to seek guidance on adaptation). At this time, fidelity measures are also refined while ensuring that the core elements are maintained. Finally, the sustainment phase involves continued use of the client and system data, which is fed back to DAP coaches on a monthly basis. A current study is testing the feasibility, acceptability, and utility of the DAP, and more information can be found in the published study protocol (Aarons et al. 2012c).

Fig. 7.2 Dynamic adaptation process to implement SafeCare

various implementation approaches in social service settings is far less robust (Landsverk et al. 2011; Novins et al. 2013; Powell et al. 2014). One of the most consistent findings documented in the literature is that the dominant way of implementing psychosocial treatments—intensive trainings and continuing education courses—is not sufficient to promote provider behavior change (Beidas and Kendall 2010; Herschell et al. 2010). Increasingly, there is consensus that successful implementation may require multicomponent strategies that address myriad challenges and barriers (Aarons et al. 2011; Glisson and Schoenwald 2005; Solberg et al. 2000; Wensing et al. 2009). Some of these multicomponent strategies have been developed and tested in children's social service settings (e.g., Chamberlain et al. 2008;

Glisson et al. 2010, 2012, 2013; Hurlburt et al. 2014; Pipkin et al. 2013; Sosna and Marsenich 2006) Two of them are summarized in Figs. 7.3 and 7.4. An additional example, in Fig. 7.5, illustrates how to incorporate organizational stakeholder perceptions of implementation into the planning process in ways that improve the likelihood the intervention successfully addresses their needs and preferences.

Implementing EBPPs within a single setting is challenging enough, but it is even more difficult to scale-up an intervention in multiple organizations or across service systems. This difficulty is due not only to the scope of large-scale implementation efforts, but also to variations at the organizational, team, and individual levels that make it more or less difficult to implement EBPPs (Flottorp et al. 2013; Shortell 2004). The Interagency Collaborative Team model was designed to respond to these challenges and support the implementation of EBPPs in large geographic areas. Like the Dynamic Adaptation Process described above (Aarons et al. 2012c), the Interagency Collaborative Team model is also grounded in the four-phased Exploration, Preparation, Implementation, and Sustainment model (Aarons et al. 2011). The Interagency Collaborative Team model, described in detail by Hurlburt and colleagues (2014), involves a number of structured steps that are designed to overcome barriers to implementation by generating the types of structural and process supports needed to implement and sustain interventions. The process begins by identifying and convening stakeholders with interests in a shared improvement effort (e.g., preventing child neglect). This generally includes funders, administrators, and service delivery organizations. The next step is to seek relevant expertise required to address the central question of the improvement effort and to generate as much data as possible about potential EBPP options. Once a commitment is made to pursue the implementation of a given EBPP, interagency seed teams are developed. Seed teams intentionally include employees from a number of different organizations in order to build broad investment, commitment, and enhance communication pertaining to the change effort. Seed teams are responsible for learning the EBPP, conducting the initial delivery of the EBPP, training local EBPP practitioners, liaising with EBPP developers, monitoring and providing feedback regarding the quality of EBPP delivery, communicating a commitment to quality EBPP delivery, and communicating implementation progress to all stakeholders. Moreover,the seed teams train additional interagency training teams that will deliver the EBPP, provide feedback to the seed team, and share information with one another about implementation challenges and progress.Eventually, there is a phased reduction in EBPP developer involvement as seed and interagency teams continue to deepen their expertise in the EBPP (Hurlburt et al. 2014).

The Interagency Collaborative Team model is particularly promising in that it is inherently participatory and strengthens collaborative ties between organizations. Indeed, the "cross-organizational membership on the seed team contributes to ensuring a continuing locus of expertise available to all organizations within the Interagency Collaborative Team partnership, reducing the kinds of expertise loss that regularly occur within individual organizations due to staff turnover and organizational changes" (Hurlburt et al. 2014, p. 4). Perhaps most importantly, the model provides a much needed opportunity for organizations to learn from one another, mitigating potential barriers associated with implementing EBPPs without the benefit of role models (Powell et al. 2013a).

Fig. 7.3 Interagency collaborative team model for implementing SafeCare

The Getting to Outcomes model is a framework developed to help organizations plan, implement, and evaluate prevention programs (Chinman et al. 2004). It has recently been used to implement an evidence-based case management model (Solution-Based Casework) in Washington state (Pipkin et al. 2013). The Getting to Outcomes model involves ten steps: identifying needs and resources; setting goals and objectives to meet the needs; selecting an EBPP; ensuring that the EBPP fits the organization; assessing what capacities are needed to implement the program; creating and implementing a plan; evaluating the quality of implementation; evaluating how well the EBPP worked; determining how a continuous quality improvement process could improve EBPP delivery; and taking steps to ensure sustainability (Pipkin et al. 2013).

This type of model (and other active frameworks for implementation, e.g., Metz et al. 2014) can serve to ensure that implementation is not an afterthought and that clear processes are in place to plan, execute, and evaluate implementation processes in a transparent manner. Pipkin and colleagues (2013) attest to the value of such a framework and nicely illustrate the utility of a using the Getting to Outcomes framework to manage the complexity of large-scale implementation efforts.

Fig. 7.4 Using the getting to outcomes framework to implement an evidence-based casework model

Sustainment

The literature focusing on the sustainability of EBPPs has been characterized as "fragmented and underdeveloped" (Wiltsey Stirman et al. 2012, p. 15). However, recent reviews of the literature have enhanced conceptual clarity in this area, providing a foundation for more rigorous prospective studies of sustainability. For instance, Wiltsey Stirman and colleagues (2012) reviewed 125 studies and found that across fields, sustainability was generally related to four core factors: context (e.g., policies, legislation, culture, and structure); the innovation itself (e.g., fit, adaptability, and effectiveness); implementation processes (e.g., fidelity monitoring, evaluation, etc.); and the capacity to sustain (e.g., funding, resources, workforce characteristics, etc.). Within these broad categories of factors, the authors also note that the key elements identified varied considerably (Wiltsey Stirman et al. 2012). More recently, researchers from the Center for Public Health Systems Science conducted a study that included a comprehensive literature review, input from an expert panel, and concept mapping to identify core constructs for a conceptual framework for program sustainability in public health (Kane and Trochim 2007; Schell et al. 2013). They identified nine constructs that affect an EBPP's capacity for sustainability: funding stability, political support, partnerships, organizational capacity, program adaptation, program evaluation, communications, public health impacts, and strategic planning. They also developed a free online assessment that allows stakeholders to assess the sustainability capacity of programs and practices (Center for Public Health Systems Science 2012). Clearly, there is a need

To successfully integrate EBPPs, implementation strategies will not only need to be effective, but also feasible, acceptable, sustainable, and scalable (Mittman 2012). Thus, it is imperative that efforts to identify and develop implementation strategies be grounded by a thorough understanding of real world service systems as well as organizational stakeholders' preferences for particular strategies. In other words, there is a need for a better understanding of usual care settings, and in particular, what constitutes "implementation as usual." Powell and colleagues (2013) are conducting a mixed methods multiple case study in six children's social service organizations to identify and characterize the implementation strategies used in community-based children's social service settings; explore how organizational leaders make decisions about which treatments and programs to implement and how to implement them; assess stakeholders' (organizational leaders and clinicians) perceptions of the effectiveness, relative importance, acceptability, feasibility, and appropriateness of implementation strategies; and examine the relationship between organizational context (culture and climate) and implementation strategy selection, implementation decisionmaking, and perceptions of implementation strategies. By shedding light on "implementation as usual," this study will inform efforts to develop and tailor strategies that are responsive to stakeholder preferences and move the field toward the ideal of evidence-based implementation. Results of this study are forthcoming, though a detailed description of the methods and rationale can be found in the study protocol (Powell et al. 2013b).

Fig. 7.5 Implementation strategy use and stakeholder perceptions in usual care settings

for more empirical study of sustainability, and Wiltsey Stirman et al. (2012) call for prospective studies that clearly define sustainability, lend more attention to the types of modifications that occur, and assess sustainability over several years rather than at a single time point.

Contextual Factors That Influence Implementation Processes

It would be ideal if interventions found to be efficacious and effective could be readily implemented in real world settings or if implementation strategies could be identified that are effective irrespective of the EBPP, context, or individuals involved in a given change effort. However, research has demonstrated that there are no implementation strategies that are universally effective (Oxman et al. 1995). Rather, the research has shown that the effectiveness of both EBPPs and the strategies used to implement them are mediated and moderated by a host of contextual factors (Glisson 2007; Lee and Mittman 2012; Luke 2004). In the following sections we discuss a number of factors at the "inner setting" (i.e., the organizational or system level) and "outer setting" (i.e., the economic, political, and social context) levels that can play a large role in determining implementation success or failure (Damschroder et al. 2009).

Inner Setting Factors

The inner setting, or organizational or system level, plays a critical role in promoting or inhibiting the implementation of EBPPs. Palinkas and Soydan (2012) describe the organizational level as "an ideal focus for examining the context of research translation" (p. 105) because organizations serve as the most proximal context in which EBPPs are delivered. Embedded within a broader set of influences represented in policies, funding, client demand, and other factors, organizations are a critical unit of analysis to consider when examining the processes that affect how a program or practice is implemented. Here we discuss a number of organizational factors that can impact implementation efforts, including organizational structure, organizational culture and climate, implementation climate, organizational readiness for change, staff turnover, and communication patterns. Figure 7.6 presents one example of how organization factors can impact implementation.

New work by Bosk (forth coming) investigates the intersection of organizational, cultural, and individual factors in the adoption and implementation of an EBPP intended to improve the consistency and accuracy of decision making in child protective service work. Using qualitative research methods (observation and semi-structured interviews), Bosk provides insight into the complexity of translating practice innovations into real world settings. By examining the implementation of the same program (the Structured Decision-Making Model) in two settings, Bosk (forth coming) observes how distinctly an intervention meant to standardize child welfare practice across organizations and individuals can play out in practice.

Approaches to the intervention varied greatly based on organizational context. In one setting, workers approached the intervention as being designed for agency administrators and reported that it had little practical influence on their routine decision making. In the second setting, the majority of workers reported that the intervention played a central role in their decision making and everyday practice. Differences in the implementation of the intervention across two settings demonstrated that "whether a standardized tool achieves a standardizing function is not a consequence of the validity or reliability of the tool itself but the social and structural context in which a tool is introduced and utilized" (Bosk forth coming).

While practice innovations hold promise for improving the quality of service provision, it is important to remember that environmental, organizational, and individual factors can mean that the same intervention will function differently in distinct settings. Rather than trying to tightly retrofit organizations or workers to carry out interventions in mechanistic ways, effectively implementing interventions into real world child welfare settings requires having ways to incorporate possibilities for variation into the interventions themselves.

Fig. 7.6 Emerging research related to the inner setting

Organizational Structure The literature identifies several aspects of organizational structure that are critical to innovation. As noted by Proctor and colleagues (2014), Damanpour's (1991) meta-analysis of organizational studies in both for profit and nonprofit organizations revealed positive associations between innovation and specialization (specialties or role complexities in an organization), functional differentiation (number of different units in terms of structure, department, or hierarchy), professionalism (education, training, and experience of staff), managerial attitudes toward change, technical knowledge resources, administrative intensity (ratio of administration and managers to total staff), slack resources, and external and internal communication. A negative association was found between innovation and centralization (dispersed or concentrated authority and decision making)—the more centralized the decision making, the less innovative the practice.[2] Some determinants of innovation are much less mutable (e.g., slack resources and managerial tenure) than others (e.g., internal communication); however, there may be opportunities to consider these structural characteristics and to work toward ensuring that they facilitate rather than complicate EBPP implementation. Data on elements of the organizational infrastructure—such as program operations, staffing patterns, supervisory practices, electronic technologies for tracking services, and the content of services—are often not publicly available (Hoagwood and Kolko 2009). This leads many implementers and researchers to launch their efforts without knowing the types of strategies and processes they will need to employ in order to implement a given EBPP well. Research that systematically documents the strengths and weaknesses of the infrastructure for implementing effective services is sorely needed.

Organizational Culture and Climate Organizational culture (i.e., the way things are done in an organization) and climate (i.e., the way people perceive their environment; see Verbeke et al. 1998) also may affect the adoption, implementation, and sustainability of EBPPs. More constructive or positive organizational cultures and climates are associated with more positive staff morale (Glisson 2007), reduced staff turnover (Glisson et al. 2008), increased access to mental health care (Glisson and Green 2006), improved service quality and outcomes (Glisson and Hemmelgarn 1998; Glisson 2007), and greater sustainability of new programs (Glisson et al. 2008). Additionally, organizational culture may facilitate (or hinder) implementation by promoting more positive attitudes toward EBPPs. Aarons and Sawitzky (2006) found that constructive organizational cultures were associated with more positive attitudes toward EBPPs. Implementation research not only investigates the links between climate and culture but also uncovers what being part of a "good" or "positive" organizational culture means. By investigating the meanings associated with "good" or "positive organizational culture," research in this area attempts to map out what makes the implementation of an EBPP successful.

---

[2] Damanpour (1991) provides a helpful table that specifies the theoretical justification for these associations (pp. 1990–1991) and a more recent article details approaches to measuring these aspects of organizational structure (Kimberly and Cook 2008).

Implementation Climate Implementation climate, defined as "targeted employees' shared summary perceptions of the extent to which their use of a specific innovation is rewarded, supported, and expected within their organization" (Klein and Sorra 1996, p. 1060), is an emerging construct that may be critical to consider. According to Klein and Sorra, strong implementation climates encourage the use of innovations by ensuring employees are adequately skilled in its use, incentivizing employees to use the innovation and eliminating any disincentives, and removing any structural barriers that may block the innovation's use. Development of measures to accurately assess implementation climate specific to health and social service settings is currently underway (Aarons et al. 2012a; Jacobs et al. 2014; Weiner et al. 2011). Once established and validated, such measures will go a long way in generating evidence regarding this construct's relationship to implementation, service system, and clinical outcomes (Proctor et al. 2011).

Organizational Readiness for Change Organizational readiness for change can be defined as "the extent to which organizational members are psychologically and behaviorally prepared to implement organizational change" (Weiner et al. 2008, p. 381). Four beliefs related to organizational readiness to change may be particularly important to assess:

- change valence (i.e., "whether employees think the change being implemented is beneficial or worthwhile for them personally");
- change efficacy (i.e., "the degree to which employees think they are capable of implementing a change");
- discrepancy (i.e., "an employee's belief that organizational change is needed due to a gap between the organization's current state and some desired end state"); and
- principal support (i.e., "formal leaders and opinion leaders in the organization are committed to the successful implementation of a given change"(Aarons et al. 2012d, pp. 138–139).

High levels of organizational readiness for change may translate into individuals who are more invested in the implementation effort, expend more effort in the process, and persist in the face of implementation barriers and other setbacks (Weiner et al. 2008).

Turnover Organizational turnover at the staff and administrator level has been identified as a major barrier to successful program implementation (Isett et al. 2007; Manuel et al. 2009; Rapp et al. 2010; Woltmann et al. 2008). Recent findings from the children's social services literature suggest staff turnover can be reduce by improving organizational culture and climate (Glisson et al 2006, 2008). More central to this discussion, researchers are also finding that careful implementation of EBPPs accompanied by consistent feedback to staff on findings from routine fidelity monitoring (framed as supportive consultation) can also can decrease staff turnover (Aarons et al. 2009).

Communication Patterns Finally, it is important to acknowledge the critical role that communication patterns play in organizational change (Damschroder et al. 2009; Greenhalgh et al. 2004). Assessing intra-organizational communication patterns, including communication between direct service providers and upper management, can be an important first step toward attaining the implementation of change. Implementing new practices is essentially a "human" endeavor. As Kotter and Cohen (2002) remind us, ". . .the core of the matter is always about changing the behavior of people, and behavior change happens in highly successful situations mostly by speaking to people's feelings" (p. xii). Ensuring that lines of communication are open and that the environment is "psychologically safe" for the personal risk taking that change efforts inevitably entail is essential (Edmondson 1999).

Outer Setting Factors

The outer setting is comprised of the broader economic, political, and social context in which prevention and treatment services take place (Damschroder et al. 2009). The outer setting of implementation has garnered considerably less attention than provider-level and inner setting factors (Powell et al. 2014; Raghavan et al. 2008). Evidence concerning barriers and facilitators related to the administrative, policy, and funding context is largely anecdotal but speaks to the importance of taking stock of these issues in assessing barriers and facilitators to implementation. For example, adequate finances are necessary to support successful implementation, as there are costs associated with both the EBPPs and the implementation strategies required to ensure their institutionalization in routine care (Raghavan et al. 2008; Raghavan, 2012). Many scholars have noted financial resources as being a facilitator or barrier and have emphasized the need for specific strategies to obtain funding for EBPPs (e.g., Bruns and Hoagwood 2008; Ganju 2003; Hoagwood 2003; Isett et al. 2007; Magnabosco 2006). It is likely that EBPPs will be more readily implemented and sustained if they are reimbursable, perverse incentives (i.e., incentives not well aligned with quality of care or the best interests of children and families) are removed, financial incentives are integrated, and the marginal costs of EBPPs are supported (Raghavan et al. 2008).

Similarly, Isett and colleagues (2007) catalogued barriers and facilitators to implementing EBPPs in mental health settings related to financing and regulations, leadership and politics, and training and quality. Challenges related to financing and regulations included high start-up costs, issues related to reimbursement for services, and the need for prospective payments to cover various aspects such as lag time costs, adequate rate structures, and supplemental funding. Leadership imperatives involved tasks such as ensuring that the EBPPs were not seen as coercive and were responsive to differences between rural and urban populations, facilitating consensus building early on, and managing the coordination of services across agency boundaries. Finally, Isett and colleagues identified a number of challenges pertinent to training and quality, such as having to retrain existing teams, the need for high standards and ongoing monitoring, and properly aligning incentives (Isett et al. 2007). While many barriers and facilitators associated with the outer setting are not likely to be easily altered, ignorance of their existence can exacerbate other implementation difficulties.

Core Pathways to Progress

The field of implementation research is rapidly advancing; however, there are a number of improvements that could further strengthen the practical utility of this line of research. Overall, there is a need for more comparative effectiveness research testing a wider range of dissemination and implementation strategies (Institute of Medicine 2009a; Landsverk et al. 2011; Novins et al. 2013; Powell et al. 2014), and for rigorous studies of contextual elements that influence patient, provider, and organizational behavior (Eccles et al. 2009). Within those broad priorities we discuss eight key areas for improvement and document promising advances in the hopes of spurring innovation and progress.

Use Partnered Research Approaches to Understand and Address Complex Problems

Implementation research is inherently a partnered endeavor and advancing the field will require an engagement in transdisciplinary problem solving and a commitment to participatory approaches. The primary impetus for transdisciplinary collaboration is derived from the recognition that multiple disciplinary perspectives are required to better understand and ameliorate complex problems (Stokols et al. 2008). Interdisciplinary collaboration has the potential to enhance the creativity, rigor, and (ultimately) the impact of research. Interdisciplinary collaboration has also become a pragmatic necessity in order to obtain federal research funding (Landsverk, 2009). Similarly, as Chambers and Azrin (2013) note, translation from research to practice is no longer viewed as a "handoff from one world to another," but rather, researchers and practitioners are embracing a more blended view of the research, policy, and practice worlds. Furthermore, implementation research must involve the engagement of a wide range of stakeholders including children, youth, and families; caseworkers, clinicians, and other providers; organizational leaders; funders; policymakers; and other relevant stakeholders (Birkel et al. 2003; Institute for the Advancement of Social Work Research 2007; Kirchner et al. 2014; Wiltsey Stirman et al. 2009). Thus, community-based participatory research, or research in which "community stakeholders are full participants in research design, conduct of the research, analysis, interpretation, conclusions, and communication of results," is particularly relevant to the advancement of the field (Alegria et al. 2012, pp. S1–9).

Integrate Conceptual Models and Theories to Build Generalizable Knowledge

There is a need for better integration of conceptual models and (perhaps more importantly) theory in implementation research. There are a number of conceptual models and theories that can potentially guide this work in research and practice (Grol et al. 2007; Tabak et al. 2012); however, they are drastically underutilized, as the vast majority of published implementation studies do not report the explicit use of a conceptual model or theory (Colquhoun et al. 2013; Davies et al. 2010; Powell et al. 2014). This limits our understanding of how implementation strategies exert their effects, how contextual variables mediate or moderate implementation and clinical outcomes, and ultimately limits the generation of a generalizable body of knowledge that informs how to implement EBPPs effectively (Powell et al. 2014). Researchers should report the implementation model(s) and theory(ies) used and discuss how they were used to guide the design, conduct, analysis, and interpretation of study results (Michie et al. 2009; Proctor et al. 2012).

Develop a Wide Range of Valid and Reliable Measures

The development of process and outcome measures for key implementation constructs has been prioritized by leaders in the field (Eccles et al. 2009; Proctor et al. 2011, 2014; Rabin et al. 2012). Efforts to catalogue measures and rate them according to their reliability, validity, and "real world" utility have recently emerged through the Seattle Implementation Research Collaborative (2011) and the Grid Enabled Measures Project at the National Cancer Institute (2013). Recent examples of innovative measure development related to implementation in child welfare settings include the Stages of Implementation Completion (SIC) measure (Chamberlain et al. 2011) and the associated Cost of Implementing New Strategies (COINS) measure (Saldana et al. 2013). The SIC can be used to compare the effectiveness of different implementation strategies in driving implementation processes, and the COINS measure can be used to estimate the costs of different implementation strategies—something we know very little about (Goldhaber-Fiebert et al. 2011; Raghavan 2012; Vale et al. 2007). Opportunities abound to develop measures in virtually all areas of implementation science. This is true even for constructs that may initially seem well-developed, such as "organizational readiness for change" (Weiner et al. 2008).

Use Multiple Research Methods to Capture the Complexity of Implementation Processes

There has been a call for the use of mixed methods to study the processes and outcomes of implementation (Aarons et al. 2012b; Berwick 2008; Institute of Medicine 2007; Palinkas et al. 2011a), and qualitative and ethnographic methods have been touted as being essential for capturing the complexity of implementation processes and generating a deeper knowledge about how complex, multifaceted implementation strategies exert their effects (Alexander and Hearld 2012; Berwick 2008). There are also a number of advanced quantitative techniques that have been utilized to varying extents, and those may hold an expanded role as the field advances. For instance, increasingly sophisticated methods of research synthesis, such as network meta-analyses, are critical in determining which EBPPs are most likely to be effective in real world contexts (Caldwell et al. 2005; Wilen et al. 2012). The centrality of contextual influences in implementation necessitates the use of analytic approaches that take contextual variations into account (Luke 2005). For instance, the use of multilevel (or hierarchical linear) modeling (Luke 2004) is necessary to account for the hierarchical nature of data in which variation at the client level may be influenced by variation at higher levels such as the provider or agency level (Bhattacharyya and Zwarenstein 2009). The fact that the effects of implementation strategies are often mediated or moderated by contextual elements also necessitates the use of methods such as structural equation modeling, which allows for the estimation of multiple and interrelated dependence relationships (Lee and Mittman 2012). Finally, "systems science" approaches, including the use of network analysis (e.g., Palinkas et al. 2013; Valente 2012), system dynamics (e.g., Hovmand and Gillespie 2010), and simulation models (e.g., Goldhaber-Fiebert et al. 2012) have been used to model the complexity of implementation processes. Unfortunately, there is evidence to suggest that several of the aforementioned methods are underutilized (Luke, 2005); thus, it will be important to expand their use to improve implementation science and practice.

Develop and Use Reporting Guidelines to Improve the Quality of Published Research

A continued barrier to the communication of implementation research findings is the idiosyncratic use of terminology and the poor reporting of implementation studies (Brouwers et al. 2011; McKibbon et al. 2010; Michie et al. 2009). The terminology used to describe implementation research, strategies, and outcomes has been characterized as a "Tower of Babel" (McKibbon et al. 2010). To make matters worse, implementation strategies and clinical interventions are often poorly described and differentiated, and are presented without reference to an explicit theoretical justification or program logic (Davies et al. 2010; Michie et al. 2009). From a research standpoint, the inconsistent use of terminology and poor descriptions of implementation research limit opportunities for scientific replication and hinder the synthesis of knowledge by complicating efforts to generate systematic reviews and meta-analyses in implementation research. Organizational leaders and other would-be implementers of EBPPs who turn to the literature to learn about effective implementation approaches will undoubtedly be frustrated by a lack of clear guidance on what to do and how to do it. Reporting needs to be more detailed and better organized, and there has been a call for the development of a suite of implementation-specific reporting guidelines (Eccles et al. 2009) similar to those developed for other types of research (Equator Network 2014).

There are a few resources currently available that have the potential to improve the reporting of implementation research. The WIDER Recommendations aim to enhance the detail in which the content of behavior change interventions, including implementation strategies and other clinical interventions, are reported (Albrecht et al. 2013; Workgroup for Intervention Development and Evaluation Research 2008). Similarly, Proctor et al. (2013) have recently advanced recommendations for specifying and reporting implementation strategies, urging researchers to clearly name and define component implementation strategies, and to operationalize them by specifying the associated actors, actions, action targets, temporality (i.e., sequence of component strategies), dose, implementation outcome affected, and justification (theoretical, empirical, or pragmatic, or a combination of these). There are also a number of resources developed in the closely related field of quality improvement that may be of use to those conducting or consuming implementation research (e.g., Davidoff et al. 2008; Davidoff and Batalden 2005; Fan et al. 2010). Nevertheless, there remains room to develop guidelines that will enhance the quality, consistency, and usability of published research that can inform the improvement of prevention and intervention programs for children and families.

Harness Technology to Increase the Reach and Effectiveness of Implementation Efforts

Technological advances stand to benefit implementation science in many ways. First, technology may increase the reach of prevention and treatment interventions (e.g., delivering interventions by telemedicine; see Funderburk et al. 2008). Second, technologies such as smart phone applications and web-based training and supervision tools may reduce the cost of some implementation strategies. For example, Aarons et al. (2012c) examine whether automated telephone technology or wireless netbooks are efficient and reliable ways of monitoring fidelity to the SafeCare intervention. Technology also holds tremendous promise for promoting intra- and inter-organizational communication and collaboration, both of which have been identified as critical to implementation success (Damschroder et al. 2009; Palinkas et al. 2014). Nickerson (2010) provides a good example of this through a method called ChangeCasting, in which short videos of organizational leaders coupled with anonymous feedback systems are used to facilitate communication between leaders and other members of the organization. This admittedly broad area is ripe for further innovations that could improve the implementation and sustainment of EBPPs.

Improve Methods for Selecting and Tailoring Strategies to Overcome Barriers

As we have discussed above, a number of factors can serve as barriers or facilitators to implementation (Flottorp et al. 2013). There is growing recognition that implementation strategies should be thoughtfully applied to overcome barriers and leverage facilitators unique to specific implementation contexts (Baker et al. 2010; Mittman 2012; Wensing et al. 2009). For example, if an assessment of barriers and facilitators reveals a lack of provider knowledge, then training may an appropriate implementation strategy. Likewise, if barriers related to a poor organizational culture and climate are identified, it may be necessary to apply implementation strategies to improve the organization's social context prior to (or concurrent with) implementing an EBPP (Glisson et al. 2010, 2012, 2013). Though matching implementation strategies to identified barriers is intuitive, there is a need for reliable methods that can facilitate the process of selecting strategies to address identified barriers. Indeed, published reports often indicate mismatches between identified barriers and strategies (e.g., identifying barriers at the organizational level and using primarily provider-focused strategies in an implementation effort; see Bosch et al. 2007).

The fact that most implementation efforts involve the use of multiple implementation strategies (e.g., Magnabosco 2006; Pipkin et al. 2013) further complicates the matter, elevating the importance of having methods and frameworks in place to ensure that relevant barriers and facilitators are addressed or leveraged. Several of the examples we provided above (e.g., the Dynamic Adaptation Process, Getting to Outcomes framework, and the Interagency Collaborative Teams model) represent efforts to be more thoughtful about how implementation strategies are selected. Additionally, Powell and colleagues (forthcoming) have proposed several potential methods that could be used to match implementation strategies to identified barriers and facilitators, such as the use of logic models (see Goeschel et al. 2012) and intervention mapping (Bartholemew et al. 2011).

It is beyond the scope of this chapter to discuss these methods in detail; however, they represent a means of ensuring that implementation strategies are systematically selected based upon relevant theory and identified barriers and facilitators. It remains to be seen how effective, reliable, and feasible these methods are in real world practice. But these methods hold promise and may ensure that we do not default to what Martin Eccles refers to as the ISLAGIATT principle, making an implementation decision because, "it seemed like a good idea at the time" (Grimshaw 2012).

Develop "Learning Organizations" Capable of Implementing Numerous EBPPs Well

Child welfare systems and social service organizations are tasked with not just implementing one, but a number of new prevention and treatment approaches. Since evidence does not stop accumulating over time, it also means that organizations will have to "exnovate," or get rid of interventions that are obsolete or no longer effective (Glied 2012; Prasad and Ioannidis 2014). Thus, Chambers (2012) projects that the future of implementation science will need to be dedicated to the ". . .sustainable integration of interventions within dynamic health care delivery systems and the implementation of evidence-based systems of care rather than the individual intervention" (p. ix).

March (1991) has described the mutual learning process that occurs in organizations. Organizations accumulate knowledge over time as they learn from their members and individuals are, in turn, socialized into the organization's beliefs and culture. Mechanisms for obtaining, utilizing, and generating knowledge within organizations can be formal (e.g., academic partnerships, research departments, use of scholarly literature) or informal (e.g., interpersonal networks, practice-based evidence). According to Grol and colleagues (2007), learning organizations are typified by an experimental mindset, curiosity about trying new things, open climates, acceptance of debate and conflict, a commitment to education and development, and engaged leaders. Implementation strategies that encourage organizations to become more data driven, develop capacity for leadership, and encourage intra- and interorganizational communication may improve organizations' capacity for learning and continuous growth. Furthermore, some implementation strategies (e.g., training and supervision structures, quality monitoring systems) may need to be institutionalized within organizations and systems to enable continuous quality improvement (Powell et al. 2013a, b).

Conclusion

At its core, implementation science is simply about "making the right thing to do, the easy thing to do" (Clancy and Slutsky 2007, p. 747). It is about equipping service systems, organizations, and providers with the tools that they need to succeed, and, more importantly, it is about ensuring that children and families receive the best possible chance of benefiting from intervention and preventive services. Clearly, both challenges and opportunities associated with implementing EBPPs in community settings abound. Through the continued advancement of implementation science and practice, we can improve the utilization and implementation of EBPPs for the prevention and treatment of child maltreatment, and ultimately, contribute to the promotion of child well-being.

Reflection: Reflections on Implementation Science and Child Welfare

Lawrence A. Palinkas
University of Southern California, Los Angeles, CA, USA

In the past 10 years, there have been three specific developments that have significantly enhanced our ability to address the paucity of evidence-based practice (EBP) in general and evidence-based practices (EBPs), interventions, and treatments in child welfare. The first development has been the transition from conducting largely observational studies of the barriers and facilitators to developing, testing, and implementing evidence-based strategies to implementing and sustaining effective and accepted evidence-based program models. When I first began in the field of implementation science, our primary goal was to understand why only 10 % of youth-serving agencies, including child welfare systems, were using evidence-based service models. Since then, we have learned much about the barriers to successful and sustainable implementation and incorporated what we have learned into developing effective *implementation* interventions. Some of these interventions, like the Institute for Healthcare Improvement's learning collaboratives model and Glasgow's RE-AIM model, were developed in the broader context of health services. Others, like the Availability, Responsiveness, Continuity (ARC) intervention developed by Charles Glisson or the Dynamic Adaptation Process (DAP) and Interagency Collaborative Teams (ICT) interventions developed by Greg Aarons, were specifically tailored to child welfare and child mental health settings.

The second development has been a greater appreciation within child welfare of the value and potential of evidence-based practice. Ten years ago, many child welfare leaders and case managers were reluctant to adopt specific models out of concerns that the models deprived them of control over services delivery, were too expensive to implement, and were not validated with populations that mirrored their own clients. These attitudes have changed, in part, due to the increasing evidence of the successful outcomes these programs can achieve, the realization that child welfare workers liked them because they offered structure and a scientific rationale to what they had been doing previously, and because many child welfare workers are graduating from educational programs that have given greater emphasis to the teaching evidence-based practice and practices as the preferred approach to service delivery. My own research has demonstrated an increased use of web-based clearinghouses like the California Evidence-Based Clearinghouse for Child Welfare and the Substance Abuse and Mental Health Services Administration's (SAMHSA) National Registry of Evidence-Based Programs and Practices to identify and select service models that address the specific needs of child welfare-involved youth and families. Child welfare systems leaders also make extensive use of personal and professional networks to acquire information and resources to support the implementation of evidence-based models most relevant to the needs of their communities and client populations.

The third development has been the improvement in the methods used to both implement evidence-based programs and to understand and facilitate the *implementation process*. In the past 10 years, there has been greater use of qualitative and quantitative methods together in mixed methods designs. These designs have enabled investigators to answer the same question using different methods (through convergence) or answer related questions simultaneously or sequentially (though complementarity, expansion, development, and sampling). There has been greater use of hybrid designs where studies of practice effectiveness and implementation are conducted simultaneously or sequentially. Such designs are cost effective and help document the inherent linkage between effectiveness and implementation. In addition, researchers are making greater use of alternatives to traditional randomized controlled trial, including randomized encouragement trials, randomized fractional factorial designs, and sequential multiple assignment randomized trials. These designs promise strong external validity at reduced expense. Child welfare workers also are more likely to participate in research that does not require them to provide their clients with less than optimal care or delay access to optimal care.

As to whether these three developments alter the way institutions and organizations select and integrate specific interventions into their overall operation or represent a major new advancement in child welfare, only time will tell. However, it is clear to me that they are actively being used to support a drive for greater accountability and greater innovation in child welfare. These developments have also led to greater collaboration between researchers and child welfare practitioners. Such partnerships are leading to the creation and application of knowledge that is directly relevant to the needs of child welfare systems and the communities they serve.

References

Aarons, G. A., & Sawitzky, A. C. (2006). Organizational culture and climate and mental health provider attitudes toward evidence-based practice. *Psychological Services, 3*(1), 61–72. doi:10.1037/1541-1559.3.1.61.

Aarons, G. A., Sommerfeld, D., Hecht, D. B., Silovsky, J. F., & Chaffin, M. J. (2009). The impact of evidence-based practice implementation and fidelity monitoring on staff turnover: Evidence for a protective effect. *Journal of Consulting and Clinical Psychology, 77*(2), 270–280.

Aarons, G. A., Hurlburt, M., & Horwitz, S. M. (2011). Advancing a conceptual model of evidence-based practice implementation in public service sectors. *Administration and Policy in Mental Health and Mental Health Services Research, 38*, 4–23.

Aarons, G. A., Ehrhart, M., & Dlugosz, L. (2012a). *Implementation climate and leadership for evidence-based practice implementation: Development of two new scales.* Presented at the NIH Conference on the Science of Dissemination and Implementation, Bethesda.

Aarons, G. A., Fettes, D. L., Sommerfeld, D. H., & Palinkas, L. A. (2012b). Mixed methods for implementation research: Application to evidence-based practice implementation and staff turnover in community-based organizations providing child welfare services. *Child Maltreatment, 17*(1), 67–79.

Aarons, G. A., Green, A. E., Palinkas, L. A., Self-Brown, S., Whitaker, D. J., Lutzker, J. R., et al. (2012c). Dynamic adaptation process to implement an evidence-based child maltreatment intervention. *Implementation Science, 7*(32), 1–9.

Aarons, G. A., Horowitz, J. D., Dlugosz, L. R., & Ehrhart, M. G. (2012d). The role of organizational processes in dissemination and implementation research. In R. C. Brownson, G. A. Colditz, & E. K. Proctor (Eds.), *Dissemination and implementation research in health: Translating science to practice* (pp. 128–153). New York: Oxford University Press.

Albrecht, L., Archibald, M., Arseneau, D., & Scott, S. D. (2013). Development of a checklist to assess the quality of reporting of knowledge translation interventions using the Workgroup for Intervention Development and Evaluation Research (WIDER) recommendations. *Implementation Science, 8*(52), 1–5.

Alegria, M., Wong, Y., Mulvaney-Day, N., Nillni, A., Proctor, E. K., Nickel, M., et al. (2012). Community-based partnered research: New directions in mental health services research. *Ethnicity & Disease, 21,* S1-8–S1-16.

Alexander, J. A., & Hearld, L. R. (2012). Methods and metrics challenges of delivery-systems research. *Implementation Science, 7*(15), 1–11.

Baker, R., Cammosso-Stefinovic, J., Gillies, C., Shaw, E. J., Cheater, F., Flottorp, S., & Robertson, N. (2010). Tailored interventions to overcome identified barriers to change: Effects on professional practice and health care outcomes. *Cochrane Database of Systematic Reviews, 3 Art. No.: CD005470,* 1–77.

Bartholemew, L. K., Parcel, G. S., Kok, G., & Gottlieb, N. H. (2011). *Planning health promotion programs: An intervention mapping approach.* San Francisco: Jossey-Bass, Inc.

Beidas, R. S., & Kendall, P. C. (2010). Training therapists in evidence-based practice: A critical review of studies from a systems-contextual perspective. *Clinical Psychology: Science and Practice, 17*(1), 1–30.

Beidas, R. S., & Kendall, P. C. (Eds.). (2014). *Dissemination and implementation of evidence-based practices in child and adolescent mental health.* New York: Oxford University Press.

Bernal, G. E., & Domenech Rodriguez, M. M. (2012). *Cultural adaptations: Tools for evidence-based practice with diverse populations.* Washington, DC: American Psychological Association.

Berwick, D. M. (2008). The science of improvement. *Journal of the American Medical Association, 299*(10), 1182–1184.

Bhattacharyya, O., & Zwarenstein, M. (2009). Methodologies to evaluate effectiveness of knowledge translation interventions. In S. Straus, J. Tetroe, & I. D. Graham (Eds.), *Knowledge translation in health care* (pp. 249–260). Hoboken: Wiley-Blackwell.

Birkel, R. C., Hall, L. L., Lane, T., Cohan, K., & Miller, J. (2003). Consumers and families as partners in implementing evidence-based practice. *Psychiatric Clinics of North America, 26,* 867–881.

Bloom, M., Fischer, J., & Orme, J. G. (2006). *Evaluating practice: Guidelines for the accountable professional* (5th ed.). Boston: Allyn and Bacon.

Bosch, M., van der Weijden, T., Wensing, M., & Grol, R. (2007). Tailoring quality improvement interventions to identified barriers: A multiple case analysis. *Journal of Evaluation in Clinical Practice, 13,* 161–168.

Bosk, E. A. (Forthcoming). *No longer neglecting neglect: Moving from intervention to prevention.*

Brouwers, M. C., De Vito, C., Bahirathan, L., Carol, A., Carroll, J. C., Cotterchio, M., et al. (2011). What implementation interventions increase cancer screening rates? A systematic review. *Implementation Science, 6*(111), 1–17.

Brownson, R. C., Colditz, G. A., & Proctor, E. K. (Eds.). (2012). *Dissemination and implementation research in health: Translating science to practice.* New York: Oxford University Press.

Bruns, E. J., & Hoagwood, K. E. (2008). State implementation of evidence-based practice for youths, part I: Responses to the state of the evidence. *Journal of the American Academy of Child and Adolescent Psychiatry, 47*(4), 369–373.

Bushman, B. J., & Wang, M. C. (2009). Vote counting procedures in meta-analysis. In H. Cooper, L. V. Hedges, & J. C. Valentine (Eds.), *The handbook of research synthesis and meta-analysis* (pp. 207–220). New York: The Russell Sage Foundation.

Cabassa, L. J., & Baumann, A. A. (2013). A two-way street: Bridging implementation science and cultural adaptations of mental health treatments. *Implementation Science, 8*(90), 1–14.

Caldwell, D. M., Ades, A. E., & Higgins, J. P. T. (2005). Simultaneous comparison of multiple treatments: Combining direct and indirect evidence. *British Medical Journal, 331*, 897–900.

Center for Public Health Systems Science. (2012). *Program sustainability assessment tool*. http://sustaintool.org. Accessed 27 May 2013.

Chamberlain, P., Brown, C. H., Saldana, L., Reid, J., Wang, W., Marsenich, L., et al. (2008). Engaging and recruiting counties in an experiment on implementing evidence-based practice in California. *Administration and Policy in Mental Health and Mental Health Services Research, 35*, 250–260.

Chamberlain, P., Brown, C. H., & Saldana, L. (2011). Observational measure of implementation progress in community based settings: The stages of implementation completion. *Implementation Science, 6*(116), 1–8.

Chambers, D. A. (2012). Foreword. In R. C. Brownson, G. A. Colditz, & E. K. Proctor (Eds.), *Dissemination and implementation research in health: Translating science to practice* (pp. vii–x). New York: Oxford University Press.

Chambers, D. A., & Azrin, S. T. (2013). Partnership: A fundamental component of dissemination and implementation research. *Psychiatric Services, 64*(16), 509–511.

Chambless, D. L., Baker, M. J., Baucom, D. H., Beutler, L. E., Calhoun, K. S., Crits-Christoph, P., et al. (1998). Update on empirically validated therapies, II. *The Clinical Psychologist, 51*(1), 3–16.

Chinman, M., Imm, P., & Wandersman, A. (2004). *Getting to outcomes 2004: Promoting accountability through methods and tools for planning, implementation, and evaluation*. Santa Monica: Rand Health.

Clancy, C. M., & Slutsky, J. R. (2007). Guidelines for guidelines: We've come a long way. *CHEST, 132*(3), 746–747.

Colquhoun, H. L., Brehaut, J. C., Sales, A., Ivers, N., Grimshaw, J., Michie, S., et al. (2013). A systematic review of the use of theory in randomized controlled trials of audit and feedback. *Implementation Science, 8*(66), 1–8.

Concato, J. (2004). Observational versus experimental studies: What's the evidence for a hierarchy? *NeuroRx: The Journal of the American Society for Experimental NeuroTherapeutics, 1*(3), 341–347.

Damanpour, F. (1991). Organizational innovation: A meta-analysis of effects of determinants and moderators. *The Academy of Management Journal, 34*(3), 555–590.

Damschroder, L. J., Aron, D. C., Keith, R. E., Kirsh, S. R., Alexander, J. A., & Lowery, J. C. (2009). Fostering implementation of health services research findings into practice: A consolidated framework for advancing implementation science. *Implementation Science, 4*(50), 1–15.

Davidoff, F., & Batalden, P. (2005). Toward stronger evidence on quality improvement. Draft publication guidelines: The beginning of a consensus project. *Quality and Safety in Health Care, 14*, 319–325.

Davidoff, F., Batalden, P., Stevens, D., Ogrinc, G., & Mooney, S. (2008). Publication guidelines for quality improvement in health care: Evolution of the SQUIRE project. *Quality and Safety in Health Care, 17*(Supplement 1), i3–i9.

Davies, P., Walker, A. E., & Grimshaw, J. M. (2010). A systematic review of the use of theory in the design of guideline dissemination and implementation strategies and interpretation of the results of rigorous evaluations. *Implementation Science, 5*(14), 1–6.

Doris Duke Charitable Foundation. (2010). *Child abuse prevention*. http://www.ddcf.org/Child-Abuse-Prevention/. Accessed 21 Apr 2012.

Durlak, J. A., & DuPre, E. P. (2008). Implementation matters: A review of research on the influence of implementation on program outcomes and the factors affecting implementation. *American Journal of Community Psychology, 41*, 327–350.

Eccles, M. P., & Mittman, B. S. (2006). Welcome to Implementation Science. *Implementation Science, 1*(1), 1–3.

Eccles, M. P., Armstrong, D., Baker, R., Cleary, K., Davies, H., Davies, S., et al. (2009). An implementation research agenda. *Implementation Science, 4*(18), 1–7.

Edmondson, A. C. (1999). Psychological safety and learning behavior in work teams. *Administrative Science Quarterly, 44*(2), 350–383.

Equator Network. (2014). *Equator network*. http://www.equator-network.org/. Accessed 11 Jan 2014.

Fan, E., Laupacis, A., Pronovost, P. J., Guyatt, G. H., & Needham, D. M. (2010). How to use an article about quality improvement. *Journal of the American Medical Association, 304*(20), 2279–2287.

Flottorp, S. A., Oxman, A. D., Krause, J., Musila, N. R., Wensing, M., Godycki-Cwirko, M., et al. (2013). A checklist for identifying determinants of practice: A systematic review and synthesis of frameworks and taxonomies of factors that prevent or enable improvements in healthcare professional practice. *Implementation Science, 8*(35), 1–11.

Fonagy, P., & Target, M. (2001). *The history and current status of outcome research at the Anna Freud Centre*. London: The Anna Freud Centre.

Fraser, M. W., Richman, J. M., Galinsky, M. J., & Day, S. H. (2009). *Intervention research: Developing social programs*. New York: Oxford University Press.

Funderburk, B. W., Ware, L. M., Altshuler, E., & Chaffin, M. (2008). Use and feasibility of telemedicine technology in the dissemination of parent–child interaction therapy. *Child Maltreatment, 13*(4), 377–382.

Ganju, V. (2003). Implementation of evidence-based practices in state mental health systems: Implications for research and effectiveness studies. *Schizophrenia Bulletin, 29*(1), 125–131.

Garland, A. F., Brookman-Frazee, L., Hurlburt, M. S., Accurso, E. C., Zoffness, R. J., Haine-Schlagel, R., & Ganger, W. (2010). Mental health care for children with disruptive behavior problems: A view inside therapists' offices. *Psychiatric Services, 61*(8), 788–795.

Gibbs, L. E. (2003). *Evidence-based practice for the helping professions*. Pacific Grove: Brooks/Cole.

Glied, S. (2012). *Opening plenary*. Presented at the NIH Conference on the Science of Dissemination and Implementation, Bethesda.

Glisson, C. (2007). Assessing and changing organizational culture and climate for effective services. *Research on Social Work Practice, 17*, 736–747.

Glisson, C., & Green, P. (2006). The effects of organizational culture and climate on the access to mental health care in child welfare and juvenile justice systems. *Administration and Policy in Mental Health and Mental Health Services Research, 33*(4), 433–448.

Glisson, C., & Hemmelgarn, A. (1998). The effects of organizational climate and interorganizational coordination on the quality and outcomes of children's service systems. *Child Abuse & Neglect, 22*(5), 401–421.

Glisson, C., & Schoenwald, S. K. (2005). The ARC organizational and community intervention strategy for implementing evidence-based children's mental health treatments. *Mental Health Services Research, 7*(4), 243–259.

Glisson, C., Dukes, D., & Green, P. (2006). The effects of the ARC organizational intervention on caseworker turnover, climate, and culture in children's service systems. *Child Abuse & Neglect, 30*(8), 855–880.

Glisson, C., Schoenwald, S. K., Kelleher, K., Landsverk, J., Hoagwood, K. E., Mayberg, S., & Green, P. (2008). Therapist turnover and new program sustainability in mental health clinics as a function of organizational culture, climate, and service structure. *Administration and Policy in Mental Health and Mental Health Services Research, 35*(1–2), 124–133.

Glisson, C., Schoenwald, S., Hemmelgarn, A., Green, P., Dukes, D., Armstrong, K. S., & Chapman, J. E. (2010). Randomized trial of MST and ARC in a two-level evidence-based treatment implementation strategy. *Journal of Consulting and Clinical Psychology, 78*(4), 537–550.

Glisson, C., Hemmelgarn, A., Green, P., Dukes, D., Atkinson, S., & Williams, N. J. (2012). Randomized trial of the availability, responsiveness, and continuity (ARC) organizational intervention with community-based mental health programs and clinicians serving youth. *Journal of the American Academy of Child & Adolescent Psychiatry, 51*(8), 780–787.

Glisson, C., Hemmelgarn, A., Green, P., & Williams, N. J. (2013). Randomized trial of the availability, responsiveness and continuity (ARC) organizational intervention for improving youth outcomes in community mental health programs. *Journal of the American Academy of Child & Adolescent Psychiatry, 52*(5), 493–500.

Goeschel, C. A., Weiss, W. M., & Pronovost, P. J. (2012). Using a logic model to design and evaluate quality and patient safety improvement programs. *International Journal for Quality in Health Care, 24*(4), 330–337.

Goldhaber-Fiebert, J. D., Snowden, L. R., Wulczyn, F., Landsverk, J., & Horwitz, S. M. (2011). Economic evaluation research in the context of child welfare policy: A structured literature review and recommendations. *Child Abuse & Neglect, 35*, 722–740.

Goldhaber-Fiebert, J. D., Bailey, S. L., Hurlburt, M. S., Zhang, J., Snowden, L. R., Wulczyn, F., et al. (2012). Evaluating child welfare policies with decision-analytic simulation models. *Administration and Policy in Mental Health and Mental Health Services Research, 39*(6), 466–477. doi:10.1007/s10488-011-0370-z.

Grant, E. S., & Calderbank-Batista, T. (2013). Network meta-analysis for complex social interventions: Problems and potential. *Journal of the Society for Social Work and Research, 4*(4), 406–420.

Greenhalgh, T. (1997). How to read a paper. Getting your bearings (deciding what the paper is about). *BMJ, 315*(7102), 243–246.

Greenhalgh, T., Robert, G., Macfarlane, F., Bate, P., & Kyriakidou, O. (2004). Diffusion of innovations in service organizations: Systematic review and recommendations. *The Milbank Quarterly, 82*(4), 581–629.

Grimshaw, J. M. (2012). *Practical methodology of implementation.* Presented at the Knowledge Translation Canada Summer Institute, Ottawa.

Grimshaw, J. M., Eccles, M. P., Lavis, J. N., Hill, S. J., & Squires, J. E. (2012). Knowledge translation of research findings. *Implementation Science, 7*(50), 1–17.

Grol, R., Bosch, M. C., Hulscher, M. E. J., Eccles, M. P., & Wensing, M. (2007). Planning and studying improvement in patient care: The use of theoretical perspectives. *The Milbank Quarterly, 85*(1), 93–138.

Grol, R., Wensing, M., Eccles, M., & Davis, D. (Eds.). (2013). *Improving patient care: The implementation of change in health care* (2nd ed.). Chichester: Wiley.

Harris, J. K., Luke, D. A., Zuckerman, R. B., & Shelton, S. C. (2009). Forty years of secondhand smoke research: The gap between discovery and delivery. *American Journal of Preventive Medicine, 36*(6), 538–548.

Herschell, A. D., Kolko, D. J., Baumann, B. L., & Davis, A. C. (2010). The role of therapist training in the implementation of psychosocial treatments: A review and critique with recommendations. *Clinical Psychology Review, 30*, 448–466.

Hoagwood, K. E. (2003). The policy context for child and adolescent mental health services: Implications for systems reform and basic science development. *Annals of the New York Academy of Sciences, 1008*, 140–148.

Hoagwood, K. E., & Kolko, D. J. (2009). Introduction to the special section on practice contexts: A glimpse into the nether world of public mental health services for children and families. *Administration and Policy in Mental Health and Mental Health Services Research, 36*, 35–36.

Hovmand, P. S., & Gillespie, D. F. (2010). Implementation of evidence-based practice and organizational performance. *Journal of Behavioral Health Services & Research, 37*(1), 79–94.

Hurlburt, M., Aarons, G. A., Fettes, D., Willging, C., Gunderson, L., & Chaffin, M. J. (2014). Interagency collaborative team model for capacity building to scale-up evidence-based practice. *Children and Youth Services Review, 39*(4), 160–168.

Institute for the Advancement of Social Work Research. (2007). *Partnerships to integrate evidence-based mental health practices into social work education and research.* http://www.socialworkpolicy.org/publications/iaswr-publications/partnerships-to-integrate-evidence-based-mental-health-practices-into-social-work-education-and-research.html. Accessed 9 May 2012.

Institute of Medicine. (2007). *The state of quality improvement and implementation research: Workshop summary.* Washington, DC: The National Academies Press.

Institute of Medicine. (2009a). *Initial national priorities for comparative effectiveness research.* Washington, DC: The National Academies Press.

Institute of Medicine. (2009b). *Preventing mental, emotional, and behavioral disorders among young people: Progress and possibilities.* Washington, DC: National Academies Press.

Institute of Medicine and National Research Council. (2013). *New directions in child abuse and neglect research.* Washington, DC: The National Academies Press.

Isett, K. R., Burnam, M. A., Coleman-Beattie, B., Hyde, P. S., Morrissey, J. P., Magnabosco, J., et al. (2007). The state policy context of implementation issues for evidence-based practices in mental health. *Psychiatric Services, 58*(7), 914–921.

Jacobs, S. R., Weiner, B. J., & Bunger, A. C. (2014). Context matters: Measuring implementation climate among individuals and groups. *Implementation Science, 9*(46), 1–14.

Kane, M., & Trochim, W. M. K. (2007). *Concept mapping for planning and evaluation.* Thousand Oaks: Sage.

Kimberly, J. R., & Cook, J. M. (2008). Organizational measurement and the implementation of innovations in mental health services. *Administration and Policy in Mental Health and Mental Health Services Research, 35*, 11–20.

Kirchner, J. E., Kearney, L. K., Ritchie, M. J., Dollar, K. M., Swensen, A. B., & Schohn, M. (2014). Lesson's learned through a national partnership between clinical leaders and researchers. *Psychiatric Services, 65*(5), 577–579.

Klein, K. J., & Sorra, J. S. (1996). The challenge of innovation implementation. *Academy of Management Review, 21*(4), 1055–1080.

Kohl, P. L., Schurer, J., & Bellamy, J. L. (2009). The state of parent training: Program offerings and empirical support. *Families in Society, 90*(3), 247–254.

Kotter, J. P., & Cohen, D. S. (2002). *The heart of change: Real-life stories of how people change their organizations.* Boston: Harvard Business Review Press.

Landsverk, J. (2009). Creating interdisciplinary research teams and using consultants. In A. R. Stiffman (Ed.), *The field research survivors guide* (pp. 127–145). New York: Oxford University Press.

Landsverk, J., Brown, C. H., Rolls Reutz, J., Palinkas, L. A., & Horwitz, S. M. (2011). Design elements in implementation research: A structured review of child welfare and child mental health studies. *Administration and Policy in Mental Health and Mental Health Services Research, 38*, 54–63.

Lee, M. L., & Mittman, B. S. (2012). *Quantitative approaches for studying context-dependent, time-varying, adaptable complex social interventions.* Los Angeles: Presented at the VA HSR&D Cyberseminars.

Luke, D. A. (2004). *Multilevel modeling.* Thousand Oaks: Sage.

Luke, D. A. (2005). Getting the big picture in community science: Methods that capture context. *American Journal of Community Psychology, 35*(3/4), 185–200.

Lutzker, J. R., Bigelow, K. M., Doctor, R. M., & Kessler, M. L. (1998). Safety, health care, and bonding within an ecobehavioral approach to treating and preventing child abuse and neglect. *Journal of Family Violence, 13*(2), 163–185.

Magnabosco, J. L. (2006). Innovations in mental health services implementation: A report on state-level data from the U.S. evidence-based practices project. *Implementation Science, 1*(13), 1–11.

Manuel, J. I., Mullen, E. J., Fang, L., Bellamy, J. L., & Bledsoe, S. E. (2009). Preparing social work practitioners to use evidence-based practice: A comparison of experiences from an implementation project. *Research on Social Work Practice, 19*(5), 613–627.

March, J. G. (1991). Exploration and exploitation in organizational learning. *Organizational Science, 2*(1), 71–87.

McKibbon, K. A., Lokker, C., Wilczynski, N. L., Ciliska, D., Dobbins, M., Davis, D. A., et al. (2010). A cross-sectional study of the number and frequency of terms used to refer to knowledge translation in a body of health literature in 2006: A tower of babel? *Implementation Science, 5*(16), 1–11.

Metz, A., Bartley, L., Ball, H., Wilson, D., Naoom, S., & Redmond, P. (2014). Active implementation frameworks for successful service delivery: Catawba county child wellbeing project. *Research on Social Work Practice*, 1–8.

Michie, S., Fixsen, D. L., Grimshaw, J. M., & Eccles, M. P. (2009). Specifying and reporting complex behaviour change interventions: The need for a scientific method. *Implementation Science, 4*(40), 1–6.

Mittman, B. S. (2012). Implementation science in health care. In R. C. Brownson, G. A. Colditz, & E. K. Proctor (Eds.), *Dissemination and implementation research in health: Translating science to practice* (pp. 400–418). New York: Oxford University Press.

National Cancer Institute. (2013). *GEM-dissemination and implementation initiative (GEM-D&I).* http://www.gem-beta.org/GEM-DI. Accessed 27 May 2013.

National Institutes of Health. (2013). *Dissemination and implementation research in health (R01).* http://grants.nih.gov/grants/guide/pa-files/PAR-13-055.html. Accessed 30 Jan 2013.

Nickerson, J. (2010). *Leading change in a web 2.1 world.* Washington, DC: Brookings Institution Press.

Norcross, J. C., Beutler, L. E., & Levant, R. F. (2006). *Evidence-based practices in mental health.* Washington, DC: American Psychological Association.

Novins, D. K., Green, A. E., Legha, R. K., & Aarons, G. A. (2013). Dissemination and implementation of evidence-based practices for child and adolescent mental health: A systematic review. *Journal of the American Academy of Child & Adolescent Psychiatry, 52*(10), 1009–1025.e18.

Oxman, A. D., Thomson, M. A., Davis, D. A., & Haynes, B. (1995). No magic bullets: A systematic review of 102 trials of interventions to improve professional practice. *Canadian Medical Association Journal, 153*(10), 1424–1431.

Palinkas, L. A., & Soydan, H. (2012). *Translation and implementation of evidence-based practice.* New York: Oxford University Press.

Palinkas, L. A., Aarons, G. A., Horwitz, S., Chamberlain, P., Hurlburt, M., & Landsverk, J. (2011a). Mixed methods designs in implementation research. *Administration and Policy in Mental Health and Mental Health Services Research, 38*, 44–53.

Palinkas, L. A., Horwitz, S. M., Chamberlain, P., Hurlburt, M. S., & Landsverk, J. (2011b). Mixed-methods design in mental health services research: A review. *Psychiatric Services, 62*(3), 255–263.

Palinkas, L. A., Holloway, I. W., Rice, E., Brown, C. H., Valente, T. W., & Chamberlain, P. (2013). Influence network linkages across implementation strategy conditions in a randomized controlled trial of two strategies for scaling up evidence-based practices in public youth-serving systems. *Implementation Science, 8*(133), 1–11.

Palinkas, L. A., Fuentes, D., Finno, M., Garcia, A. R., Holloway, I. W., & Chamberlain, P. (2014). Inter-organizational collaboration in the implementation of evidence-based practices among public agencies serving abused and neglected youth. *Administration and Policy in Mental Health and Mental Health Services Research, 41*, 74–85.

Pipkin, S., Sterrett, E. M., Antle, B., & Christensen, D. N. (2013). Washington state's adoption of a child welfare practice model: An illustration of the getting-to-outcomes implementation framework. *Children and Youth Services Review, 35*(12), 1923–1932.

Powell, B. J., McMillen, J. C., Proctor, E. K., Carpenter, C. R., Griffey, R. T., Bunger, A. C., et al. (2012). A compilation of strategies for implementing clinical innovations in health and mental health. *Medical Care Research and Review, 69*(2), 123–157.

Powell, B. J., Hausmann-Stabile, C., & McMillen, J. C. (2013a). Mental health clinicians' experiences of implementing evidence-based treatments. *Journal of Evidence-Based Social Work, 10*(5), 396–409.

Powell, B. J., Proctor, E. K., Glisson, C. A., Kohl, P. L., Raghavan, R., Brownson, R. C., et al. (2013b). A mixed methods multiple case study of implementation as usual in children's social service organizations: Study protocol. *Implementation Science, 8*(92), 1–12.

Powell, B. J., Proctor, E. K., & Glass, J. E. (2014). A systematic review of strategies for implementing empirically supported mental health interventions. *Research on Social Work Practice, 24*(2), 192–212.

Powell, B. J., Beidas, R. S., Lewis, C. C., Aarons, G. A., McMillen, J. C., Proctor, E. K., & Proctor, E. K. (revise & resubmit). Methods to improve the selection and tailoring of implementation strategies. *Journal of Behavioral Health Services and Research.*

Prasad, V., & Ioannidis, J. P. A. (2014). Evidence-based de-implementation for contradicted, unproven, and aspiring healthcare practices. *Implementation Science, 9*(1), 1–5.

Proctor, E. K., Silmere, H., Raghavan, R., Hovmand, P., Aarons, G. A., Bunger, A., et al. (2011). Outcomes for implementation research: Conceptual distinctions, measurement challenges, and research agenda. *Administration and Policy in Mental Health and Mental Health Services Research, 38*(2), 65–76.

Proctor, E. K., Powell, B. J., Baumann, A. A., Hamilton, A. M., & Santens, R. L. (2012). Writing implementation research grant proposals: Ten key ingredients. *Implementation Science, 7*(96), 1–13.

Proctor, E. K., Powell, B. J., & McMillen, J. C. (2013). Implementation strategies: Recommendations for specifying and reporting. *Implementation Science, 8*(139), 1–11.

Proctor, E. K., Powell, B. J., & Feely, M. (2014). Measurement in dissemination and implementation science. In R. S. Beidas & P. C. Kendall (Eds.), *Dissemination and implementation of evidence-based practices in child and adolescent mental health* (pp. 22–43). New York: Oxford University Press.

Rabin, B. A., Purcell, P., Naveed, S., Moser, R. P., Henton, M. D., Proctor, E. K., et al. (2012). Advancing the application, quality and harmonization of implementation science measures. *Implementation Science, 7*(119), 1–11.

Raghavan, R. (2007). Administrative barriers to the adoption of high-quality mental health services for children in foster care: A national study. *Administration and Policy in Mental Health and Mental Health Services Research, 34,* 191–201.

Raghavan, R. (2012). The role of economic evaluation in dissemination and implementation research. In R. C. Brownson, G. A. Colditz, & E. K. Proctor (Eds.), *Dissemination and implementation research in health: Translating science to practice* (pp. 94–113). New York: Oxford University Press.

Raghavan, R., Bright, C. L., & Shadoin, A. L. (2008). Toward a policy ecology of implementation of evidence-based practices in public mental health settings. *Implementation Science, 3*(26), 1–9.

Raghavan, R., Inoue, M., Ettner, S. L., & Hamilton, B. H. (2010). A preliminary analysis of the receipt of mental health services consistent with national standards among children in the child welfare system. *American Journal of Public Health, 100*(4), 742–749.

Rapp, C. A., Goscha, R. J., & Carlson, L. S. (2010). Evidence-based practice implementation in Kansas. *Community Mental Health Journal, 46,* 461–465.

Rogers, E. M. (2003). *Diffusion of innovations* (5th ed.). New York: Free Press.

Roth, A., & Fonagy, P. (2005). *What works for whom? A critical review of psychotherapy research.* New York: Guilford.

Sackett, D. L., Rosenberg, W. M. C., Gray, J. A. M., Haynes, R. B., & Richardson, W. S. (1996). Evidence-based medicine: What it is and what it isn't. *BMJ, 312*(7023), 71–72.

Saldana, L., Chamberlain, P., Bradford, W. D., Campbell, M., & Landsverk, J. (2013). The cost of implementing new strategies (COINS): A method for mapping implementation resources using the stages of implementation completion. *Children and Youth Services Review, 39,* 177–182.

Scheirer, M. A. (2013). Linking sustainability research to intervention types. *American Journal of Public Health.* doi:10.2105/AJPH.2012.300976.

Schell, S. F., Luke, D. A., Schooley, M. W., Elliott, M. B., Herbers, S. H., Mueller, N. B., & Bunger, A. C. (2013). Public health program capacity for sustainability: A new framework. *Implementation Science, 8*(15), 1–9.

Seattle Implementation Research Conference. (2011). *SIRC measures project.* http://www.seattle-implementation.org/sirc-projects/sirc-instrument-project/. Accessed 10 Sept 2013.

Shapiro, C. J., Prinz, R. J., & Sanders, M. R. (2012). Facilitators and barriers to implementation of an evidence-based parenting intervention to prevent child maltreatment: The triple P-positive parenting program. *Child Maltreatment, 17*(1), 86–95.

Shortell, S. M. (2004). Increasing value: A research agenda for addressing the managerial and organizational challenges facing health care delivery in the United States. *Medical Care Research Review, 61,* 12S–30S.

Solberg, L. I., Brekke, M. L., Fazio, C. J., Fowles, J., Jacobsen, D. N., Kottke, T. E., et al. (2000). Lessons from experienced guideline implementers: Attend to many factors and use multiple strategies. *Journal on Quality Improvement, 26*(4), 171–188.

Sosna, T., & Marsenich, L. (2006). *Community development team model: Supporting the model adherent implementation of programs and practices.* Sacramento: California Institute for Mental Health.

Soydan, H., Mullen, E. J., Alexandra, L., Rehnman, J., & Li, Y. P. (2010). Evidence-based clearinghouses in social work. *Research on Social Work Practice, 20*(6), 690–700.

Stokols, D., Misra, S., Moser, R. P., Hall, K. L., & Taylor, B. K. (2008). The ecology of team science: Understanding contextual influences on transdisciplinary collaboration. *American Journal of Preventative Medicine, 35*(2S), S96–S115.

Straus, S., Tetroe, J., & Graham, I. D. (Eds.). (2013). *Knowledge translation in health care: Moving from evidence to practice* (2nd ed.). Chichester: Wiley.

Tabak, R. G., Khoong, E. C., Chambers, D. A., & Brownson, R. C. (2012). Bridging research and practice: Models for dissemination and implementation research. *American Journal of Preventive Medicine, 43*(3), 337–350.

The California Evidence-Based Clearinghouse for Child Welfare. (2014). Retrieved April 27, 2014, from http://www.cebc4cw.org/

Vale, L., Thomas, R., MacLennan, G., & Grimshaw, J. (2007). Systematic review of economic evaluations and cost analyses of guideline implementation strategies. *European Journal of Health Economics, 8,* 111–121.

Valente, T. W. (2012). Network interventions. *Science, 337*(39), 49–53.

Verbeke, W., Volgering, M., & Hessels, M. (1998). Exploring the conceptual expansion within the field of organizational behavior: Organizational climate and organizational culture. *Journal of Management Studies, 35*(3), 303–329.

Weiner, B. J., Amick, H., & Lee, S.-Y. D. (2008). Conceptualization and measurement of organizational readiness for change: A review of the literature in health services research and other fields. *Medical Care Research and Review, 65*(4), 379–436.

Weiner, B. J., Belden, C. M., Bergmire, D. M., & Johnston, M. (2011). The meaning and measurement of implementation climate. *Implementation Science, 6*(78), 1–12.

Weissman, M. M., Verdeli, H., Gameroff, M. J., Bledsoe, S. E., Betts, K., Mufson, L., et al. (2006). National survey of psychotherapy training in psychiatry, psychology, and social work. *Archives of General Psychiatry, 63,* 925–934.

Wensing, M., Bosch, M., & Grol, R. (2009). Selecting, tailoring, and implementing knowledge translation interventions. In S. Straus, J. Tetroe, & I. D. Graham (Eds.), *Knowledge Translation in health care: Moving from evidence to practice* (pp. 94–113). Oxford: Wiley-Blackwell.

Westen, D., Novotny, C. M., & Thompson-Brenner, H. (2004). The empirical status of empirically supported psychotherapies: Assumptions, findings, and reporting in controlled clinical trials. *Psychological Bulletin, 130*(4), 631–663.

Wilen, J. S. (2014). *A systematic review and network meta-analysis of psychosocial interventions for adults who were sexually abused as children.* ProQuest dissertations & theses, Bryn Mawr College.

Wilen, J. S., Littell, J. H., & Salanti, G. (2012). Psychosocial interventions for adults who were sexually abused as children (protocol). *Cochrane Database of Systematic Reviews, 9,* 1–22.

Wiltsey Stirman, S., Buchhofer, R., McLaulin, J. B., Evans, A. C., & Beck, A. T. (2009). The beck initiative: A partnership to implement cognitive therapy in a community behavioral health system. *Psychiatric Services, 60*(10), 1302–1304.

Wiltsey Stirman, S., Kimberly, J., Cook, N., Calloway, A., Castro, F., & Charns, M. (2012). The sustainability of new programs and innovations: A review of the empirical literature and recommendations for future research. *Implementation Science, 7*(17), 1–19.

Wiltsey Stirman, S., Calloway, A., Toder, K., Miller, C. J., DeVito, A. K., Meisel, S. N., et al. (2013a). Community mental health provider modifications to cognitive therapy: Implications for sustainability. *Psychiatric Services, 64*(10), 1056–1059.

Wiltsey Stirman, S., Miller, C. J., Toder, K., & Calloway, A. (2013b). Development of a framework and coding system for modifications and adaptations of evidence-based interventions. *Implementation Science, 8*(65), 1–12.

Woltmann, E. M., Whitley, R., McHugo, G. J., Brunette, M., Torrey, W. C., Coots, L., et al. (2008). The role of staff turnover in the implementation of evidence-based practices in mental health care. *Psychiatric Services, 59*(7), 732–737.

Workgroup for Intervention Development and Evaluation Research. (2008). *WIDER recommendations to improve reporting of the content of behaviour change interventions.* http://www.biomedcentral.com/content/supplementary/1748-5908-7-70-S4.pdf. Accessed 18 Aug 2014.

Zima, B. T., Hurlburt, M. S., Knapp, P., Ladd, H., Tang, L., Duan, N., et al. (2005). Quality of publicly-funded outpatient specialty mental health care for common childhood psychiatric disorders in California. *Journal of the American Academy of Child and Adolescent Psychiatry, 44*(2), 130–144.

Byron J. Powell is a postdoctoral researcher at the Center for Mental Health Policy and Services Research, Department of Psychiatry, Perelman School of Medicine, University of Pennsylvania. Dr. Powell's research focuses on efforts to improve the quality of mental health and social services that are provided in community settings. Specifically, he is working to develop a better understanding of the types of strategies that can be used to implement effective services, and the organizational and systemic factors that can facilitate or impede implementation and quality improvement. Dr. Powell received a B.A. in psychology from Taylor University, an AM in social work from the University of Chicago, and a Ph.D. in social work from Washington University in St. Louis where he was a National Institute of Mental Health Pre-Doctoral Fellow (T32MH19960). The Doris Duke Charitable Foundation, Fahs-Beck Fund for Research and Experimentation, and National Institute of Mental Health (F31MH098478) have supported his research.

Emily A. Bosk is a doctoral candidate in social work and sociology at the University of Michigan. Emily's research examines how high-risk children, youth and families intersect with and experience multiple social service systems. Her dissertation research focuses on understanding how child protective service workers decide which families investigated for neglect will be offered legal versus social service interventions in the context of tools intended to standardize the decision-making process. Previously, Ms. Bosk received her B.A. from Vassar College and her M.S.W. from the University of Michigan. The Doris Duke Charitable Foundation, Fahs-Beck Fund for Research and Experimentation, and the National Science Foundation's Dissertation Research Improvement Grant in Law and Social Science have supported her work.

Jessica S. Wilen currently coordinates special projects for the Office of the Vice Chancellor for Students at Washington University. In this role, she manages a university-wide sexual assault and relationship violence task force, develops and implements diversity and inclusion initiatives, and creates systems for at-risk students. Dr. Wilen received her doctoral degree in social work from Bryn Mawr College of Social Work and Social Research, where her research focused on treatment for adult survivors of childhood sexual abuse and research synthesis. Dr. Wilen's dissertation work was supported by the *Doris Duke Fellowships for the Promotion of Childhood Well-Being.* Previously, Dr. Wilen worked as a clinical social worker with both survivors and perpetrators of sexual and domestic violence.

Christina M. Danko is a postdoctoral fellow in the Division of Pediatric Psychology and Neuropsychology at Mt. Washington Pediatric Hospital. Her research has focused on investigating evidence-based interventions and programs to promote the well-being of young children in foster care and prevent child maltreatment recidivism. Previously, Dr. Danko received a B.A. in psychology from the University of Virginia, an M.A. in clinical psychology from the University of Colorado Denver, and a Ph.D. in clinical psychology from DePaul University. She completed her pre-doctoral internship in clinical psychology at the Louisiana State University Health Sciences Center. Her research has been supported by the Doris Duke Charitable Foundation.

Amanda Van Scoyoc is a doctoral student in clinical psychology at the University of Oregon. Amanda's research focuses on promoting child well-being and preventing family disruption by addressing maternal addiction in pregnancy. Specifically, her doctoral research identifies pregnant women's common experiences and behavioral patterns while abusing substances in pregnancy. This project aims to identify protective behaviors that women engage in due to concerns about the developing fetus and determine whether these behaviors predict seeking treatment. Amanda has a documentary studies background and a strong interest in the dissemination of research findings beyond academia. Amanda received a B.A. in psychology from University of Pennsylvania and an M.S. in psychology from University of Oregon. Her research has been supported by the Doris Duke Charitable Foundation and the Lewis Hine Documentary Fellows Program.

Aaron Banman is a doctoral candidate in social work at the University of Chicago, School of Social Service Administration. His research interests include involving fathers in early home visiting programs, child abuse and neglect prevention, measuring father involvement, and implementation of evidence based practices. His current research involves implementing a father engagement intervention within existing home visiting programs while studying organizational and worker factors involved in engaging those fathers. Previously Mr. Banman received a B.A. in social work from St. Olaf College and an M.S.W. from Columbia University, School of Social Work.

Chapter 8
Scaling Up: Replicating Promising Interventions with Fidelity

Kristen D. Seay, Kaela Byers, Megan Feely, Paul Lanier, Kathryn Maguire-Jack, and Tia McGill

Chapter 8 in Brief

Context

- While a number of evidence-based interventions have been developed, insufficient attention has been given to insuring these highly specified programs are implemented as intended.

K.D. Seay (✉)
College of Social Work, DeSaussure College, University of South Carolina,
Columbia, SC 29208, USA
e-mail: kdseay@mailbox.sc.edu

K. Byers
School of Social Welfare, University of Kansas, Lawrence, KS 66045, USA
e-mail: kaela@ku.edu

M. Feely
Brown School of Social Work, Washington University in St. Louis,
1 Brookings Drive, Campus Box 1196, St. Louis, MO 63130, USA
e-mail: mfeely@wustl.edu

P. Lanier
School of Social Work, University of North Carolina at Chapel Hill,
325 Pittsboro Street, CB # 3550, Chapel Hill, NC 27599, USA
e-mail: planier@email.unc.edu

K. Maguire-Jack
College of Social Work, The Ohio State University,
1947 College Rd., Columbus, OH 43210, USA
e-mail: maguirejack.1@osu.edu

T. McGill
School of Public Health, Center for Healthy Development, Georgia State University,
34 Peachtree Street, Suite 1700, Atlanta, GA 30303, USA
e-mail: tiamcgill@gsu.edu

© Springer International Publishing Switzerland 2015
D. Daro et al. (eds.), *Advances in Child Abuse Prevention Knowledge*,
Child Maltreatment 5, DOI 10.1007/978-3-319-16327-7_8

- There is general agreement that fidelity is an important component of implementing interventions; less consensus exists on how to meet individual client needs while adhering to core intervention components.
- Data gathered during fidelity monitoring has important implications in research settings and can guide decision making in practice.

Strategies for Moving Forward

- Simple strategies to ensure fidelity are available and can be utilized by researchers and practitioners to document implementation and improve replication quality.
- When adaptations are required to meet the needs of a specific or emerging target population, primary attention should be placed on insuring the fidelity of an intervention's core components.

Implications for Research

- Include fidelity monitoring in the initial design and testing of an intervention to ensure that program content and the service delivery process are adequately measured and monitored.
- When there is not a systematic way to monitor fidelity, determine the usefulness and feasibility of developing a fidelity monitoring system.

Introduction[1]

The recent Institute of Medicine and National Research Council report identified fidelity as a strategy to enhance the impact of interventions for individuals in the child welfare system (Institute of Medicine and National Research Council 2013). Fidelity is an important component of service provision to families at risk for abuse or neglect. At its most basic level, fidelity refers to the process of ensuring that a program or intervention is implemented as designed (Dumas et al. 2001; Dusenbury et al. 2003). However, fidelity can also include assessing if the treatment conditions in a study were provided with the intended variation of the treatment, determining

[1] This work is supported by *Doris Duke Fellowships for the Promotion of Child Well-Being* to all authors, the National Institute on Drug Abuse (K. Seay; F31DA034442, 5T32DA015035), the National Institute on Mental Health (M. Feely, P. Lanier; T32MH19960), the National Institutes of Health (M. Feely; UL1 TR000448, TL1 TR000449), the Kansas Department of Aging and Disability Services (K. Byers), and a Fahs-Beck Doctoral Dissertation Grant (K. Seay). The content is solely the responsibility of the authors and does not necessarily represent the official views of the National Institutes of Health. Gratitude is expressed to Katy Miller, Drs. John R. Lutzker, Daniel J. Whitaker, Shannon Self-Brown, Caroline Roben, and Mary Dozier for their willingness to share fidelity insights on the ABC and SafeCare interventions.

if recipients obtained the knowledge or treatment intended, and determining if recipients used the skills learned (Bellg et al. 2004; Lichstein et al. 1994; Moncher and Prinz 1991).

Monitoring the fidelity of manualized interventions (i.e., interventions standardized by written protocols for implementation) is an important step in determining effectiveness in research studies and maintaining quality control in practice. The results of fidelity measurement have many practical functions, including comparing the degree to which fidelity was obtained with client outcomes across a number of domains and providing feedback for practitioner training. These comparisons can yield important information for agencies or researchers. For example, an intervention provided with low fidelity that leads to ineffective outcomes does not necessarily indicate that the intervention should no longer be provided to clients. In this situation, a first step might involve agency directors working with providers to ensure higher fidelity in the future, with the hopes that this will improve client outcomes. In order to be able to examine the relationship between how an intervention was implemented and client outcomes, fidelity data must be collected in a detailed and systematic manner.

One illustrative example of the importance of considering the relationship between fidelity and program outcomes involves the examination of Intensive Family Preservation Services. Early evaluations of the Intensive Family Preservation Services program indicated that the services were not effective at reducing out-of-home placements of children. However, subsequent analyses indicated that Intensive Family Preservation Services that maintained fidelity to the Homebuilders Intensive Family Preservation Services program model were effective at decreasing out-of-home placements (Washington State Institute for Public Policy 2006). As illustrated in this case, by considering fidelity to the model, providers and researchers were able to unpack important aspects related to program effect and use this information to inform the program model and practice decisions.

The importance of fidelity is well-supported in the literature (Bellg et al. 2004). However, disagreement exists in the field about the extent to which interventions can be adapted to meet client needs while maintaining the key components of an intervention that are documented as effective (Kendall and Beidas 2007). In this chapter, we will examine the role of fidelity in both practice and research, provide an in-depth examination of fidelity monitoring in two programs, and highlight innovations around fidelity.

Balancing Fidelity and Flexibility

In the research setting, fidelity measurement is currently implemented inconsistently despite the recognition in the literature that fidelity monitoring is an important part of intervention research (Bellg et al. 2004; Hasson 2010; Institute of Medicine and National Research Council 2013). Within social work research, the amount of quantitative data collected to monitor fidelity has been quite low in the past. Less than 10% of 128 social work outcome studies published from 1990 to 1999 discuss treatment fidelity, treatment adherence, or treatment integrity (Tucker and Blythe 2008). From that review, Tucker and Blythe concluded that these low rates may be attributable to the cost of assessment and the limited published examples of how to assess treatment fidelity. The Treatment Fidelity Workgroup of the National Institutes of Health Behavior Change Consortium developed specific recommendations—applicable to both practice and research—to increase fidelity in five domains: study design, training providers, delivering treatment, receipt of treatment, and enactment of treatment skills (Bellg et al. 2004). These recommendations provide a detailed list of best practices and simple strategies to increase fidelity that can be employed in research or practice settings. For example, when one goal of ensuring fidelity is "minimize 'drift' in provider skills," Bellg et al. propose seven strategies, including booster sessions, weekly supervision, and client interviews to determine if the intervention components were delivered (2004, p. 447).

In addition to serving as an indicator of whether or not a program is being provided as initially designed, information gathered from the fidelity monitoring process has other practical applications at the provider and agency levels. These data can be utilized to make decisions about the quality of services provided by staff, thereby informing employment decisions; to determine if specific services should continue to be funded or provided; to report back to clients or funders about the extent to which a program was provided as designed; and to inform the clinical supervision of providers (Schoenwald 2011). As the purpose of fidelity is extended to include a more extensive monitoring and feedback system, the need to assure accuracy in the measure of fidelity increases.

Strategies utilized by the Oregon Model of Parent Management Training (Forgatch et al. 2005) and Nurse Family Partnership (Olds et al. 2002) to insure model fidelity illustrate the importance of systematic training and monitoring. In the case of the Oregon Model of Parent Management Training, the Fidelity of Implementation Rating System is used to appraise provider skills on five critical aspects: knowledge, structure, teaching skill, clinical skill, and overall effectiveness. During the assessment of fidelity, practitioners are video recorded conducting sessions and trained fidelity providers evaluate the videotapes on a 9-point scale. Fidelity coders receive 40 h of training to ensure reliability before conducting fidelity assessments. Similarly, the Nurse Family Partnership (NFP) requires their agency providers to complete contractual agreements to deliver the program as designed and to maintain consistency with 18 separate model elements (Olds et al. 2002; Olds et al. 2013). To insure compliance with this agreement, NFP's National Service Office provides agencies and practitioners (i.e., the front line service providers) with access to supports including an online network of providers, provider education and training, program marketing services, and a standardized management information system (Olds et al. 2013).

Practitioners come to their positions with a variety of strengths, challenges, and preferences, which can sometimes translate into adapting programs to meet their individual strengths and the needs of their clients. Therefore, practitioners may be hesitant to adopt a new program with fidelity due to concerns about inflexibility for local adaptation (Botvin 2004). Practitioners may also experience concerns about the added burden of completing fidelity monitoring processes or maintaining records on fidelity. Programs cannot be implemented with fidelity if these practitioner concerns are ignored. In response, researchers have recognized the need to build flexibility into their interventions to allow for some adaptation to meet the perceived needs of different client populations.

Mazzucchelli and Sanders (2010) have suggested a framework to promote flexibility within interventions. First, they recommend separating interventions into core components which are easier to implement than a highly structured program. Blase and Fixsen (2013) explain that as the push for evidence-based practice grows, researchers must learn not only whether an intervention works, but what specific components are essential for achieving intended outcomes. They recommend applying usability testing to help operationalize a program and understand its core components. This strategy includes implementing an identified core component on a small number of participants, assessing results, making changes as necessary, and then repeating this process until the program is producing "credible proximal or short-term outcomes related to the tested core components and associated active ingredients" (Blase and Fixsen 2013, p. 8). Through usability testing, researchers will be able to better articulate the specific core components that are necessary for program success, which will then assist practitioners in implementing the program with the right balance between flexibility and fidelity.

Mazzucchelli and Sanders (2010) also stress the importance of training practitioners on the principles of the intervention with explicit instructions to be flexible when necessary. Specifically, they state, "Knowing the difference between an appropriate modification and one that eliminates, or even contradicts, a key feature of the program requires a thorough understanding of the underlying principles of the intervention" (Mazzucchelli and Sanders 2010, p. 247). They also recommend training practitioners on a variety of possible situations and how to respond, using positive and negative teaching examples (i.e., what to do versus what not to do when delivering the intervention), varying different aspects of the training setting to allow for the transfer to a real world setting, and facilitating feedback between practitioners and researchers to prevent practitioners from experimenting with different aspects of the intervention on their own (Mazzucchelli and Sanders 2010).

By explicitly training practitioners to be flexible in their delivery of the intervention, the researcher acknowledges the reality of providing an intervention in practice and promotes a continuous feedback loop between practitioners and researchers to improve interventions. Although it is much more difficult to train someone to know what is an appropriate versus an inappropriate adaptation of a program than to train on a traditional manualized intervention, it is a key strategy for striking a balance between adaptation and nonadherence. In order to prevent unintentional drift beyond the intended adaptation, the fidelity monitors must check in regularly with practitioners. To reinforce this concept, Sanders, the developer of Triple P, a parenting program focused on parenting behaviors and preventing child behavior problems, incorporates flexibility within the manualized intervention. For example, program components can be addressed in a different order or at slower or faster a pace that is appropriate for the individual client. Also, practitioners are trained in a number of different parenting strategies. However, rather than requiring that all parents learn the same set of strategies, practitioners can use their judgment to decide which strategies are appropriate for a particular family (Mazzucchelli and Sanders 2010). It is currently unknown if this is something that can be incorporated into a wider array of interventions in the mental health and social services fields.

Case Examples

To better illustrate the incorporation of fidelity monitoring within the context of manualized interventions, two case examples are presented: Attachment and Biobehavioral Catch-Up (ABC) and SafeCare. The fidelity monitoring systems for these interventions provide two examples of how these models have defined fidelity and have integrated fidelity monitoring systems into ongoing practice.

Attachment and Biobehavioral Catch-Up

Core Components

Attachment and Biobehavioral Catch-Up (ABC) is a 10-week, manualized, parent–child intervention developed by Dr. Mary Dozier at the University of Delaware, originally for use with foster families (Bernard et al. 2012; Dozier et al. 2006, 2008, 2009). ABC is delivered by home-based providers of early childhood services (i.e., Early Head Start programs, child protective services, family service organizations, and infant therapeutic treatment teams) through ten weekly sessions in the home. The intervention is intended for families with children between 6 and 30 months old. The purpose of the intervention is to help caregivers identify and reinterpret child behavior and override their own responses to the child in order to provide safe, stable, nurturing care that promotes development of child regulatory capabilities (Dozier et al. 2011). To meet these goals, ABC consists of two core components: target content areas and in-the-moment commenting.

The target content areas are nurturance, synchrony, delight in the child, and frightening behavior (Infant Caregiver Lab 2013). These four target areas are taught to the parent through delivery of the manualized curriculum and then reinforced through in-the-moment commenting by the provider, which is a key component of the intervention (Meade and Dozier 2012). In-the-moment provider comments are intended to describe the parent behavior, identify the target behavior it is associated with, and describe what the child learns from the parent using that behavior. Providers offer these comments in order to validate, teach, and reinforce use of the intervention targets for the parent (Infant Caregiver Lab 2013).

Evidence Base

ABC has been evaluated in randomized clinical trials with children in foster care. Evaluation findings support the use of this intervention in targeting children's regulatory capabilities, as evidenced by lower and more normative diurnal cortisol values, decreased avoidance behaviors, fewer disorganized attachments, and reduced behavioral concerns among the intervention groups (Bernard et al. 2012; Dozier et al. 2006; Dozier et al. 2008, 2009). Follow-up studies with preschool-aged children have also demonstrated support for the long term efficacy of this intervention (Lewis-Morrarty et al. 2012). Additionally, ABC is currently being implemented and tested in Early Head Start sites throughout the United States, as well as with families who adopt internationally, to expand the types of programs in which ABC can be implemented. It is also being modified for use with preschool-aged children to expand the age range for which this intervention is appropriate.

Staff Training

Implementation begins with screening potential providers for eligibility to deliver the ABC intervention. Eligibility screening consists of a short interview that incorporates a modification of the Brief Adult Attachment Interview and assessment using video vignettes to evaluate capacity for making in-the-moment comments (Infant Caregiver Lab 2012). This screening procedure was developed by Dr. Dozier and her colleagues to promote success in dissemination of the model. Their preliminary findings have demonstrated that success in this screening activity predicts use of commenting during weekly sessions, and that frequency of commenting is associated with increased parent synchrony and sensitivity (Meade and Dozier 2012; Dozier et al. 2013; Meade et al. 2013). Therefore, careful screening of potential ABC providers is considered an essential component for dissemination of this model.

Although evidence-supported screening is a major strength of the model, it may also limit the pool of potential providers, which could be especially restrictive in rural areas or small agencies. Despite this limitation, this process helps ensure that limited available resources are allocated to training providers with the most capacity to deliver the intervention reliably, thus maximizing the impact on targeted outcomes and reducing the need to replace staff who perform poorly.

Following screening, selected providers are trained to deliver ABC. The training workshop takes place in person over two days. It is followed by provider participation in 12 months of supervision and fidelity monitoring activities with the trainers in order to be evaluated for certification and rostering for the ABC intervention.

Coaching

All intervention sessions—which are held in the family's home—are video recorded by providers. The videos are uploaded in their entirety online for review by an assigned ABC supervisor. Providers are then required to participate in one hour of content supervision per week via video conference with their supervisor and a small group of other providers. Supervisors are research staff on the ABC team who have either been involved in the development of this intervention or have been trained by the developers to deliver and supervise delivery of ABC. Supervision time is used to discuss delivery of the manual content and receive qualitative feedback on provider performance. Providers also participate in 30 min of weekly individual coding supervision to evaluate use of in-the-moment commenting. To prepare for weekly coding supervision, providers are routinely assigned a 5-min video clip from their previous session to review and code for their use of comments. Weekly supervision consists of a comparison of provider and supervisor coding of in-the-moment commenting, providing quantitative feedback on interactions with the family, and establishing commenting goals for future sessions.

Staff Certification

Providers are evaluated on performance in delivering the ABC intervention during the final 2 months of their supervision period. During the final evaluation period, providers must: reach 80 % adherence to manual content delivered during the assessment period; reach ABC coding thresholds for how often coaches make comments, how often comments relate to the four target areas, and the number of commenting components that are included in provider comments on average; and reliably code in-the-moment comments. Provider performance is assessed based on seven out of the last ten 5-min video segments submitted for supervision. If providers reach the acceptable performance threshold at the end of the evaluation period, they are added to the ABC roster of certified parent coaches. In order to remain active, providers must submit video tape of one complete ABC case (ten videotaped sessions) every 2 years for evaluation by the ABC team.

Scaling Up and Fidelity

Extensive use of technology in implementation adds to the feasibility of scaling up with fidelity as it makes time-intensive, long-distance supervision possible. Use of a secure online dropbox and videoconferencing capabilities ensures that data is exchanged efficiently and securely, facilitates establishment of effective supervisory relationships by enabling face-to-face meetings, and facilitates provision of quality coaching with qualitative and quantitative feedback that is based directly on provider performance. This coaching is usually conducted via a joint viewing and critique of session videos. However, extensive use of technology also presents some challenges. Agencies that have a more rural location may encounter slow and unstable internet connections, presenting a barrier to uploading video. Also, differences in technical acumen and capacity among participating providers may require varying degrees of training and technical assistance to ensure success.

The two-pronged focus of the supervision and fidelity monitoring to emphasize both manual content and dose delivered via in-the-moment commenting promotes methodical skill-building on what is delivered and how it is delivered. This long-term and intentional skill development helps ensure that the model is delivered precisely as intended, thus increasing the likelihood of achieving intended outcomes and decreasing the likelihood of long-term model drift.

SafeCare

Core Components

The SafeCare model for the intervention and prevention of child maltreatment is one of the oldest evidence-based, ecobehavioral practices in child maltreatment prevention in the United States. Developed from Project 12-Ways (Lutzker and Rice 1984) by Dr. John Lutzker, SafeCare was designed for and evaluated with multiproblem families to address proximal behaviors of child maltreatment, reduce child neglect, and improve parent–child interactions (Aarons et al. 2009; Gershater-Molko et al. 2002; Lutzker and Bigelow 2002). Succinct and disseminable, SafeCare is ideal for use with children up to 5 years old. Parent training sessions are delivered in the home, over the course of approximately 18 weeks, as a package of three modules: Parent–child Interactions, Home Safety, and Child Health. These topics were selected based on the evidence supporting the relationship between these positive parenting behaviors and risk for child maltreatment. SafeCare is manualized, structured, and uses classic behavioral intervention techniques (e.g., ongoing measurement of observable behaviors, skill modeling, direct skill practice with feedback, training skills to criterion) (Aarons et al. 2009). To date, SafeCare sites operate in 16 states and in two additional countries (Belarus and the UK). As of this writing, new states (Pennsylvania and Montana) and countries (Spain, Israel, and Canada) are slated to receive training (National SafeCare Training and Research Center 2013).

Evidence Base

In addition to the single-case work used to develop and validate SafeCare, quasi-experimental evaluations, randomized trials, and cost-benefit analyses have been conducted. This expansive research has resulted in robust evidence that SafeCare, when implemented with fidelity, produces consistent positive observable results in the behavioral domains proximal to child maltreatment and reduces child maltreatment and recidivism. Research also has demonstrated that replicating SafeCare with fidelity facilitates employee retention and cost effectiveness (Aarons et al. 2009; Chaffin et al. 2012; Gershater-Molko et al. 2002; Jabaley et al. 2011; Lee et al. 2012; Lutzker et al. 1984; Silovsky et al. 2011).

Staff Training

In 2007, the National SafeCare Training and Research Center (NSTRC) was founded with support from the Doris Duke Charitable Foundation. Among other notable advancements in SafeCare implementation, the NSTRC allowed for the development of the train-the-trainer model. Consistent with this model, program training specialists train home visitors, coaches, and external trainers to implement the SafeCare curriculum with fidelity at each level. Training for SafeCare begins by establishing staff readiness. These sessions are facilitated through an online or in-person SafeCare webinar. Once readiness is established, didactic instruction is given. Staff knowledge and skills are measured and demonstrated through quizzes. To achieve field certification, providers must answer correctly 85 % of the questions about manual content delivered during the assessment period. Knowledge is assessed using home visitor, coach, and trainer checklists.

Staff Certification

Upon completion of training, SafeCare home visitors, coaches, and trainers receive regular feedback through coaching support and technical assistance as they complete the steps required for full certification. It is important to note that the train-the-trainer model is hierarchical, requiring successful training and certification at previous levels to advance to the next. That is, one must be successfully certified as a home visitor prior to seeking coach training and certification and must be certified as a coach before applying to become a trainer. Home visitor certification requires that three sessions in each parenting module be implemented with at least 85 % fidelity Coach certification requires at least 85 % fidelity on two coaching sessions for each module and at least 85 % reliability with trainer fidelity on coinciding home visitor sessions for each module. Trainer certification requires at least 85 % fidelity on the trainer skills evaluation on introduction or Communication/Problem-Solving components, along with completion of two SafeCare parenting curriculum modules.

Coaching

Direct practice observation by coaches, at both the agency and center level, is SafeCare's gold standard for fidelity monitoring—a choice that is empirically shown to produce benefits for model implementation and the implementers themselves (Aarons et al. 2009; Chaffin et al. 2012). Periodic fidelity monitoring is conducted as a part of standard SafeCare coaching to ensure that skills are maintained over time and to avoid implementation drift. Fidelity monitoring is also generally conducted in a hierarchical supervisory structure where home visitor fidelity is monitored by coaches, coach fidelity is monitored by trainers, and trainer fidelity is monitored by national Safe Care staff (Chaffin et al. 2012; Henggeler et al. 2002). Once certification has been achieved at each level, monthly fidelity monitoring and coaching is conducted either onsite, using a combination of video and conference calling, or through audio monitoring. In cases where a staff member has performed below 85 % fidelity to the model, feedback is provided and practice conducted until the staff member's skills allow them to reach 85 % mastery. Although fidelity monitoring and coaching by national SafeCare staff is required for the duration of service delivery, the frequency of coaching sessions is gradually reduced to a quarterly schedule. Though this process might seem labor and resource intensive, this level of support has been associated with greater staff retention, higher self-efficacy, mastery, competency, and a deeper understanding of the curriculum and how to apply it with flexibility (Aarons et al. 2009). It also has lowered training costs as compared to services as usual without fidelity monitoring (Lee et al. 2012).

Scaling Up and Fidelity

SafeCare implementation in scaled-up community services systems requires quality control to avoid diminishing returns, which are often experienced when models are expanded (Chaffin et al. 2012). Over the course of SafeCare's existence, there have been several adaptations to coaching and fidelity, which have been necessary to support widespread dissemination. While most fidelity monitoring is delivered in person by coaches and trainers, in a number of cases, video and audio technology have been used to deliver SafeCare coaching and fidelity monitoring in real-time as well as through recordings.

The national SafeCare office also has utilized technological advances to address issues of distance. In 2009, the program rolled out the SafeCare portal to facilitate the inducting and training of users. The portal tracks the status of trainees as they complete training requirements for each level (home visitor, coach, trainer) and works as a platform to exchange information (such as audiotaped sessions) for fidelity monitoring and scoring. Currently, the portal connects 64 sites, 357 home visitors, 17 coaches, and 9 trainers, providing an organized method of meeting coaching and fidelity requirements. The center has also piloted I-technology, using FaceTime to provide live coaching and fidelity monitoring to home visitors during home visits. Challenges to this method have included limitations due to internet access, the cost of requiring additional hardware, and the need for additional training and technical support regarding how to operate the technology.

Research and implementation of SafeCare remains dynamic and iterative, with the goal of consistently improving to ensure the best possible outcomes to provide quality staff training, exemplary support through coaching, and ensure model fidelity; all towards the goal of reducing rates of child maltreatment.

Cross Model Lessons

When examining the ABC intervention and SafeCare, a few common characteristics emerged as key components of scaling up intervention models with fidelity. First, both models demonstrate emphasis on methodical selection of providers through provider screening, evaluation of readiness, or both. Though this selection can be achieved in many ways, consideration of whether there are particular skills, qualifications, or characteristics that should be required of providers is a key concern to address in fidelity protocol development. Both models are also manualized and highly structured. Though this level of structure may limit opportunity for individual adaptation, it also promotes ease in measuring provider performance, which often directly relates to child and family outcomes. Model drift represents another such threat to good child and family outcomes. Model effectiveness and a commitment to implementation of evidence-supported interventions requires a long-term commitment of resources to ensure the model is delivered as designed and achieves intended outcomes. Both of the highlighted models provide an example of how to effectively address model drift through the inclusion of long-term coaching and how to address fidelity monitoring through certification and the duration of model implementation. Another common characteristic demonstrated by both models is the integrated use of technology to increase access and streamline training and fidelity protocols. Technology offers many advantages that support large-scale dissemination of promising intervention models. However, it is also important to consider the barriers and limitations of technology for a wide variety of populations and geographical areas when employing these resources. There are many aspects that must be considered in the development and implementation of fidelity protocol for any model. These case examples serve as an illustration of how two prominent models operationalized key characteristics of fidelity and executed protocol for model scale up.

Improving Fidelity Monitoring Systems and Program Quality

The availability of evidence-based, manualized interventions to prevent child abuse represents major progress for the field. In order for these programs to be replicated with quality and to achieve results found in the original trials, however, programs must be delivered with fidelity to the tested model. This focus on fidelity to a manualized or standardized intervention brings tensions to the field that must be resolved. The tension that is borne out of a focus on fidelity is the need to balance opposing forces or values, such as flexibility versus rigidity, autonomy versus accountability, client- or practitioner-driven versus model-driven services, and demand for fidelity versus innovation. A shift in practice and policy towards an outcomes-based orientation and increased uptake of evidence-based models places increased demands on providers and practitioners. An emphasis on results demands high fidelity. In turn, high fidelity demands organizational investment in monitoring and supporting fidelity as well as practitioner buy-in. Research on dissemination and implementation is still in development and there is not as much focus at organizational and policy levels on how to increase the perceived value of fidelity. The final section of this chapter will discuss these issues from the perspective of the practitioner, administrator, policymaker, and researcher.

Practitioners

The individual delivering the intervention is at the nexus of these tensions. Practitioners with varying levels of experience are being asked to implement evidence-based practices with high fidelity, yet their prior experience and clinical training may not align well with the agency-selected intervention's orientation towards practice. In social work education particularly, there is an ongoing debate as to what evidence-based practice is (Thyer 2004), and how to distinguish between "evidence-based practice" and "evidence-based practices" (Adams et al. 2009). The difference is subtle, but extremely important. In the evidence-based practice model, the pursuit of best practice is a process of critically appraising the research literature and incorporating the best evidence with experience, the client system, and social context. A focus on evidence-based practices (alternatively referred to as empirically supported treatments or evidence-based interventions) is squarely limited to selecting and employing a specific intervention or protocol based on a hierarchy of research evidence or a list of approved interventions selected by a governing body. One perspective characterizes the evidence-based practice process model as a "mutual decision-making process occurring between the clinician and client" juxtaposed with collecting lists of specific interventions or programs and "urging that social workers select their psychotherapies from such lists" (Thyer and Pignotti 2011, p. 328; a more detailed discussion of this process is provided in Chap. 7).

The evidence-based practice process model that is taught in many schools of social work allows for flexibility and autonomy in practitioner interactions and intervention planning with clients (Gibbs 2003). The use of manualized interventions is discussed, but the manner in which a model is selected and implemented is decided by the practitioner and the client. There are several issues given the value placed on model fidelity. First, if a practitioner does not select a specific model, there is no prescribed framework to follow, and as such, the concept of fidelity does not apply. Second, a practitioner may select components of a model, combine several different models, stray from one model while adhering completely to another, or choose to augment one approach with another. Although some prevention models build flexibility into their content and service delivery methods, practitioners are given a mixed message when asked to replicate a model as closely as possible to the intended delivery while at the same time being asked to use professional discretion when working with their clients (Barth et al. 2012).

The pursuit of fidelity may also create a situation in which the quality of clinical services and the effectiveness of a program may actually be diminished. In describing the tension that may occur when replicating an intervention in a new context, Morrison et al. (2009) suggest that "slavish fidelity may result in an intervention that is faithful to the form, but not the spirit, of the original" (p. 129). In many cases, a practitioner is deploying an intervention with a population or individual family for whom the program has not been tested or evidence of effectiveness is not conclusive. Deferring to fidelity may come at a cost to successful adaptation given the specific context. Valuing fidelity may stifle practitioner creativity and, at worst, could lead to a situation where potentially beneficial services or interventions are withheld because it does not fit with the model.

Research has suggested several causes that might account for the gap between the "nonevidence-based practices" commonly used by service providers and "evidence-based practices" (Aarons and Palinkas 2007). Some have suggested that this gap is partially attributable to the provider attitudes about adopting such interventions (Aarons and Palinkas 2007). The implication of much of this research is that practitioners must be sufficiently convinced about the effectiveness of the interventions and can be motivated to adopt these models given ample organizational support. However, more experienced practitioners are attempting to adapt to a new practice landscape and must evolve to accept evidence-based practices generally. New practitioners may also be confronted with a practice arena that looks very different from the process model promised in their graduate studies. Practitioners are oftentimes not involved in agency- or policy-level decisions regarding which models will make it on the "list" of what they can practice.

When presented with a practice arrangement that includes fidelity monitoring, practitioners may feel threatened or unsure about what it means for them. Practitioners may wonder how they will benefit by documenting fidelity and participating in coaching or other strategies to sustain fidelity. They may wonder whether it will actually improve effectiveness or help develop their competence as a practitioner. In some cases, particularly when fidelity is monitored "in house," practitioners may confuse fidelity monitoring with performance review. Sustaining fidelity is an ongoing process where deviations from the intended model can be corrected with additional supervision and coaching. One must consider whether the benefits of achieving fidelity consistently outweigh the costs of potentially creating a more stressful and fearful work environment. Moving forward, methods to address these concerns could include the following:

- To address initial resistance among practitioners, either to evidence-based practice in general or to a particular evidence-based practice, additional information and education about these practices, their efficacy, and the practitioners' role should be offered.
- To increase adoption and adherence, practitioners should receive clear, consistent and ongoing guidance on how to balance model fidelity and flexibility in addressing the needs of their program's participants.
- When introducing an evidence-based model to staff, agency managers should highlight the benefits of such programs, such as improving the consistency and quality of what is provided clients, providing staff with specific strategies for addressing challenging cases, and stronger anticipated benefits for families.

Administrators

The bulk of the responsibility to ensure fidelity in practice is shouldered by practitioners. However, there are aspects of fidelity that have organizational components that must be addressed to support process and content delivery. The tensions of fidelity are felt by agency leaders and administrators tasked with successfully implementing a model with fidelity across a team of practitioners. In most cases, small- and medium-sized organizations must implement at least one specific evidence-based intervention to be competitive for funding and to advertise that their program indeed delivers an evidence-based treatment approach. Yet, most evidence-based models have not been fully tested within the context of community-based or public agency settings. Such models are more commonly implemented within the context of a clinical study or in situations in which the fidelity monitoring system has been part of the research design and, therefore, the cost of fidelity monitoring has been fully funded by the research study. In contrast, local agencies seeking to adopt these models often need to build fidelity monitoring systems into their organization.

Creating such a system can represent significant financial investments. As such, administrators must consider both the cost of the model itself (license fees, training, and other elements) as well as the cost to develop an appropriate fidelity monitoring system, perhaps as part of a larger continuous quality improvement system. Such systems generally include a data collection strategy and a process for using the information generated by this system in a timely manner when deviations in fidelity surface. Core fidelity indicators commonly tracked in such systems, such as caseloads and number of service contacts, can have significant impacts on staffing strategies. Further, the reality of an agency's budget situation or the need to retain current staff may require administrators to reduce dosage, increase caseloads, or alter the provider credentials prescribed by the model. If an organization is committed to delivering a specific model for a long period of time, the opportunity to hire more appropriate staff may exist, providing program participants certain benefits that may only exist if the services are provided by the trained and experienced practitioners. Such staff may bring certain "intangibles" to the clinical process that may not be replicated with a less skilled or experienced practitioner. In maximizing the benefits of evidence-based models, agency managers might consider the following strategies:

- If a fidelity system needs to be developed by an agency for use in their setting, careful attention should be paid to including the costs of developing and maintaining such systems when estimating the financial commitment required to adopt an evidence-based program.
- Agency managers should use all available evidence to identify what aspects of an intervention are critical for achieving strong outcomes for their specific client population. These might include required staff qualifications as well as initial and ongoing training. Administrators may consider strategies to incentivize model adherence and fidelity monitoring among practitioners.

Policy can be used to design systems that are supportive of well-implemented evidence-based interventions. To encourage the adoption and effective implementation of evidence-based interventions, policymakers need to design policies that require ongoing consideration of model fidelity and provide adequate financial support for the fidelity process. If either piece of the policy is lacking, the chances for implementation with high fidelity, and the corresponding strong effects, are lessened.

Policymakers

Requiring that fidelity be incorporated and considered throughout the implementation of the intervention will help bridge the gap between what policymakers expect to happen and the reality of implementation at the agency level. Different policy mechanisms could be employed to accomplish this goal. One example policymakers can use to increase adherence to program models is Maryland's Mental Hygiene Administration and Department of Rehabilitation Services. Under this collaborative project, the agency implemented a reward system for maintaining program fidelity across all of its implementation sites. Based on the level of fidelity and proficiency in core competencies demonstrated during biannual visits by state level officials, individual program sites will be eligible to bill for their services at a higher rate. Such reward systems establish clear financial incentives for program sites to adopt a new practice with fidelity.

To achieve the positive and enduring results promised through the adoption of evidence-based programs, policymakers need to consider—and fund—the costs associated with measuring and maintaining program fidelity. In addition to the costs associated with initial training in the model, ongoing training for both direct service providers as well as supervisors will require additional resources. Beyond training costs, there are the program development and equipment costs associated with building robust fidelity monitoring systems. Furthermore, agencies might have to recruit, train, and support additional staff to accommodate lower caseloads, ensure funding to train new people in the intervention as attrition occurs, and potentially recruit workers with specialized training. These additional tasks are likely to increase the cost estimate of adopting a new intervention.

To develop accurate program cost estimates, all costs associated with fidelity monitoring must be identified. Some interventions have built the components of monitoring fidelity into the program, such as Parent Management Training Oregon Model (PMTO) (Forgatch et al. 2005). The ABC intervention and SafeCare, both profiled in this chapter, have also built fidelity monitoring into their programs. In these interventions, fidelity is not an add-on but was designed by the developers and is integrated into the program's administration. The systems for monitoring fidelity are slightly different in each intervention, demonstrating that there are multiple ways to incorporate fidelity. Failing to include these and other additional expenses (such as the need to hire more experienced direct service providers) when estimating the total cost of implementing a new evidence-based model can greatly underestimate the true level of resources needed to achieve full operation of the model as designed. Once included, the total estimate for adopting these strategies may make evidence-based models appear significantly more expensive than service as usual. However, continuing with an existing option or selecting a less expensive alternative could be a false economy. Policies which require the documentation of all costs associated with replication efforts, as well as the potential benefits of such models, would be more transparent and facilitate accurate comparisons between evidence-based programs and their alternatives.

To overcome this tension between cost and limited resources, policymakers must be convinced of the importance of funding such program improvements at a level sufficient to ensure model fidelity. With this goal in mind, policymakers should be encouraged to base their decision on the full costs associated with implementing such programs with fidelity. These costs may include ongoing training, workforce changes and development, appropriate staffing levels and a system to monitor fidelity. Policy makers should weigh both the total costs and anticipated benefits of implementing evidence-based programs in comparing these options with their alternatives.

Researchers

Researchers often develop and test interventions with the goal of improving people's lives. However, the impacts achieved during clinical trials often are not replicated, in part, because these programs are not replicated with fidelity. In some cases, deviation from a program model reflects an appropriate adaptation given the context in which it is being implemented. In other cases, these deviations reflect a change that violates a core component of the program. An important line of research going forward is developing fidelity monitoring systems that will assist practitioners in balancing the tension between core components and strict adherence to the model. As successful interventions are integrated into practice settings, researchers have an opportunity and obligation to consider fidelity monitoring and maintenance in that setting. Developing an intervention that cannot be accurately replicated in usual care reduces the model's capacity to achieve positive results across a broad range of settings.

There are two different ways that intervention researchers develop and scale up their programs. These two approaches have different foci for fidelity development. In one scenario, researchers develop an intervention, test it from initial development through effectiveness trials, and then manage dissemination into usual care settings. In the second scenario, researchers test interventions that have been developed by others. Such testing may occur in efficacy trials with new populations or effectiveness trials within usual care (e.g., Chaffin et al. 2004). Both groups of researchers have to consider fidelity to the intervention and the overall quality of the delivery. Ideally, a functional fidelity monitoring system would be developed concurrently with the intervention. This gives the program developer maximum control over the implementation process and allows them to determine how core components should be measured and if fidelity requires strict adherence to a manual. If the intervention has already been developed without an embedded fidelity monitoring system and is now being tested in an effectiveness study, the researcher testing the intervention will have to determine how to best measure fidelity and create a system for monitoring and maintaining it.

Regardless of whether a researcher is the original program developer, researchers evaluating interventions have a responsibility to consider how to monitor and maintain model fidelity so that its effects can be accurately measured and interpreted.

Researchers have suggested frameworks for assessing fidelity (Bellg et al. 2004) and for developing a fidelity assessment for research studies and practice (Schoenwald et al. 2011). Additionally, for some established interventions, such as motivational interviewing, fidelity measures have been developed (Madson and Campbell 2006). However, unless the intervention is a permutation of an existing treatment that already has a system for measuring fidelity, such as motivational interviewing, identifying a system that accurately measures the developers' original model can be difficult.

To increase the likelihood of fidelity being monitored and maintained, intervention developers should conceptualize fidelity monitoring as part and parcel of their intervention rather than as a separate or optional component. This would not only enhance the chances of a fidelity system being used but increase the possibility of sustained effects being achieved. This process has been followed by the Oregon Social Learning Center in its scale-up of Parent Management Training-Oregon Model and by the SafeCare and ABC interventions highlighted in this chapter.

In contrast, researchers testing already-developed interventions in an effectiveness trial have different challenges. They must determine what and how to measure and then develop a system that is feasible within the constraints of the study. Some researchers may choose to develop a system that can also be used in practice (Schoenwald et al. 2011). This can add a layer of complexity to the study but it is an important step to prepare for wider utilization in usual care. The costs and time of developing a system should be considered when designing the research study.

Fidelity monitoring and maintenance for an intervention should not end with efficacy trials. Fidelity should be a consideration from the beginning of the development process and balance the quality of the intervention with the feasibility for the end-user. Monitoring fidelity through the adoption into usual care provides an opportunity for researchers to study the intervention in the field and to continue maintaining the quality and success of the intervention. Moving forward, there are two strategies researchers might consider. One, those researchers developing interventions should include fidelity monitoring in their original design. They should also conduct testing to ensure that content and process domains are adequately measured. Two, if the intervention that lacks a systematic way to monitor fidelity, researchers, as part of their study design, should develop a monitoring system that will meet the study's needs as well as provide a realistic monitoring for those implementing the practice in usual care settings.

Conclusion

Maintaining fidelity is an essential step towards achieving sustained change for individuals and communities. The development of a system of ongoing monitoring can be challenging on many levels, but the tensions between expediency and success must be reconciled if evidence-based interventions are to achieve the level of success that has been promised and that communities need. There are real challenges for practitioners, administrators, policymakers and researchers in maintaining high fidelity to the intervention. However, the challenges are not insurmountable. Clarifying the tensions for each role is the first step in identifying solutions. Moreover, it should be recognized that these roles are interconnected. For example, if policymakers design policies that include adequate training and ongoing support for frontline staff, it will be easier for administrators to maintain and measure fidelity. Monitoring and maintaining fidelity may not be the glamorous part of the process of human services, but it is an essential component of delivering the quality, results-oriented interventions that families deserve.

Reflections: Scaling Up Evidence-Based Programs with Fidelity

Lucy Berliner
Harborview Center for Sexual Assault and Traumatic Stress
University of Washington, Seattle, WA, USA

In recent years, a science of dissemination and implementation of evidence-based programs (EBPs) has come into its own. Frameworks have been developed, relevant factors identified, and research conducted that has confirmed organizational variables associated with the successful adoption of these efforts. Among the key factors driving successful implementation are organizational leadership and commitment, training and expert consultation from the model developers, ongoing supervision, and ongoing monitoring. Various studies have now shown that under favorable organizational circumstances and with external financial support, real world organizations can deliver EBPs and achieve strong outcomes.

While this all is very good news, it is also clear that outcomes in typical real world environments tend not to be as good as those in the more structured contexts, except when organizations can replicate the conditions of the controlled research. It is no coincidence that the best results occur in funded research studies or for proprietary programs where external funding is maintained and ongoing monitoring is required. However, in our work in public mental health the biggest question put to us is how to sustain EBPs with fidelity when community programs are expected to cover the associated costs out of their usual operating budgets. The research has shed little light on this question so far.

Another consideration is that the extant research has focused almost exclusively on programs that target a single outcome (recidivism, parenting skills, or abuse prevention). The typical community-based programs, however, serve a diverse clientele seeking help for multiple problems. In our experience, individual brand name programs do an excellent job of providing support and resources that can be purchased for their specific program addressing their specific outcome. They are not concerned, understandably, with helping organizations manage the problem of delivering multiple EBPs with fidelity. It is unrealistic to expect that community-based organizations can manage multiple intervention-specific supervision structures or separate quality assurance methods. The research needs to identify practical strategies that can be integrated into usual care contexts offering EBPs to all of their clients, not just a few subgroups.

The science is clear that fidelity, monitored in some way, is important to get the desired outcomes. But it turns out that fidelity is defined and measured in many different ways. For example, an important distinction is between adherence to program characteristics versus competent delivery of specific clinical content. From the perspective of real world organizations, the methods have to be feasible to implement because fidelity monitoring consumes organizational resources. For example, if adherence to organizational characteristics is connected to outcomes across different EBPs, this would be very attractive to organizations.

It is our observation, at least in public mental health, that the value of EBP is no longer challenged. What organizations are asking is how to do it within the reality of their practice settings and fiscal constraints. If the goal is to scale up and extend the reach of these programs, then the research has to begin addressing these real world exigencies.

References

Aarons, G. A., & Palinkas, L. A. (2007). Implementation of evidence-based practice in child welfare: Service provider perspectives. *Administration and Policy in Mental Health and Mental Health Services Research, 34*(4), 411–419.

Aarons, G. A., Sommerfeld, D. H., Hect, D. B., & Silovsky, J. F. (2009). The impact of evidence-based practice implementation and fidelity monitoring on staff turnover: Evidence for a protective effect. *Journal of Consulting and Clinical Psychology, 77*(2), 270–280.

Adams, K. B., Matto, H. C., & LeCroy, C. (2009). Limitations of evidence-based practice for social work education: Unpacking the complexity. *Journal of Social Work Education, 45*(2), 1–22.

Barth, R. P., Lee, B. R., Lindsey, M. A., Collins, K. S., Strieder, F., Chorpita, B. F., et al. (2012). Evidence-based practice at a crossroads: The timely emergence of common elements and common factors. *Research on Social Work Practice, 22*(1), 108–119.

Bellg, A. J., Borrelli, B., Resnick, B., Hecht, J., Minicucci, D. S., Ory, M., et al. (2004). Enhancing treatment fidelity in health behavior change studies: Best practices and recommendations from the NIH behavior change consortium. *Health Psychology, 23*(5), 443–451.

Bernard, K., Dozier, M., Bick, J., Lewis-Morrarty, E., Lindhiem, O., & Carlson, E. (2012). Enhancing attachment organization among maltreated children: Results of a randomized clinical trial. *Child Development, 83*(2), 623–636.

Blase, K., & Fixsen, D. (2013). Core intervention components: Identifying and operationalizing what makes programs work. ASPE Research Brief. Office of the Assistant Secretary for Planning and Evaluation. http://files.eric.ed.gov/fulltext/ED541353.pdf. Accessed 18 Aug 2014.

Botvin, G. (2004). Advancing prevention science and practice: Challenges, critical issues, and future directions. *Prevention Science, 5*(1), 69–72.

Chaffin, M., Silovsky, J. F., Funderburk, B., Valle, L. A., Brestan, E. V., Balachova, T., et al. (2004). Parent–child interaction therapy with physically abusive parents: Efficacy for reducing future abuse reports. *Journal of Consulting and Clinical Psychology, 72*, 500–510.

Chaffin, M., Hecht, D., Bard, D., Silovsky, J. F., & Howard, W. (2012). A statewide trial of the SafeCare home-based services model with parents in child protective services. *Pediatrics, 129*(3), 509–515.

Dozier, M., Peloso, E., Lindhiem, O., Gordon, M. K., Manni, M., Sepulveda, S., Ackerman, J., Bernier, A., & Levine, S. (2006). Developing evidence-based interventions for foster children: An example of a randomized clinical trial with infants and toddlers. *Journal of Social Issues, 62*(4), 765–783.

Dozier, M., Peloso, E., Lewis, E., Laurenceau, J., & Levine, S. (2008). Effects of an attachment-based intervention on the cortisol production of infants and toddlers in foster care. *Development and Psychopathology, 20*(3), 845–859.

Dozier, M., Lindhiem, O., Lewis, E., Bick, J., Bernard, K., & Peloso, E. (2009). Effects of a foster parent training program on young children's attachment behaviors: Preliminary evidence from a randomized clinical trial. *Child and Adolescent Social Work Journal, 26*(4), 321–332.

Dozier, M., Bick, J., & Bernard, K. (2011). Attachment-based treatment for young, vulnerable children. In J. D. Osofsky (Ed.), *Clinical work with traumatized young children* (pp. 75–95). New York: The Guilford Press.

Dozier, M., Meade, E., Wallin, A. R., & Bernard, K. (2013). *Implementing an evidence-based intervention for high-risk parents in the community: The importance of model fidelity.* Paper presented at the biennial meeting of the Society for Research on Child Development (SRCD), Seattle.

Dumas, J. E., Lynch, A. M., Laughlin, J. E., Phillips Smith, E., & Prinz, R. J. (2001). Promoting intervention fidelity: Conceptual issues, methods, and preliminary results from the early alliance prevention trial. *American Journal of Preventive Medicine, 20*(1 Suppl), 38–47.

Dusenbury, L., Brannigan, R., Falco, M., & Hansen, W. B. (2003). A review of research on fidelity of implementation: Implications for drug abuse prevention in school settings. *Health Education Research, 18*(2), 237–256.

Forgatch, M. S., Patterson, G. R., & DeGarmo, D. S. (2005). Evaluating fidelity: Predictive validity for a measure of competent adherence to the Oregon model of parent management training. *Behavior Therapy, 36*(1), 3–13.

Gershater-Molko, R., Lutzker, J. R., & Wesch, D. (2002). Using recidivism data to evaluate Project SafeCare: Teaching bonding, safety, and health care skills to parents. *Child Maltreatment, 7*(3), 277–285.

Gibbs, L. E. (2003). *Evidence-based practice for the helping professions: A practical guide with integrated multimedia* (Vol. 1). Pacific Grove: Thomson Brooks/Cole.

Hasson, H. (2010). Systematic evaluation of implementation fidelity of complex interventions in health and social care. *Implementation Science.* doi:10.1186/1748-5908-5-67.

Henggeler, S. W., Schoenwald, S. K., Liao, J. G., Letourneau, E. J., & Edwards, D. L. (2002). Transporting efficacious treatments to field settings: The link between supervisory practices and therapist fidelity in MST programs. *Journal of Clinical Child Adolescent Psychology, 31*(2), 155–167.

Infant Caregiver Lab. (2012). *Screening parent coaches.* Unpublished interview guide.

Infant Caregiver Lab. (2013). *Attachment and biobehavioral catch-up for infants who have experienced early adversity (ABC-I).* Intervention manual, Unpublished.

Institute of Medicine & National Research Council. (2013). *New directions in child abuse and neglect research.* Washington, DC: The National Academies Press.

Jabaley, J. J., Lutzker, J. R., Whitaker, D. J., & Self-Brown, S. (2011). Using iPhones to enhance and reduce face-to-face home safety sessions with SafeCare, an evidence-based child maltreatment prevention program. *Journal of Family Violence, 26*(5), 377–385.

Kendall, P. C., & Beidas, R. S. (2007). Smoothing the trail for dissemination of evidence-based practices for youth: Flexibility within fidelity. *Professional Psychology: Research and Practice, 38*(1), 13–20.

Lee, S., Aos, S., Drake, E., Pennucci, A., Miller, M., & Anderson, L. (2012). *Return on investment: Evidence based options to improve statewide outcomes, April 2012. (Document No. 12-04-1201).* Olympia: Washington State Institute for Public Policy.

Lewis-Morrarty, E., Dozier, M., Bernard, K., Terracciano, S. M., & Moore, S. V. (2012). Cognitive flexibility and theory of mind outcomes among foster children: Preschool follow-up results of a randomized clinical trial. *Journal of Adolescent Health, 51*(2), s17–s22.

Lichstein, K. I., Riedel, B. W., & Grieve, R. (1994). Fair tests of clinical trials: A treatment imple-mentation model. *Advances in Behavior Research and Therapy, 16*, 1–29.

Lutzker, J. R., & Bigelow, K. M. (2002). *Reducing child maltreatment: A guidebook for parent services.* New York: Guilford Publications.

Lutzker, J. R., & Rice, J. M. (1984). Project 12-ways: Measuring outcome of a large in-home ser-vice for treatment and prevention of child abuse and neglect. *Child Abuse and Neglect, 8*(4), 519–524.

Lutzker, J. R., Campbell, R. V., & Watson-Perczel, M. (1984). Using the case study method to treat several problems in a family indicated for child neglect. *Education and Treatment of Children, 7*(4), 315–333.

Madson, M. B., & Campbell, T. C. (2006). Measures of fidelity in motivational enhancement: A systematic review. *Journal of Substance Abuse Treatment, 31*(1), 67–73.

Mazzucchelli, T. G., & Sanders, M. R. (2010). Facilitating practitioner flexibility within an empiri-cally supported intervention: Lessons from a system of parenting support. *Clinical Psychology: Science and Practice, 17*(3), 238–252.

Meade, E., & Dozier, M. (2012). *In the moment: Commenting: A fidelity measurement and active ingredient in a parent training program.* Unpublished manuscript, University of Delaware.

Meade, E., Roben, C., & Dozier, M. (2013). *Using screening interviews to predict therapist performance in the attachment and biobehavioral catch-up intervention.* Unpublished manuscript.

Moncher, F. J., & Prinz, F. J. (1991). Treatment fidelity in outcome studies. *Clinical Psychology Review, 11*, 247–266.

Morrison, D. M., Hoppe, M. J., Gillmore, M. R., Kluver, C., Higa, D., & Wells, E. A. (2009). Replicating an intervention: The tension between fidelity and adaptation. *AIDS Education and Prevention, 21*(2), 128–140.

National SafeCare Training and Research Center. (2013). *SafeCare sites.* http://safecare.publichealth.gsu.edu/safecare/safecare-sites/. Accessed 10 Dec 2013.

Olds, D. L., Robinson, J., O'Brien, R., Luckey, D. W., Pettitt, L. M., Henderson, C. R., Jr., et al. (2002). Home visiting by paraprofessionals and by nurses: A randomized controlled trial. *Pediatrics, 110*(3), 486–496.

Olds, D., Donelan-McCall, N., O'Brien, R., MacMillan, H., Jack, S., Jenkins, T., et al. (2013). Improving the nurse-family partnership in community practice. *Pediatrics, 132*(Sup 2), S110–S117.

Schoenwald, S. K. (2011). It's a bird, it's a plane, it's … fidelity measurement in the real world. *Clinical Psychology, 18*(2), 142–147.

Schoenwald, S. K., Garland, A. F., Chapman, J. E., Frazier, S. L., Sheidow, A. J., & Southam-Gerow, M. A. (2011). Toward the effective and efficient measurement of implementation fidel-ity. *Administration and Policy in Mental Health and Mental Health Services Research, 38*(1), 32–43.

Silovsky, J. F., Bard, D., Chaffin, M., Hecht, D., Burris, L., Owora, A., et al. (2011). Prevention of child maltreatment in high-risk rural families: A randomized clinical trial with child welfare outcomes. *Children and Youth Services Review, 33*(8), 1435–1444.

Thyer, B. A. (2004). What is evidence-based practice? *Brief Treatment and Crisis Intervention, 4*, 167–176.

Thyer, B. A., & Pignotti, M. (2011). Evidence-based *practices* do not exist. *Clinical Social Work Journal, 39*, 328–333.

Tucker, A. R., & Blythe, B. (2008). Attention to treatment fidelity in social work outcomes: A review of the literature from the 1990s. *Social Work Research, 32*(3), 185–190.

Washington State Institute for Public Policy. (2006). *Intensive family preservation programs: Program fidelity influences effectiveness.* http://www.wsipp.wa.gov/rptfiles/06-02-3901.pdf. Accessed 19 Dec 2013.

Kristen D. Seay is an assistant professor at the University of South Carolina College of Social Work. Her research focuses on the impact of parental substance abuse on child and family well-being and child welfare. Her current work examines the direct and indirect pathways from care-giver problematic substance use to child harm among families involved with the child welfare system. Before obtaining her doctorate, Dr. Seay worked as an investigator for child protective services in Georgia and Alabama. She received a BSW from the University of Georgia, a MSW from Florida State University, and a Ph.D. from the Brown School of Social Work at Washington University in St. Louis.

Kaela Byers is a Ph.D. candidate in social welfare at the University of Kansas where her research focuses on early childhood toxic stress screening and intervention to promote child and family protective factors supporting healthy social-emotional development. Ms. Byers is currently a project manager at the Center for Children and Families at KU where she conducts research on the implementation and evaluation of evidenced-based interventions in community mental health, child welfare, and early childhood service settings. Ms. Byers' professional experience includes providing home and community-based early childhood mental health services and community mental health consultation. She received a B.S. in social welfare from the University of Kansas and a M.S.W. from the University of Maryland-Baltimore.

Megan Feely is a Ph.D. candidate in social work at Washington University in St. Louis. Her work focuses on the definition, measurement and status of well-being for child welfare involved children, particularly as it relates to child and young adult outcomes. She has a particular interest in the measures that are used for research and practice and the implementation of evidence-based interventions in the child welfare system.

Paul Lanier is an assistant professor at the University of North Carolina at Chapel Hill School of Social Work. He received his doctorate from the Brown School at Washington University in St. Louis. The goal of Dr. Lanier's research is to prevent child maltreatment and promote child well-being among vulnerable populations. His work focuses on early childhood interventions designed to enhance healthy parent-child relationships and prepare caregivers to meet their child's developmental needs. He is also interested in health and mental health outcomes of maltreated children. Dr. Lanier's research agenda seeks to inform both policy and practice by testing innovative interventions and improving the availability of evidence-based service strategies.

Kathryn Maguire-Jack is an assistant professor at The Ohio State University, College of Social Work. She has a B.A. in Social Welfare and Political Science, MPA, MSW, and Ph.D. from the University of Wisconsin—Madison. Dr. Maguire-Jack has experience as a fiscal analyst, working on the Wisconsin state budget at the Wisconsin Legislative Fiscal Bureau and as a program and policy analyst at the Wisconsin Children's Trust Fund. Her research interests include child maltreatment prevention, risk and protective factors for maltreatment, neighborhood research, and program evaluation.

Tia McGill is a doctoral candidate at the Georgia State University School of Public Health, with a concentration in behavioral science. Prior to her doctoral training, she worked nationally and internationally as a senior training specialist with the National SafeCare® Training and Research Center. Ms. McGill holds a B.A. in psychology from Spelman College, and an MPH from Emory University Rollins School of Public Health. Ms. McGill has been awarded several honors including the Hebrew University's Haruv Institute International Ph.D. Workshop on Child Maltreatment in Jerusalem, Israel. Tia's research interests include child abuse and neglect prevention; implementation of evidence-based models for the prevention of child maltreatment; the relationship between mental health variables and engagement, uptake, and outcomes of behavioral parent training interventions.

Chapter 9
Promoting Protective Factors and Strengthening Resilience

Tova B. Walsh, Sandra Nay McCourt, Whitney L. Rostad, Kaela Byers, and Kerrie Ocasio

Chapter 9 in Brief

Context

- Resilience, protective factors, and strategies for achieving them are topics of growing interest across fields and disciplines.
- Partnering with families to identify and enhance protective factors is seen as an important new approach to prevention, offering a more acceptable framework to families than programs focusing solely on risks and deficits.
- Evidence-based protective factors linked to lower incidence of child abuse and neglect include parental resilience, social connections, knowledge of parenting

T.B. Walsh (✉)
Robert Wood Johnson Foundation Health & Society Scholars Program,
University of Wisconsin-Madison, Madison, WI 53711, USA
e-mail: tbwalsh@wisc.edu

S.N. McCourt
Social Science Research Institute, Duke University, Durham, NC 27708, USA
e-mail: sandra.nay@duke.edu

W.L. Rostad
National SafeCare Training and Research Center (NSTRC), Georgia State University,
Atlanta, GA 30302, USA
e-mail: wrostad@gsu.edu

K. Byers
School of Social Welfare, University of Kansas, Lawrence, KS 66045, USA
e-mail: kaela@ku.edu

K. Ocasio
School of Social Work, Rutgers, The State University of New Jersey,
New Brunswick, NJ 08901, USA
e-mail: kocasio@ssw.rutgers.edu

© Springer International Publishing Switzerland 2015
D. Daro et al. (eds.), *Advances in Child Abuse Prevention Knowledge*,
Child Maltreatment 5, DOI 10.1007/978-3-319-16327-7_9

and child development, concrete support in times of need, and social and emotional competence of children.

Strategies for Moving Forward

- Foster partnerships with parents and parent organizations to increase opportunities to promote protective factors through all parenting improvement and parent support programs.
- Use professional development and training opportunities to increase a shared approach, set of goals, language, and knowledge base across disciplines around this topic.
- Coordinate and integrate efforts across all stakeholders.

Implications for Research

- Expand use of community-based participatory research to enhance the evidence base for resilience-focused prevention efforts.
- Develop research strategies that examine the extent to which programs implement a positive, promotional approach to better describe what these concepts look like in practice.
- Evaluate the impact of policy initiatives to promote protective factors and strengthening resilience in preventing child maltreatment.
- Conduct longitudinal research to identify the conditions most conducive to creating and sustaining protective factors and promoting resilience.

Introduction

Protective factors are qualities of individuals and conditions in families and communities that serve to preserve and promote child and family well-being. Protective factors can be external—such as access to needed informal supports and community resources—or internal—such as interpersonal coping strategies that allow parents to parent effectively, even—and especially—when confronted with stress and adversity. Protective factors function as buffers, mitigating risk for child abuse and neglect and promoting resilience. Resilience is the ability to successfully and positively adapt to "challenging or threatening circumstances" (Yates and Masten 2004, p. 522). Even when exposed to significant adversity, resilient parents avoid negative behaviors toward their children and children can demonstrate healthy development (see, for example, Luthans and Jensen 2005; Luthans and Youssef 2004; Luthans et al. 2007). The concept of resilience also can be embedded in groups of individuals and community contexts. Across fields and disciplines, protective factors and resilience—and strategies for achieving them—are topics of considerable and growing interest.

In this chapter, we draw on literature from within and beyond the field of child maltreatment to present findings that can inform prevention efforts. We begin by exploring the emergence of a focus on protective factors and resilience in general and discussing the growing evidence of the concept's importance for child maltreatment prevention. We then present several examples of innovative programming and research efforts that specifically focus on strengthening families by promoting protective factors and enhancing resilience. We conclude with a discussion of how these types of promotional approaches can be taken to scale and highlight research and policy initiatives with the potential to inform program planning.

Interest in Protective Factors and Resilience

There is growing evidence to support the existence of protective factors that moderate the negative effects of exposure to risk (Pollard et al. 1999). Beginning with investigations of mental illness and extending to investigations of other stressors, including child maltreatment, researchers have attempted to understand why some individuals adapt better under adverse conditions than others (Cicchetti and Garmezy 1993; Luthar et al. 2000). In contrast to an earlier, more singular emphasis on risk factors, symptoms, pathology, and maladaptive outcomes (Luthar et al. 2000; Masten and Powell 2003), in recent decades researchers and practitioners have begun to shift away from a deficit-based approach toward holistic models of prevention and intervention that include attention to strengths (Trout et al. 2003).

One example of this increased interest in strengths-based approaches is the emerging science of positive psychology. Launched in 1998 by Martin Seligman as one of his initiatives as president of the American Psychological Association, positive psychology is the scientific study of well-being and optimal human functioning (Seligman and Csikszentmihalyi 2000). Since its inception, positive psychology has drawn together previously disparate lines of research (e.g., resilience research and research focused on positive emotions) and created momentum for well-being research to expand exponentially. A search of the PsychINFO database conducted in January 2011 for peer-reviewed journal articles between 1900 and 2011 with the keyword "well-being" yielded a total of 24,369 articles. Only 2,935 of these articles were published prior to 1998 (see Mitchell et al. 2010). Positive psychology research has yielded persuasive evidence that techniques that build positive traits and positive subjective experiences can be effective in prevention efforts (Seligman et al. 1999). By identifying distal buffers, such as personal strengths and social connections, the application of positive psychology techniques represents an untapped and potentially powerful tool in improving outcomes at the individual and population levels (Keyes and Lopez 2002). These conclusions are borne out empirically in the realm of child maltreatment. As reported by Daro and Cohn-Donnelly (2002), efforts to provide support and education to build the strengths of new parents have demonstrated more promising results (Baker et al. 1999; Daro 1988, 1993; Carter and Harvey 1996; Wolfe 1994) than efforts to intervene to reduce negative behaviors of abusive or neglectful parents (Daro and Cohn 1988).

Beginning in 2001, the Center for the Study of Social Policy (CSSP) set out to examine the evidence and develop a framework for building strengths within families as a means to prevent child abuse and neglect (Horton 2011). This effort emerged from recognition that families are often resistant to programs and services that target them as being "at risk." A framework that defines the service relationship as a "partnership" with families and targets the promotion of resilience offers an important new approach to prevention and presents supportive services in a manner more acceptable to potential participants.

In defining its framework, CSSP identified five evidence-based protective factors for individuals that are linked to a lower incidence of child abuse and neglect, based on its review of extant research (see Horton 2011). These factors include parental resilience, social connections, knowledge of parenting and child development, concrete support in times of need, and social and emotional competence of children. Building on the work of CSSP, the Administration on Children, Youth & Families (ACYF) within the US Department of Health & Human Services commissioned a comprehensive literature review of protective factors associated with children who have already experienced abuse or neglect (i.e., considered "in-risk," such as those targeted by ACYF programs and policies). The aim of the literature review was to develop a theoretical framework that could be applied to ACYF-funded programs (see http://www.dsgonline.com/ACYF). The review discerned multiple variables at the individual, relationship, and community levels—many of which overlap with those detected by CSSP—with moderate to strong evidence of protecting children who have experienced maltreatment from negative outcomes. For example, factors with the strongest evidence for their protective function include self-regulation, relational and problem solving skills, parenting competence and parent or caregiver well-being, positive peer relationships, and a stable living situation. However, it is important to consider that our review found that much of the evidence on the impact of these factors has been limited to adolescence; much less is known about how protective factors function with children at other developmental stages.

After developing a new conceptual framework for the prevention of child abuse and neglect, CSSP sought to apply and test the framework. Seven states piloted the model, each attempting to enhance policies and practices by emphasizing parent engagement and collaboration across service sectors such as early childhood and child protective services (Daro and Dodge 2009). Among the strategies employed for engaging parents was the introduction of "Parent Cafés," structured small group conversations in which parents come together to share their concerns and ideas about how to prevent child maltreatment and promote child well-being. At the Parent Cafés, parents are welcomed as part of the "team" seeking to promote healthy outcomes for children and families in their communities. CSSP identified several core elements of cafés that promote building protective factors and leadership among parents, including: bringing parents and other community members together to foster positive relationships and strengthen families and communities; maintaining a safe, welcoming, and respectful environment that encourages diverse viewpoints and meaningful conversations in both large and small groups; eliciting, sharing, and recording the group's ideas and insights; allowing parents to serve as primary participants, organizers, hosts, and leaders; and training parent hosts in the Protective Factors framework and the café approach (Center for the Study of Social Policy 2014). A recent evaluation conducted by Be Strong Families/Strengthening Families Illinois that included over 4,000 parent café participants indicated that over 85 % of participants who responded reported greater awareness and knowledge of protective factors after participating in a café experience, and almost all participants found the café helpful (99 %), planned to attend a future café (97 %), and would recommend the café experience to a friend or family member (98 %) (Be Strong Families 2014).

Through partnerships with early care and education centers, CSSP sought to embed the Protective Factors framework within existing "primary supports," augmenting children's services with direct support for parents (Daro and Dodge 2009). Following a two-year pilot phase (2005–2007), CSSP launched the Strengthening Families National Network, which has grown to include 40 states, each implementing the protective factors approach in its own way, often within sectors including early childhood, home visiting, and child welfare, and often with a host of partner organizations, such as the United Way (see http://www.cssp.org/reform/strengthening-families/). The next section of this chapter will examine protective factors in greater detail and discuss the extension of the protective factors/resilience perspective from individuals to families and communities.

Evidence Supporting Protective Factors

Parental Resilience

Parental resilience is the ability of parents to cope with stresses and continue to parent effectively. There are multiple components of parental resilience, including the parent's developmental history and mental health. Parents with strong emotional skills play an important role in protecting potential victims of child abuse and neglect from negative outcomes (Administration on Children, Youth and Families 2013). Indeed, research suggests that the most influential component may be the capacity to be empathetic to oneself and to others, including the capacity for attunement to the child's perspective and needs (Egeland et al. 2002; Fraiberg et al. 1975). Other key factors that contribute to the resilience of parents include flexibility, use of social support, high expectations, self-efficacy, and self-esteem (Earvolino-Ramirez 2007; Luthar 2006). While multiple, chronic stressors may undermine parental resilience, research suggests that internal resources such as flexibility and self-esteem can mitigate the effects of exposure to stress and support continued effective parenting.

Social Connections

The network of people—family, friends, neighbors, and coworkers—that families can turn to in times of need for emotional and practical support are considered social connections. Whereas feelings of isolation and the absence of a support network is linked to greater risk of child abuse and neglect, the presence of a reliably supportive social network has long been recognized as a protective factor (see, for example, Kempe 1977). Similarly, the ACYF literature review (2013) identified relationships with, and support from, positive peers as an important source of protection from substance use, antisocial behavior, and suicide for children who have already experienced abuse or neglect. Involvement in positive activities, particularly within the school environment, also was identified as a key source of protection.

Prevention and intervention programs have identified social connections as a modifiable protective factor and have sought to reduce the social isolation of vulnerable families and increase positive social connections within the community. Importantly, research has established that *quality*, and not simply *quantity*, of social connections determines the capacity of social connections to serve as a protective factor against maltreatment (Beeman 1997). The ability to increase positive social connections has been documented as an outcome in at least one home visiting program (e.g., Nurse Family Partnership, see Olds et al. 1986, 1994, 1997). Increasing the positive social connections of families can contribute to increased "social capital," or an enhanced environment of social support, connection, and civic engagement across the community. Increased social capital has been associated with reduced risk of neglectful and psychologically harsh parenting (Zolotor and Runyan 2006).

Knowledge of Parenting and Child Development

Children thrive when parents understand and can provide caregiving to facilitate healthy development (Shonkoff and Phillips 2000). This includes balancing rules and structure with warmth and caring, and having the capacity to adapt parenting in developmentally-sensitive ways. Indeed, parenting competence, such as parents' use of consistent discipline practices and establishment of clear expectations about children's behavior, is strongly related to an array of more positive outcomes for children who have been victims of abuse and neglect (ACYF 2013). Efforts to increase knowledge about parenting and child development as a means of strengthening families and preventing maltreatment have taken many forms. Research on a range of parent education programs has identified some key characteristics of effective programs. Programs have been most successful when services are available for an extended period of time, when programs and providers are culturally sensitive, when participation offers a supportive community of peers in similar life circumstances, and when the quality of relationships between and among parents and providers is recognized as important for facilitating learning (Carter and Harvey 1996; Daro 2002; Hoelting et al. 1996; Reppucci et al. 1997).

Concrete Supports in Times of Need

Another important protective factor is sufficient income and access to necessary material resources. There is widespread agreement that helping families access needed material resources (i.e., food, clothing, housing, and transportation) is an essential and promising strategy for preventing maltreatment. For example, Cancian et al. (2010) manipulated a random assignment experiment to generate differences in family income in order to measure the effect of income on the risk of maltreatment reported to the child welfare system. They found that increasing income—through the provision of additional child support—reduced the risk of child maltreatment. Conversely, poverty is the risk factor most strongly correlated with child maltreatment, and the association between poverty and child maltreatment has been repeatedly demonstrated in the literature (e.g., Drake and Pandey 1996; Sedlak and Broadhurst 1996; Sedlak et al. 2010; Trickett et al. 1991).

Social and Emotional Competence of Children

Children's social and emotional competence—or the development of skills, such as communication skills, that provide the foundation for strong relationships—can be considered a protective factor against maltreatment because difficult child behaviors can contribute to a spiral of negative parent–child interactions (Ammerman 1991; Shonkoff and Phillips 2000). Children's behaviors are not a cause of maltreatment, but can be a "red flag" and suggest the need for family-focused intervention. Among children who have already experienced maltreatment, interpersonal skills such as the ability to self-regulate emotions and thought processes are strongly linked to reductions in psychopathology, fewer disruptions in out-of-home placements, and overall social and emotional well-being (ACYF 2013). Supporting children's early social-emotional competence may thus prevent direct harm or mitigate harm incurred to a child's development. Social competence, problem solving, autonomy, and sense of future and purpose have all been found to promote resilience in children (Benard 1991; Berndt and Ladd 1989; Garmezy 1974; Masten 1989; Werner and Smith 1989).

Nurturing and Attachment

The experience of a nurturing relationship with one or more parents or caregivers provides a context within which children learn to relate to others and within which children's development unfolds. These bonds influence the child's early behavior and development as well as outcomes across the lifecourse. The Safe, Stable, and Nurturing Relationships and Environments framework (Centers for Disease Control and Prevention 2013) holds that the parent–child relationship is a key factor in the promotion of health and well-being of all children. When children are provided with relationships characterized by safety (i.e., no physical or psychological harm), stability (i.e., predictability and consistency), and nurturance (i.e., sensitive and consistent response from a caregiver), health and well-being can be optimized and the risk of child maltreatment can be reduced. At the same time, the environments in which children live must also be characterized by safety, stability, and nurturance. When child maltreatment occurs, the health promoting function of the parent–child relationship is disrupted and places the child at risk for maladaptive outcomes. The Safe, Stable, and Nurturing Relationships and Environments framework is a form of primary prevention in that it attempts to build protection before maltreatment occurs. That is not to suggest that protection cannot be built or fostered for children who have already experienced abuse. Indeed, the development of safe, stable, and nurturing relationships within and outside the family system can be integral in fostering resilience for children who experience maltreatment.

Processes of nurturing and attachment have been the targets of numerous interventions to enhance positive parenting and strengthen early parent–child relationships (see, e.g., Lieberman et al. 2006; Marvin et al. 2002; Slade et al. 2005). A review of meta-analyses of interventions targeting parental sensitivity, child attachment security, or both concluded that short-term, targeted, behavioral interventions are more effective in addressing these targets than long-term, broadband approaches (van Ijzendoorn et al. 2005). Factors such as warm relationships with a partner, sibling, mother, and father relationships, positive communication, and relationship satisfaction have all been identified as serving a protective function (Conger et al. 2013; Herrenkohl et al. 2013; Jaffee et al. 2013; Thornberry et al. 2013). Additional research is needed to more clearly understand the specific aspects of relationships (i.e., safety, stability, nurturance) that may serve a protective function. At the same time, defining and understanding the role of safe, stable, and nurturing environments provides promise for creating contexts in which children can thrive.

Protective Factors and Resilience at the Level of Families and Communities

The ACYF-sponsored research review to inform the development of a protective factors framework identified protective factors at the levels of family and community (http://www.dsgonline.com/ACYF). At the family level, factors include caring adults, positive relationships, and social connections. At the community level, factors include community social and economic resources and opportunities, available services, and school characteristics and environment. Several authors have applied the concept of resilience to the ability of the family and community systems to minimize the negative consequences of adversity. For example, Walsh (1998) identified three sets of factors that promote family resilience: family belief systems, organizational patterns, and communication processes. Walsh further specified that "resilient families are typically oriented towards making meaning out of adversity, maintaining a positive outlook on life, and being grounded in some set of transcendent or spiritual beliefs." Other researchers have identified collaborative goal setting and problem solving, strong relationships, emotion regulation, and stress management skills as important contributors to family resilience (Saltzman et al. 2011; Simon et al. 2005).

In the field of national security, including national health security, there is a growing emphasis on community resilience (Obama 2010; U.S. Department of Health & Human Services 2009; U.S. Department of Homeland Security 2010) as a strategy to help communities, as independent entities, "withstand and recover from adversity (e.g., economic stress, influenza pandemic, man-made or natural disasters)" (RAND Corporation 2011, p. 1). This concept of community resilience can be usefully applied to the realm of child maltreatment to reflect the substantial need for communities that are "prepared for, protected from, and able to respond to and recover from" incidents of maltreatment (RAND Corporation 2011, p. 1).

Building resilience at the community level encompasses the development and enhancement of resources and supports that individuals and families can utilize when they encounter stressful situations and challenges. In some communities, community-level strategies to prevent child abuse and neglect have included efforts to inculcate a belief in collective responsibility to protect children from harm and to expand supports and services available to families (Schobera et al. 2012; Zielinski and Bradshaw 2006).

The Centers for Disease Control and Prevention developed the Essentials for Childhood framework to guide state and local efforts to promote healthy relationships for all children and families. The framework incorporates four integrated goals that, when addressed on a macro scale, can facilitate the promotion of safe, stable, and nurturing relationships at the community and state level (Centers for Disease Control and Prevention 2013). The framework embodies four primary goals:

- to raise community awareness and commitment to promote safe, stable, and nurturing relationships and to prevent child abuse and neglect;
- to use data to inform prevention programming decisions;
- to create the context for healthy children and families through norms change and programs; and
- to create the context for healthy children and families through policy and legislation.

Figure 9.1 provides greater detail on each of these goals.

By addressing the conditions and contexts in which children develop, the Essentials for Childhood framework seeks to promote population-based health and well-being for all children and families, not just those at high-risk for child abuse and neglect. By addressing the contexts in which all children develop, community supports may be enhanced for those children who are recovering from the experience of abuse or neglect.

Goal 1: To raise community awareness and commitment to promote safe, stable, and nurturing relationships and to prevent child abuse and neglect

Building community awareness and support for child maltreatment prevention requires communities to establish a clear vision for local child maltreatment prevention and to disseminate this vision across the community. In addition, support for child maltreatment prevention must also expand beyond the human services sector and must begin to engage with nontraditional partners. For example, developing collaborative relationships with the business sector may expand the reach and possibility for child maltreatment prevention at the community level.

Goal 2: To use data to inform prevention programming decisions

It is critical for communities to explore existing data sources (e.g., child welfare records, birth records, and emergency room records) to identify community needs and strengths and to develop new data collection strategies to fill current data gaps. Again, this goal requires cooperation and collaboration among agencies in the broader community to share resources and to partner in future data collection efforts.

Goal 3: To create the context for healthy children and families through norms change and programs

Currently, there is a great deal of stigma surrounding parenting programs for new parents. At times, families turn away needed services, not because the services are not wanted or valued, but because asking for help with child rearing is not an acceptable norm in our society. Addressing the stigma associated with help-seeking behavior is imperative if families are to be engaged in effective, evidence-based parenting programs. Further, the responsibility for creating supportive environments where children can thrive is not just the responsibility of parents. Everyone can help create safe, stable, and nurturing environments where children and families can succeed. From this perspective, when all children have the opportunity to succeed, all children benefit.

Goal 4: To create the context for healthy children and families through policy and legislation

Many policies already exist to support children and families and the identification of these policies is a crucial first step. Evaluation of current child and family policies allows communities to support effective streams of legislation and to identify the need for additional child and family policies in an effort to create the conditions and contexts for children and families to thrive.

Fig. 9.1 Essentials for childhood framework goals
Centers for Disease Control and Prevention

Summary

The Protective Factors framework developed by the CSSP has been widely adopted, and protective factors, along with risk factors, are central to the current prevention and intervention agenda of the Office on Child Abuse and Neglect (OCAN), situated within the U.S. Department of Health and Human Services Administration for Children and Families. In addition, the ACYF study of protective factors (2013) among children and youth who have already experienced abuse or neglect, and thus are considered "in-risk," provides a useful framework to improve and test interventions and enhance the well-being of those targeted by ACYF strategies. Research, practice, and policy increasingly focus on understanding and addressing the interactions between risk and protective factors within the complex contexts of families and communities. In the next section of this chapter we turn our focus to empirical investigations of programs that aim to promote protective factors and enhance individual and family resilience.

Programs Utilizing a Protective Factors Framework

Growing emphasis on promoting protective factors and strengthening resilience as a promising approach to prevent child abuse has necessitated the need for research to establish its efficacy. Careful and rigorous evaluations of practices and programs built around a protective factors framework are essential for ensuring that dissemination efforts and investment decisions focus on the most effective options (Prinz et al. 2009; Wald 2009). In the context of limited resources, stakeholders face questions about whether to invest in programs that intervene with at-risk populations or programs that promote protective factors for all families, and how to balance investment in treatment and investment in prevention (Wald 2009).

ACYF has identified several challenges faced by researchers and interventionists seeking to take a protective factors approach to promoting child well-being to scale (ACYF 2013). One of the limitations of research on protective factors to date is that many different definitions and measures of protective factors have been used across studies, making it difficult to integrate and generalize findings. Also, the relative strength of evidence supporting the effects of protective factors varies, and effect sizes have not been reported consistently. ACYF noted that individual- and family-level factors have received far greater attention than community-level factors, and little research has focused on specific mechanisms of change or the possible mediating, moderating, and cumulative effects of protective factors. In addition, research typically has not taken into account specific cultural- and gender-specific factors that may influence effects. ACYF encouraged researchers to develop and implement interventions that incorporate protective factors with a moderate-to-strong evidence base and test their effects; continue to conduct research on protective factors for which the evidence base is promising but not yet strong; evaluate the psychometric properties of instruments used to measure protective factors; and investigate interactions among protective factors across individual, relational, and community levels (Administration on Children, Youth and Families 2013).

In this section, we examine the potential of seven interventions or practice reforms that focus on strengthening protective factors and building participant resilience. Two of the interventions have been found to be effective in randomized clinical trials; five of the interventions are at earlier stages in their research. All of these efforts are focused on building family strengths and helping participants not merely survive, but thrive. The specific examples highlighted in this chapter represent efforts that one or more of the authors have direct experience in implementing or evaluating. As such, these programs may not be representative of the full range of interventions utilizing this framework.

Programs Subject to Recent Randomized Trials

Two of the interventions we examined have demonstrated an ability to strengthen positive parental behavior with two very different populations. The first, Minding the Baby, is an intensive home visiting intervention designed for first-time mothers and their infants in an urban community. The program builds upon and combines intervention components from other empirically supported early intervention programs, such as the Nurse-Family Partnership (Olds et al. 2007) and infant-parent psychotherapy (Lieberman et al. 1999). Its logic model is built on the premise that a multidisciplinary approach to intervention allows diverse goals to be targeted within a single, integrated program and that broader impacts can be achieved by drawing upon different professions to address families' multiple needs. Specifically, Minding the Baby uses the expertise of public health nurses to target health outcomes for mothers and children, as well as the specialized skills of mental health professionals to address parenting skills and attachment. This intervention directly targets first-time mothers' capacity for reflective functioning. Reflective functioning, or reflective parenting, is a parent's ability to engage in mentalization of her own and her baby's internal experiences, such as feelings, thoughts, and intentions, and understand her baby's behavior in the context of underlying mental states (Sadler et al. 2013).

Investigators at the Yale Child Study Center and the Yale School of Nursing recently conducted a pilot randomized controlled trial of the Minding the Baby intervention using data from 105 families attending prenatal care groups at an urban community health center. The intervention group also received intensive home visiting services (Sadler et al. 2013). Despite relatively small sample sizes and high attrition levels, some encouraging results were found in this pilot investigation. With respect to health outcomes, families in the intervention group were more likely to be on track with well-child visits and immunizations at when their child was 12 months old. Intervention group mothers were significantly less likely to have experienced rapid subsequent childbearing than control group mothers. There also was a trend toward fewer referrals to child protective services for families in the intervention group. With respect to parent–child relationship outcomes, there were promising indications of program effects, including a significantly higher percentage of securely attached children and a significantly lower percentage of disorganized attachment among intervention dyads than control dyads. Mothers in the intervention group who had very low scores on the initial reflective functioning measure during pregnancy also experienced significant improvement in reflective functioning.

The second program, the Mothers and Toddlers Program (MTP), is an individual psychotherapy intervention designed as an adjunct intervention for mothers receiving outpatient substance abuse treatment and raising a young child. MTP is an attachment-based parenting intervention designed to enhance parent–child relationships by improving maternal reflective functioning and the quality of the mother's mental representations of the child (e.g., being flexible and balanced as opposed to inflexible and distorted). Researchers at Yale University School of Medicine recently reported the results of a pilot study involving 47 mothers who were enrolled in substance abuse treatment and caring for a child aged birth to 3 years (Suchman et al. 2010, 2011). Mothers were randomly assigned to participate in 12 weekly sessions of MTP or a comparison parenting education intervention. This pilot study found that mothers in the MTP intervention group achieved significantly higher reflective functioning abilities, greater sensitivity and coherence in the mental representations of their children, and higher levels of reflective functioning than mothers in the comparison group. In addition, higher levels of reflective functioning and higher quality of mental representations corresponded with improved caregiving behaviors following treatment.

Findings from pilot studies of both Minding the Baby and MTP indicate that strengths-focused interventions that directly target parenting capacities like reflective functioning and mental representations of the child. Improving these capacities can influence parent–child attachment and caregiving behaviors in ways that suggest a reduced risk for child maltreatment. It is anticipated that larger randomized controlled trials of these interventions will be conducted and they will be useful to confirm whether program effects are robust beyond the specific samples involved in the pilot studies.

Promising Strategies for Building Resilience

While embracing many of the characteristics embedded in the programs we just discussed, two of the interventions we reviewed are at earlier stages of examining their efficacy and effectiveness with respect to documenting their impact on resilience. Like Minding the Baby and MTP, the Circle of Security Parenting (COS) protocol focuses on promoting resilience by enhancing the ability of caregivers to think of their children as psychological agents and to understand their children's behavior in terms of underlying mental states (e.g., beliefs, feelings, intentions, thoughts, etc.)—that is, reflective functioning (Sharp and Fonagy 2008). Many programs that focus on strengthening family resilience by enhancing parent education and improving parent–child relationships can be time consuming and expensive. Moreover, many require a professional facilitator, which reduces the number of individuals qualified to deliver services. An alternative program that could potentially reach a greater number of parents is the DVD version of the Circle of Security Parenting program, which is based on a much longer and more intensive original program (Hoffman et al. 2006; Marvin et al. 2002).

The original 20-week Circle of Security program was created to promote parental resilience among high-risk parents by teaching parents basic attachment theory (Marvin et al. 2002; Powell et al. 2009). Teaching parents attachment theory improves their ability to reflect on children's behaviors in terms of underlying physical and emotional needs. In turn, their enhanced reflective functioning is expected to help them better, or more sensitively, meet their children's attachment needs. Indeed, the program has a growing evidence base that supports its potential to improve parent–child relationships and enhance the child's attachment security (Cassidy et al. 2010; Hoffman et al. 2006; Marvin et al. 2002).

In order to broaden the scope of parents the program could reach, the originators removed the use of personal video vignettes. They also modified the program to be an 8-week protocol utilizing an educational DVD, in an effort to make the intervention more accessible and available to more caregivers. The program consists of weekly sessions guided by the DVD and, like the original program, is conducted with groups of five to eight members (Hoffman et al. 2006; Marvin et al. 2002). Unlike the original COS, individuals who are not necessarily professionals but have been trained in the protocol facilitate the groups as guided by the manual, significantly increasing program availability.

Despite the less intensive, 8-week DVD program's potential to reach a large audience, rigorous studies have yet to investigate the program's effectiveness, particularly with at-risk samples. Currently, research is underway to examine the program's influence on various caregiver relational capacities, such as reflective functioning, strategies for coping with children's negative emotions, and other indicators of parent–child relationship quality (see, for example, Rostad 2014).

The second promising intervention we examined focuses specifically on military families. Forty-four percent of US service members are parents, and 37 % of the nearly two million American children who have at least one parent serving in the military are under 6 years of age (U.S. Department of Defense 2011). Children and families cycle through deployments with service members. Deployed and nondeployed parents report high levels of parenting stress during and after deployment (Bender 2008; Lincoln et al. 2008). Reunification, while often eagerly anticipated, also poses challenges for families, including the normative tasks of reestablishing relationships, roles, and routines, as well as potentially needing to accommodate physical or psychological wounds. Military families with young children face the added challenge of negotiating separations and reunions that take place during significant periods of the child's early development.

The steep rise in rates of child abuse, divorce, and suicide during and following deployment speaks clearly to the need for support for military families at these times (Gibbs et al. 2007; Goff et al. 2007). Responding to this need, STRoNG Military Families (Support To Restore, Repair, Nurture, and Grow Military Families) is a brief, tailored, group intervention to enhance positive parenting among military families with young children and strengthen the resilience of military families. The intervention integrates parent education with specific attention to the experiences of military families with young children, opportunities for supported parent–child interaction to enhance positive parenting, an introduction to self-care and stress reduction techniques to reduce mental health symptoms, a group context to increase social support, and individualized referrals to enhance connection to resources.

This novel intervention (see http://m-span.org/programs-for-military-families/strong-families/) is adapted from an existing civilian parenting program that was carefully modified in order to reflect and address concerns common to military family experience (LePlatte et al. 2012). There is an emphasis on meeting the unique needs of National Guard and Reserve members, who are more likely to experience isolation and lack of needed supports (Chandra et al. 2010). A NICHD-funded Phase 2 randomized controlled trial (PI: Rosenblum) to evaluate efficacy of the intervention for improving positive parenting and parent mental health currently is underway.

Biodevelopmental Approaches to Build Resilience

Recent developments in neurobiology establishing links between early childhood adversity and brain functioning, as well as the improved ability to measure these effects due to technological innovation, have substantial implications for implementing protective factor and resilience approaches in early childhood. Two areas of particular relevance are intervention and screening. Attachment and Biobehavioral Catch-Up (ABC) is one example of a well-established biodevelopmental intervention that integrates both neurobiological functioning as well as a protective factor framework to promote child resilience in response to adverse environmental conditions (Bernard et al. 2012; Dozier et al. 2006, 2008).

ABC is a 10-week, manualized intervention that has been shown in repeated randomized trials to strengthen protective factors of attachment and sensitive parenting. It also regulates child stress hormones and provides immediate buffering protection against the negative effects of environmental stressors (see Chap. 7 for a more detailed discussion of the ABC's implementation framework). Results of randomized controlled trials with infants and toddlers in foster care have demonstrated improvement in neuroendocrinological regulation of stress, higher rates of secure attachment, fewer behavioral problems, and less avoidant behavior among ABC treatment group children versus the control group (Bernard et al. 2012; Dozier et al. 2006, 2008, 2009). Buffering the effects of adversity supports positive development of the child's regulatory system, thus promoting positive long-term social-emotional development for the child, which in turn protects against future child maltreatment (Institute of Medicine and National Research Council 2014).

Building on ABC's strong evidence base, a research project currently is underway integrating the use of ABC into Early Head Start services (Byers et al. 2013). The purpose of this new research is to test the effects of this well-established intervention in a new service setting with children experiencing a range of types of adversity. It is an effort to promote healthy social-emotional development and to build capacity for strengthening protection for children who may be at increased risk neurobiologically due to their exposure to adversity. The hope is to build this capacity prior to the development of symptoms of social-emotional disruption.

In addition to intervention, another area in which neurobiological advancements can enhance the use of protective factor frameworks is screening for the purposes of early identification. Toxic stress is the result of prolonged stressors such as abuse, neglect, maternal depression, and poverty that chronically activate the body's stress response system in the absence of a stable and responsive adult who can offer buffering protection to the child (National Scientific Council on the Developing Child 2005; Shonkoff 2010; Shonkoff and Garner 2012). While toxic stress has been found to arise from multiple environmental risk factors and may cause immediate and measurable physiological changes, there has not been an easy method available for early screening to adequately intervene before biological changes take place that negatively impact the child's long-term trajectory.

In addition to examining the effects of ABC in an early childhood intervention setting, ongoing research also seeks to develop and neurobiologically validate a screening instrument for early identification of toxic stress risk and protective factors (Byers et al. 2013). The purpose of this research is to examine the interactive and cumulative effects of risk and protective factors and ensure that enhanced services that specifically strengthen physiological coping and resilience—such as ABC—are effectively targeted to children experiencing the greatest need.

Statewide Approaches to Address Emergent Needs and Promote Longer-Term Protective Factors

Community-based supports to strengthen families and prevent abuse and neglect have been gaining in popularity since the 1990s. At that time, child protection systems were under fire for failing to protect children in their care; there was a call for community-based prevention alternatives (Kosanovich et al. 2005; Schorr 2000). Family resource and support centers and differential responses to child maltreatment reports are two approaches developed to provide flexible supports to families through community-based organizations. In the section below, we discuss research examining protective factors associated with both of these approaches, which are currently being implemented in two states.

Since 2005, the development of family resource and support centers has been an important component of New Jersey's child welfare response. Family success centers serve as neighborhood-based gathering places where families can come to both receive and give support. A primary goal of these centers is to provide an array of services to promote several protective factors, including the provision of concrete supports, fostering social connections and deepening parenting resilience, improving parenting knowledge, and fostering child and youth development (New Jersey Department of Children and Families 2011). All services are intended to be voluntary and flexibly tailored to the needs of families and communities. Family support principles (see Everett et al. 2007) are employed in the engagement approach, with families playing an active role in identifying their needs and goals and selecting specific service options. Further, parent- and community-led advisory boards are used to identify and incorporate community strengths and needs into the overall planning of the centers (New Jersey Department of Children and Families 2011).

One of the challenges the centers have faced is engaging families at highest risk in fully participating in the center's strengths promotional activities, such as life and parenting skills workshops. While the centers can refer families with acute resource needs to other service providers designed to address these needs, the centers themselves are primarily focused on engaging families in activities to promote strengths that can buffer the negative effects of poverty (Ocasio n.d.). While providing families with immediate relief is an important activity, if the centers fail to engage participants in those activities intended to increase protective factors, their goal has been only partially realized. Specifically, a center could become so focused on meeting the concrete needs in a community that they might lose sight of their other goals. To protect against this outcome, the New Jersey Department of Children and Families is developing a logic model, self-study tool, and outcome measures to assist centers in focusing on their primary intended goals and to ensure that centers are aware they are not to engage in case management and other more intensive individualized services.

Research on the implementation of the family success centers is ongoing, with the goal of better understanding predictors for family engagement and implementation variation across the state (Ocasio n.d.). This research will provide insight into the characteristics and prior experiences of families seeking assistance from the center to better understand what predicts initial engagement and consistent service use. In addition to examining participant characteristics, this research also will focus on how the history of the community organizations implementing these centers (new versus established agencies) impacts the specific services offered and the extent to which the protective factors framework is fully embraced.

North Carolina is another state with a recently developed program to provide flexible supports to families. In an effort to improve child welfare outcomes and reduce subsequent reports of child maltreatment, North Carolina began implementing a dual track response system to respond to child abuse reports in 2002 (North Carolina Department of Health and Human Services 2003). With this system, reports were placed on either a traditional investigative track for more severe abuse allegations or cases that might require court involvement, or a new family assessment track designed to help stabilize high-risk families and address a broad range of needs that might interfere with effective parenting. Similar to the process adopted in many other states, the use of a family assessment process focuses on building upon families' existing strengths and support systems while engaging families in community services and resources that could enhance parents' abilities to care for their children safely, thereby reducing risks for future maltreatment (Casey Family Programs 2012). Evaluation studies have found program effects on reducing recurrence of maltreatment (Center for Child and Family Policy 2009; Lawrence et al. 2011). However, these studies do not address whether differential response policies enhance children's adaptive functioning, or resilience, following the experience of maltreatment.

A current study uses state birth records, maltreatment reports, and educational data to investigate whether North Carolina's strengths-based family assessment approach to intervening with at-risk children and families reported to child protective services promotes long-term resilient outcomes in maltreated children's academic and behavioral functioning (McCourt 2013). This study also investigates whether North Carolina's financial investments in increasing access to quality child care, health care, parenting supports, and other community services for children between the ages of 0 and 5 years old and their families through the Smart Start program, and improving school readiness among disadvantaged preschool children through the More at Four program, promotes maltreated children's academic and behavioral resilience. While existing evidence suggests these programs have the potential to improve the educational preparedness and academic outcomes of young children (e.g., Bryant et al. 2002, 2003; Ladd et al. 2014; Peisner-Feinberg and Schaaf 2010), evaluation studies generally have not addressed whether these broad-based community programs can enhance the adaptive functioning of children who experience maltreatment. However, these children are likely to be at particular risk for academic difficulties and school failure.

Challenges and Future Directions

The previous section highlighted emerging research on interventions designed to promote protective factors and foster resilience, including interventions being studied by this chapter's authors and other exemplary programs. In this section, we describe efforts to scale up successful programs, highlight a research design that holds promise for expanding the evidence base for implementing strengths-based practice on multiple ecological levels, and provide an example of a state policy initiative using a strengths-based approach to child maltreatment prevention.

Taking Efforts to Scale for Population Level Change

The wide scope of the promising interventions described in this chapter highlights the complexity involved in addressing child maltreatment prevention on a population level. Large-scale, strengths-based prevention efforts may require promoting protective factors and resilience across multiple domains of family functioning simultaneously. The broad range of protective factors found to strengthen families and promote child well-being reflect the varied and complex needs and competencies of families; the quality of parent–child, family, and greater community relationships; and access to material resources and concrete supports. This broad array of protective factors suggests that multiple strategies will be needed to promote resilience across domains. For example, one type of strategy may be effective in supporting parents' reflective functioning and capacity for sensitive and responsive parenting, which in turn can enhance the social and emotional competence of their children. A different approach is likely required to target family needs in the areas of employment, housing, and access to health care and social services. Yet another type of intervention may be needed to build communities that support parents and take collective responsibility for preventing maltreatment of the communities' children. Devising a comprehensive prevention program that addresses all domains of protective factors within a single family or community is likely to pose a substantial challenge.

Large-scale interventions will also likely need to engage and intervene with families situated within divergent contexts, such as urban and rural communities, military and civilian settings, and varied racial, ethnic, and cultural communities. Families themselves are widely diverse in composition, in ways such as having children at different developmental stages and one or more parents being of disparate backgrounds and parenting experiences. The diversity of families and communities intended to be reached and served through large-scale prevention efforts means that agencies, service providers, and community organizations may need to find many different ways of making initial contact with families and adopt varied and flexible means for sustaining or re-engaging families' involvement with prevention efforts. Multidisciplinary collaborations across agencies and organizations with a unified agenda to prevent child maltreatment and promote child well-being present one potential strategy for extending prevention efforts to a diverse range of families and communities, though there are likely to be logistical challenges involved in coordinating disparate intervention strategies and partnering with others from different fields.

Community-Based Participatory Research

One promising strategy for enhancing the evidence base for resilience-focused prevention efforts and supporting multidisciplinary collaboration across stakeholders is to adopt a community-based participatory research approach. There is growing interest among public health and social policy researchers in this research strategy, in which multiple stakeholders are included as collaborators at all stages of the research process (Minkler and Wallerstein 2008). Community-based participatory research provides opportunities for creating synergistic partnerships that recognize the complementary strengths and contributions of all partners. These partnerships draw equally upon the expertise of researchers in academic theory and empirical methodology as well as the practical knowledge and experience of community-based stakeholders (Cargo and Mercer 2008). The National Institutes of Health have provided support for this research approach through multiple funding and training initiatives across NIH components, and the Centers for Disease Control and multiple private foundations also have provided substantial funding (Mercer and Green 2008). The Institute of Medicine has described the community-based participatory research approach as:

> epidemiology enriched by contemporary social and behavioral science because it incorporates what we have learned about community processes and engagement, and the complex nature of interventions with epidemiology, in order to understand how the multiple determinants of health interact to influence health in a particular community (Gebbie et al. 2003, p. 7).

Adopting a community-based participatory research approach increases the likelihood that research activities target issues that are prioritized and valued by the community. This approach also provides community stakeholders with opportunities to serve as important partners in improving a community's capacity to implement system-wide changes that can improve public health outcomes. The collaborative process inherent in this approach could lead to the development of better-informed research aims and hypotheses, more effective intervention strategies, more precise and coherent translation of research results into policy and practice, and better fidelity and flexibility in implementing empirically-based interventions at a community level. In light of these benefits, community-based participatory research holds promise for bridging communication and cultural gaps between multidisciplinary partners and incorporating the diverse knowledge and skills of multiple stakeholders into the program planning and evaluation process.

One example of community-based participatory research aimed at promoting children's well-being is the Healthy Families Network, a community-university partnership intended to advance prevention research and build community capacity to promote mental health among formerly homeless children and their families. These children are at risk for child maltreatment and other adverse outcomes (Gewirtz 2007). Collaborators in the Healthy Families Network include university researchers, 17 nonprofit supportive housing agencies, and a nonprofit housing intermediary in a large metropolitan area in the Midwest. Each year the supportive housing agencies within the Healthy Families Network work with an estimated 600 families with over 1,200 children, comprising an estimated 90 % of the formerly homeless families in the target metropolitan area.

The Healthy Families Network was executed in three phases over the course of several years as outlined in Fig. 9.2. Beginning with a series of general education and training efforts regarding evidence-based practice and continuing with research agenda setting and the implementation of multiple research projects, the Healthy Families Network provided multiple opportunities to engage a wide range of stakeholders in determining research priority questions and activities. An assessment of this process found improved knowledge and practice among providers, including an enhanced understanding of the role and usefulness of research- and evidence-based practice in community settings and a greater knowledge of child development and mental health. Researchers also reported having a greater appreciation of the skills and expertise of providers working directly with families and the external pressures experienced by provider agencies, such as financial constraints (Gewirtz 2007). Reported challenges included limitations on provider resources, such as difficulty providing sufficient coverage to enable staff to attend seminars, as well as high turnover and burnout rates among staff. Another challenge was the perception of research and its acceptance among provider partners. For example, providers raised concerns that collecting data beyond self-report measures, such as observational or biological data, may be intrusive for vulnerable families and that randomized controlled trials posed potential unfairness for families in the control group. To address concerns about perceived inequity of research, the Healthy Families Network researcher and provider partners engaged in extensive dialogue and collaboration to promote the shared goals that community-based research be perceived as empowering, reflect the needs of the community, and promote better outcomes for families through sustainable practices.

Phase 1: Community Educatio n

Phase 1 involved coordinating a monthly seminar series on children's mental health, providing knowledge and training about developmental psychopathology and evidence-based practice in children's mental health as well as an idea exchange between practitioners and researchers. Most participants reported finding the training informative and helpful, and many reported sharing seminar materials with other professionals.

Phase 2: Agenda Setting

Phase 2 involved building a collaborative research and practice agenda based on an assessment of the psychosocial status of the children and families in supportive housing and the resources and needs of providers to be able to address these concerns. Based on the needs assessment data, the researcher and provider partners created practice priorities for developing strategies to prevent behavior problems, provided supportive parenting, and increased access to mental health services, especially for trauma-related treatment. The partnership also resulted in the generation of research questions involving engaging families in mental health treatment and evaluating the feasibility of and fidelity in implementing evidence-based practices.

Phase 3: Program Implementation and Assessment

Phase 3 involved adapting and implementing programs to address these practice priorities, including providing trauma-focused interventions, such as trauma-focused cognitive behavioral therapy; piloting a feasibility trial of Parenting Through Change (PTC), a parent group therapy program aimed at preventing conduct problems; and conducting a randomized effectiveness trial of the Early Risers Skills for Success program, a multicomponent program for preventing conduct problems involving child programming, parent programming, and family support and case management. This program provided a continuum of care anchored in a supportive housing community to use community partnerships to promote child well-being and strengthen protective processes such as social and peer competence, intellectual skills, and effective parenting (Masten 2001; Masten and Gewirtz 2006).

Fig. 9.2 Healthy families network
Implementation phases

Policy to Promote Protective Factors and Strengthen Resilience

As discussed above, the promotion of protective factors has considerable support from multiple organizations and federal agencies. However, much of the practice and research described in this chapter focuses on protective outcomes (i.e. resilience, social connections, and other outcomes) and not the extent to which a given program implements a protective factors or resilience approach. Research is needed to articulate what implementing a protective factors approach looks like in practice, how to determine the extent to which it is implemented, and what its contribution is to desired outcomes. Policy to support implementation also should be considered. For example, New Jersey adopted standards to guide practice with families and communities, explicitly mandating that parents should be treated as partners and that programs should use a strengths-based approach with families, in contrast to service planning based on clinical expertise and problem-oriented assessments (New Jersey Task Force on Child Abuse and Neglect 2013). The standards for prevention programs were developed by the Prevention Committee of the New Jersey Task Force on Child Abuse and Neglect in 2001 and were recently revised to incorporate new research, emerging best practice standards, and a progressive rubric that articulates the components of each level. These standards apply specifically to primary and secondary prevention efforts and guide state funding decisions. For example, agencies applying for funding from the New Jersey Children's Trust Fund support are required to address how their program meets various elements of the standards.

It should be acknowledged that implementation of a promotional approach may vary in different types of practice environments, since it will be applied in the context of the service setting. Therefore, characteristics related to training, approach, and focus of services will vary. For example, a treatment environment will undoubtedly focus considerable effort on addressing problems that have been identified and necessitated treatment. In this environment, focusing on protective factors is likely to be a secondary approach and problem-oriented language likely would be more common. Conversely, a nonclinical family support program might be designed primarily to promote protective factors and address risks as a secondary approach; in this environment, problem-oriented language is likely limited. Workers with experience or training in more clinically oriented practice may struggle to fully embrace this paradigm shift when working in a nonclinical family support environment. Adoption of a protective factor approach may require additional training for staff to build knowledge and capacity to apply the framework appropriately to their services and effectively integrate protective factors goals into traditional services.

Additionally, integration of a promotional approach into current service settings may require other administrative adjustments. Areas that may require attention include: examination and adaptation of assessment materials to ensure inclusion of strengths and protective factors; adjustment of eligibility criteria to improve access for both at-risk and in-risk clients; administrative adjustments, policy adjustments, or both to ensure services provided to families—rather than services restricted to one identified client—to promote family-level protective factors are billable; and integration into requirements for continuing education. Research is needed to assess the advantages and disadvantages to introducing a protective factors framework in diverse settings, to inform tailoring the framework to be better suited to a specific setting, to illuminate barriers to implementing a protective factors framework in diverse practice environments, and to identify strategies to reduce barriers.

Conclusion

The literature discussed in this chapter suggests a growing movement in support of approaches and programs that build protective factors and foster resilience. A focus on protective factors has expanded the scope of primary and secondary prevention of child maltreatment and introduced an important complement and counterpoint to a focus on individual, family, and community deficits. Key protective factors that have emerged include parental resilience, social connections, knowledge of parenting and child development, concrete support in times of need, and social and emotional competence of children.

Significant progress has been made in recent years in identifying and addressing the opportunity inherent in attending to child-, parent-, and family-level protective factors and resilience. Further work is needed to continue to advance the process of identifying the important elements of appropriate and effective prevention and intervention efforts to support children's optimal development and the well-being of families. In particular, research and development should be conducted to devise, implement, test, and improve community-level strategies. Establishing partnerships with parents, providing professional development for individuals that engage in the work of preventing child maltreatment and promoting well-being, and creating policies to promote and facilitate the adoption of a protective factors framework are recognized levers for change that are needed to further support this movement.

Reflections: Protective Factor Frameworks and Public Policy

Bryan Samuels
Chapin Hall at the University of Chicago, Chicago, IL, USA

The emergence of protective factor frameworks has been a significant boon for the field of child and family services. When, in 2003, the Center for the Study of Social Policy (CSSP) released its list of protective factors for strengthening families and preventing child abuse and neglect, it created a wave of momentum that helped drive a new focus on achieving positive outcomes instead of simply avoiding negative ones. The true genius of the CSSP study was the simplicity and directness of its message. Choosing to focus on five factors—parental resilience, social connections, concrete support in times of need, knowledge of parenting and child development, and social and emotional competence of children—the study gave policymakers and practitioners something accessible that could be easily transformed into powerful, targeted programs.

Now it is time that we in the child services community take the next steps towards improving these frameworks by refining our use of protective factors. Protective factors are not one-size-fits-all prescriptions to the problems facing vulnerable children and families. The literature makes clear that different problems faced by children and families may require different solutions. The original CSSP framework was intended to prevent child abuse and neglect, but for other problems or challenges—such as homeless youth—a different set of protective factors may be needed. During my time at the Administration on Children, Youth, and Families, we commissioned a report titled *Protective Factors for In-Risk Populations Served by the Administration on Children, Youth, and Families*. The report, released in 2013, showed a large variance in the evidence linking different protective factors to positive outcomes in the five populations on which the study focused. This indicated that customizing protective factor frameworks for different populations could lead to better outcomes.

But beyond simply identifying which factors apply to which populations, we also must continue to ensure that the factors we have chosen are indeed the correct ones, and that our decisions are backed up by scientific evidence. It is crucial that we take the current momentum we have built and use it to drive programs that are both effective and meticulously scrutinized. Our ACYF study followed this approach by identifying the strength of the evidence connecting each preventive factor to positive outcomes for our five targeted populations.

Protective factor frameworks should be recognized for the successes they have achieved. But they should also be seen as an opportunity, something to build upon by refining our methods and improving the quality and accuracy of our solutions. Each step we take towards crafting better-targeted and more scientifically rigorous programs is another step towards improving the lives of our country's children and their families.

References

Administration on Children, Youth and Families. (2013). *Protective factors for populations served by the Administration on Children, Youth, and Families: A literature review and theoretical framework*. Washington, DC: Author.

Ammerman, R. T. (1991). The role of the child in physical abuse: A reappraisal. *Violence and Victims, 6*(2), 87–101.

Baker, A. J. L., Piotrkowski, C. S., & Brooks-Gunn, J. (1999). The home instructional program for preschool youngsters (HIPPY). *The Future of Children, 9*(1), 116–133.

Be Strong Families. (2014). *Parent cafe results/impact*. Retrieved September 29, 2014, from http://www.bestrongfamilies.net/build-protective-factors/parent-cafes/parent-cafe-results-impact/

Beeman, S. K. (1997). Reconceptualizing social support and its relationship to neglect. *Social Service Review, 71*(3), 421–440.

Benard, B. (1991). *Fostering resiliency in kids: Protective factors in the family, school, and community*. Portland: Western Center for Drug-Free Schools and Communities.

Bender, E. (2008). APA survey documents extent of MH problems in military. *Psychiatric News, 43*(11), 2–37.

Bernard, K., Dozier, M., Bick, J., Lewis-Morrarty, E., Lindhiem, O., & Carlson, E. (2012). Enhancing attachment organization among maltreated children: Results of a randomized clinical trial. *Child Development, 83*(2), 623–636.

Berndt, T. J., & Ladd, G. W. (1989). *Peer relationships in child development*. New York: Wiley.

Bryant, D., Bernier, K., Peisner-Feinberg, E., & Maxwell, K. (2002). *Smart start and child care in North Carolina: Effects on quality and changes over time*. Chapel Hill: University of North Carolina, FPG Child Development Institute.

Bryant, D., Maxwell, K., Taylor, K., Poe, M., Peisner-Feinberg, E., & Bernier, K. (2003). *Smart start and preschool child care quality in North Carolina: Change over time and relation to children's readiness*. Chapel Hill: University of North Carolina, FPG Child Development Institute.

Byers, K., McDonald, T., & Lindeman, D. (2013). *Strengthening families to buffer toxic stress: A biobehavioral approach to screening and intervention for the promotion of child social-emotional wellbeing*. Lawrence: University of Kansas.

Cancian, M., Slack, K. S., & Yang, M. Y. (2010). *The effect of family income on risk of child maltreatment*. Institute for Research on Poverty Discussion Paper No. 1385–10. Retrieved September 29, 2014, from http://www.irp.wisc.edu/publications/dps/pdfs/dp138510.pdf

Cargo, M., & Mercer, S. L. (2008). The value and challenges of participatory research: Strengthening its practice. *Annual Review of Public Health, 29*, 325–350.

Carter, N., & Harvey, C. (1996). Gaining perspective on parenting groups. *Zero to Three, 16*(6), 3–8.

Cassidy, J., Ziv, Y., Stupica, B., Sherman, L. J., Butler, H., Karfgin, A., et al. (2010). Enhancing attachment security in the infants of women in a jail-diversion program. *Attachment & Human Development, 12*(4), 333–353.

Center for Child and Family Policy. (2009). *Multiple response system (MRS) evaluation report to the North Carolina division of social services (NCDSS)*. Durham, NC: Duke University, Center for Child and Family Policy.

Center for the Study of Social Policy. (2014). *Using café conversations to build protective factors and parent leadership*. Retrieved September 29, 2014, from http://www.cssp.org/reform/strengthening-families/2014/using-caf-conversations-to-build-protective-factors-and-parent-leadership.pdf

Centers for Disease Control and Prevention. (2013). *Essentials for childhood: Steps to create safe, stable, and nurturing relationships and environments*. Retrieved September 29, 2014, from http://www.cdc.gov/violenceprevention/pdf/essentials_for_childhood_framework.pdf

Chandra, A., Sandraluz, L. C., Jaycox, L. H., Tanielian, T., Burns, R. M., Ruder, T., & Han, B. (2010). Children on the homefront: The experience of children from military families. *Pediatrics, 125*(1), 16–25.

Cicchetti, D., & Garmezy, N. (1993). Prospects and promises in the study of resilience. *Development and Psychopathology, 5*, 497–502.

Conger, R. D., Schofield, T. J., Neppl, T. K., & Merrick, M. T. (2013). Disrupting intergenerational continuity in harsh and abusive parenting: The importance of a nurturing relationship with a romantic partner. *Journal of Adolescent Health, 53*(4, Supplement), S11–S17.

RAND Corporation. (2011). *Building community resilience to disasters: A roadmap to guide local planning*. Santa Monica: Author. Retrieved September 29, 2014, from http://www.rand.org/content/dam/rand/pubs/research_briefs/2011/RAND_RB9574.pdf.

Daro, D. (1988). *Confronting child abuse*. New York: The Free Press.

Daro, D. (1993). Child maltreatment research: Implications for program design. In D. Cicchetti & S. Toth (Eds.), *Child abuse, child development, and social policy* (pp. 331–367). Norwood: Ablex.

Daro, D. (2002). Educating and changing parents: Strengthening the primary safety net for children. In K. Browne, H. Hanks, P. Stratton, & C. Hamilton (Eds.), *Early prediction and prevention of child abuse: A handbook* (pp. 127–144). West Sussex: John Wiley & Sons.

Daro, D., & Cohn, A. (1988). Child maltreatment evaluation efforts: What have we learned? In G. Hotaling, D. Finkelhor, J. Kirkpatrick, & M. Straus (Eds.), *Coping with family violence: Research and policy perspectives* (pp. 275–287). Newbury Park: Sage.

Daro, D., & Cohn-Donnelly, A. (2002). Child abuse prevention: Accomplishments and challenges. In J. Myers, L. Berliner, J. Briere, T. Hendrix, C. Jenny, & T. Reid (Eds.), *APSAC handbook on child maltreatment* (2nd ed., pp. 431–448). Newbury Park: Sage.

Daro, D., & Dodge, K. A. (2009). Creating community responsibility for child protection: Possibilities and challenges. *Future of Children, 19*(2), 67–93.

Dozier, M., Peloso, E., Lindhiem, O., Gordon, M. K., Manni, M., Sepulveda, S., et al. (2006). Developing evidence-based interventions for foster children: An example of a randomized clinical trial with infants and toddlers. *Journal of Social Issues, 62*(4), 765–783.

Dozier, M., Peloso, E., Lewis, E., Laurenceau, J., & Levine, S. (2008). Effects of an attachment-based intervention on the cortisol production of infants and toddlers in foster care. *Development and Psychopathology, 20*(3), 845–859.

Dozier, M., Lindhiem, O., Lewis, E., Bick, J., Bernard, K., & Peloso, E. (2009). Effects of a foster parent training program on young children's attachment behaviors: Preliminary evidence from a randomized clinical trial. *Child and Adolescent Social Work Journal, 26*(4), 321–332.

Drake, B., & Pandey, S. (1996). Understanding the relationship between neighborhood poverty and specific types of child maltreatment. *Child Abuse & Neglect, 20*(11), 1003–1018.

Earvolino-Ramirez, M. (2007). Resilience: A concept analysis. *Nursing Forum, 42*(2), 73–82.

Egeland, B., Bosquet, M., & Chung, A. L. (2002). Continuities and discontinuities in the intergenerational transmission of child maltreatment: Implications for breaking the cycle of abuse. In K. Browne, H. Hanks, P. Stratton, & C. Hamilton (Eds.), *Early prediction and prevention of child abuse: A handbook* (pp. 217–232). West Sussex: John Wiley & Sons.

Everett, J. E., Homstead, K., & Drisko, J. (2007). Frontline worker perceptions of the empowerment process in community-based agencies. *Social Work, 52*(2), 161–170.

Fraiberg, S., Adelson, E., & Shapiro, V. (1975). Ghosts in the nursery: A psychoanalytic approach to the problems of impaired infant-mother relationships. *Journal of the American Academy of Child Psychiatry, 14*(3), 387–421.

Garmezy, N. (1974). The study of competence in children at risk for severe psychopathology. In E. J. Anthony & C. Koupernik (Eds.), *The child in his family: Children at psychiatric risk* (3rd ed., Vol. III, pp. 77–97). Oxford: John Wiley & Sons.

Gebbie, K., Rosenstock, L., & Hernandez, L. M. (2003). *Who will keep the public healthy?: Educating public health professionals for the 21st century.* Washington, DC: Institute of Medicine.

Gewirtz, A. H. (2007). Promoting children's mental health in family supportive housing: A community-university partnership for formerly homeless children and families. *Journal of Primary Prevention, 28*, 359–374.

Gibbs, D. A., Martin, S. L., Kupper, L. L., & Johnson, R. E. (2007). Child maltreatment in enlisted soldiers' families during combat-related deployments. *Journal of the American Medical Association, 298*, 528–535.

Goff, B. S. N., Crow, J. R., Reisbig, A. M. J., & Hamilton, S. (2007). The impact of individual trauma symptoms of deployed soldiers on relationship satisfaction. *Journal of Family Psychology, 21*, 344–353.

Herrenkohl, T. I., Klika, J. B., Brown, E. C., Herrenkohl, R. C., & Leeb, R. T. (2013). Tests of the mitigating effects of caring and supportive relationships in the study of abusive disciplining over two generations. *Journal of Adolescent Health, 53*(4, Supplement), S18–S24.

Hoelting, J., Sandell, E., LeTourneau, S., Smerlinder, J., & Stranik, M. (1996). The MELD experience with parent groups. *Zero to Three, 16*(6), 9–18.

Hoffman, K. T., Marvin, R. S., Cooper, G., & Powell, B. (2006). Changing toddlers' and preschoolers' attachment classifications: The circle of security intervention. *Journal of Consulting and Clinical Psychology, 74*(6), 1017–1026.

Horton, C. (2011). *Protective factors literature review: Early care and education programs and the prevention of child abuse and neglect.* Washington, DC: Center for the Study of Social Policy. Retrieved September 29, 2014, from http://www.cssp.org/reform/strengthening-families/resources/body/LiteratureReview.pdf

Institute of Medicine and National Research Council. (2014). *New directions in child abuse and neglect research.* Washington, DC: The National Academies Press.

Jaffee, S. R., Bowes, L., Ouellet-Morin, I., Fisher, H. L., Moffitt, T. E., Merrick, M. T., & Arseneault, L. (2013). Safe, stable, nurturing relationships break the intergenerational cycle of abuse: A prospective nationally representative cohort of children in the United Kingdom. *Journal of Adolescent Health, 53*(4, Supplement), S4–S10.

Kempe, H. (1977). Approaches to preventing child abuse: The health visitors concept. *American Journal of Diseases of Children, 130*(9), 941–947.

Keyes, C. L. M., & Lopez, S. J. (2002). Toward a science of mental health: Positive directions in diagnosis and interventions. In C. R. Snyder & S. J. Lopez (Eds.), *Handbook of positive psychology* (pp. 45–59). New York: Oxford University Press.

Kosanovich, A., Joseph, R. M., & Hasbargen, K. (2005). *Child welfare consent decrees: Analysis of thirty-five court actions from 1995–2005.* Retrieved September 29, 2014, from http://thehill.com/sites/default/files/consentdecrees_0.pdf.

Ladd, H. F., Muschkin, C. G., & Dodge, K. A. (2014). From birth to school: Early childhood initiatives and third grade outcomes in North Carolina. *Journal of Policy Analysis and Management, 33*, 162–187.

Lawrence, C. N., Rosanbalm, K. D., & Dodge, K. A. (2011). Evaluation of policy change in North Carolina's child welfare system. *Children and Youth Services Review, 33*, 2355–2365.

LePlatte, D., Rosenblum, K. L., Stanton, E., Miller, N., & Muzik, M. (2012). Mental health in primary care for adolescent parents. *Mental Health in Family Medicine, 9*(1), 39–45.

Lieberman, A. F., Silverman, R., & Pawl, J. (1999). Preventive intervention and outcome with anxiously attached dyads. *Child Development, 62*, 199–209.

Lieberman, A. F., Ghosh Ippen, C., & Van Horn, P. (2006). Child–parent psychotherapy: 6-month follow-up of a randomized control trial. *Journal of the American Academy of Child and Adolescent Psychiatry, 45*(8), 913–918.

Lincoln, A., Swift, E., & Shorteno-Fraser, M. (2008). Psychological adjustment and treatment of children and families with parents deployed in military combat. *Journal of Clinical Psychology, 64*, 984–992.

Luthans, K., & Jensen, S. M. (2005). The linkage between psychological capital and commitment to organizational mission: A study of nurses. *Journal of Nursing Administration, 35*(6), 304–310.

Luthans, F., & Youssef, C. (2004). Human, social, and now positive psychological capital management: Investing in people for competitive advantage. *Organizational Dynamics, 33*(2), 143–160.

Luthans, F., Avolio, B. J., Avey, J. B., & Norman, S. M. (2007). Psychological capital: Measurement and relationship with performance and satisfaction. *Personnel Psychology, 60*, 541–572.

Luthar, S. S. (2006). Resilience in development: A synthesis of research across five decades. In D. Cicchetti & D. J. Cohen (Eds.), *Developmental psychopathology: Risk, disorder, and adaptation* (2nd ed., Vol. 3, pp. 739–795). New York: Wiley.

Luthar, S., Cicchetti, D., & Becker, B. (2000). The construct of resilience: A critical evaluation and guidelines for future work. *Child Development, 71*(3), 543–562.

Marvin, R., Cooper, G., Hoffman, K., & Powell, B. (2002). The circle of security project: Attachment-based intervention with caregiver-pre-school child dyads. *Attachment and Human Development, 4*(1), 107–124.

Masten, A. S. (1989). Resilience in development: Implications of the study of successful adaptation for developmental psychopathology. In D. Cicchetti (Ed.), *The emergence of a discipline: Rochester symposium on developmental psychopathology* (pp. 261–294). Hillsdale: Lawrence Erlbaum Associates.

Masten, A. (2001). Ordinary magic: Resilience processes in development. *American Psychologist, 56*(3), 227–238.

Masten, A., & Gewirtz, A. (2006). Vulnerability and resilience. In D. Philips & K. McCartney (Eds.), *Blackwell handbook of early childhood development* (pp. 22–43). Oxford: Blackwell Publishing.

Masten, A. S., & Powell, J. L. (2003). A resiliency framework for research, policy and practice. In S. Luthar (Ed.), *Resiliency and vulnerability: Adaptation in the context of childhood adversity* (pp. 1–29). Cambridge: Cambridge University Press.

McCourt, S. Y. N. (2013). *The impact of state early childhood programs and child protective services policies on resilience following experiences of child maltreatment* (Doctoral dissertation). Available from ProQuest Dissertations and Theses database (UMI No. 35–90829).

Mercer, S., & Green, L. (2008). Federal funding and support for participatory research in public health and health care. In M. Minkler & N. Wallerstein (Eds.), *Community-based participatory research for health: From process to outcomes* (2nd ed., pp. 399–406). San Francisco: Jossey-Bass.

Minkler, M., & Wallerstein, N. (2008). Introduction to community-based participatory research: New issues and emphases. In M. Minkler & N. Wallerstein (Eds.), *Community-based participatory research for health: From process to outcomes* (2nd ed., pp. 5–23). San Francisco: Jossey-Bass.

Mitchell, J., Vella-Brodrick, D., & Klein, B. (2010). Positive psychology and the internet: A mental health opportunity. *Electronic Journal of Applied Psychology, 6*(2), 30–41.

National Scientific Council on the Developing Child. (2005). *Excessive stress disrupts the architecture of the developing brain: Working Paper #3*. Retrieved September 29, 2014, from http://developingchild.harvard.edu/resources/reports_and_working_papers/working_papers/wp3/

New Jersey Department of Children and Families. (2011). *Annual agency performance report, 2011.* Retrieved September 29, 2014, from http://www.nj.gov/dcf/documents/about/AnnualAgencyReport2011_110911.pdf

New Jersey Task Force on Child Abuse and Neglect. (2013). *New Jersey standards for prevention programs: Building success through family support.* Retrieved September 29, 2014, from http://www.state.nj.us/dcf/news/reportsnewsletters/taskforce/Standards.for.Prevention.Programs.pdf

North Carolina Department of Health and Human Services. (2003). North Carolina embarks on major reform of its child welfare system. *Fostering Perspectives, 7*(2). Raleigh: North Carolina Department of Health and Human Services, Division of Social Services. Retrieved September 29, 2014, from http://www.fosteringperspectives.org/fp_vol7no2/reform.htm

Obama, B. (2010). *National security strategy.* Retrieved September 29, 2014, from http://www.whitehouse.gov/sites/default/files/rss_viewer/national_security_strategy.pdf.

Ocasio, K. (n.d.). *Understanding behavioral determinants of repeat service use in a family support program* (Unpublished doctoral dissertation). New Brunswick: Rutgers University.

Olds, D. L., Henderson, C. R., Chamberlin, R., & Tatelbaum, R. (1986). Preventing child abuse and neglect: A randomized trial of nurse home visitation. *Pediatrics, 78*, 65–78.

Olds, D. L., Henderson, C. R., & Kitzman, H. (1994). Does prenatal and infancy nurse home visitation have enduring effects on qualities of parental caregiving and child health at 25 to 50 months of life? *Pediatrics, 93*(1), 89–98.

Olds, D. L., Eckenrode, J., Henderson, C. R., Kitzman, H., Powers, J., Cole, R., et al. (1997). Long-term effects of home visitation on maternal life course and child abuse and neglect: Fifteen-year follow-up of a randomized trial. *Journal of the American Medical Association, 278*(8), 637–643.

Olds, D., Sadler, L., & Kitzman, H. (2007). Programs for parents of infants and toddlers: Recent evidence from randomized trials. *Journal of Child Psychology and Psychiatry, 48*, 355–391.

Peisner-Feinberg, E. S., & Schaaf, J. M. (2010). *Long-term effects of the North Carolina more at four pre-kindergarten program: Children's reading and math skills at third grade.* Chapel Hill: The University of North Carolina, FPG Child Development Institute.

Pollard, J. A., Hawkins, J. D., & Arthur, M. W. (1999). Risk and protection: Are both necessary to understand diverse behavioral outcomes in adolescence? *Social Work Research, 23*(3), 145–158.

Powell, B., Cooper, G., Hoffman, K., & Marvin, R. (2009). The circle of security. In C. Zeanah (Ed.), *Handbook of infant mental health* (3rd ed., pp. 450–467). New York: Guilford Press.

Prinz, R. J., Sanders, M. R., Shapiro, C. J., Whitaker, D. J., & Lutzker, J. R. (2009). Population-based prevention of child maltreatment: The U.S. triple P system population trial. *Prevention Science, 10*, 1–13.

Casey Family Programs. (2012). *Comparison of experiences in differential response (DR) implementation: 10 child welfare jurisdictions implementing DR.* Seattle: Casey Family Programs.

Reppucci, N. D., Britner, P. A., & Woolard, J. L. (1997). *Preventing child abuse and neglect through parent education.* Baltimore: Paul H. Brookes.

Rostad, W. L. (2014). *Examining the effectiveness of the circle of security parenting DVD program* (Unpublished dissertation). Missoula: University of Montana.

Sadler, L. S., Slade, A., Close, N., Webb, D. L., Simpson, T., Fennie, K., & Mayes, L. C. (2013). Minding the baby: Enhancing reflectiveness to improve early health and relationship outcomes in an interdisciplinary home-visiting program. *Infant Mental Health Journal, 34*, 391–405.

Saltzman, W. R., Lester, P., Beardslee, W. R., Layne, C. M., Woodward, K., & Nash, W. P. (2011). Mechanisms of risk and resilience in military families: Theoretical and empirical basis of a family-focused resilience enhancement program. *Clinical Child and Family Psychology Review, 14*(3), 213–230.

Schobera, D. J., Fawcetta, S. B., & Be, J. (2012). The enough abuse campaign: Building the movement to prevent child sexual abuse in Massachusetts. *Journal of Child Sexual Abuse, 21*(4), 456–469.

Schorr, A. (2000). The bleak prospect for public child welfare. *Social Service Review, 74*(1), 124–138.

Sedlak, A. J., & Broadhurst, D. D. (1996). *Executive summary of the third national incidence study of child abuse and neglect*. Washington, DC: U.S. Dept. of Health and Human Services, Administration for Children and Families. Retrieved September 29, 2014, from https://www.childwelfare.gov/pubs/statsinfo/nis3.cfm.

Sedlak, A. J., Mettenburg, K., Basena, M., Petta, I., McPherson, K., Greene, A., & Li, S. (2010). *The fourth national incidence study of child abuse and neglect (NIS-4): Report to congress*. Washington, DC: U.S. Department of Health and Human Services, Administration for Children and Families.

Seligman, M. E. P., & Csikszentmihalyi, M. (2000). Positive psychology: An introduction. *American Psychologist, 55*, 5–14.

Seligman, M. E. P., Schulman, P., DeRubeis, R. J., & Hollon, S. D. (1999). The prevention of depression and anxiety. *Prevention & Treatment, 2*(1), Article 8. Retrieved September 29, 2014, from http://www.ppc.sas.upenn.edu/depprevseligman1999.pdf

Sharp, C., & Fonagy, P. (2008). The parent's capacity to treat the child as a psychological agent: Constructs, measures and implications for developmental psychopathology. *Social Development, 17*(3), 737–754.

Shonkoff, J. P. (2010). Building a new biodevelopmental framework to guide the future of early childhood policy. *Child Development, 81*(1), 357–367.

Shonkoff, J. P., & Garner, A. S. (2012). The lifelong effects of early childhood adversity and toxic stress. *Pediatrics, 129*(1), 232–246.

Shonkoff, J. P., & Phillips, D. A. (2000). *From neurons to neighborhoods: The science of early childhood development*. Washington, DC: National Academy Press.

Simon, J. B., Murphy, J. J., & Smith, S. M. (2005). Understanding and fostering family resilience. *The Family Journal: Counseling and Therapy for Couples and Families, 13*(4), 427–436.

Slade, A., Grienenberger, J., Bernbach, E., Levy, D., & Locker, A. (2005). Maternal reflective functioning and attachment: Considering the transmission gap. *Attachment and Human Development, 7*, 283–292.

Suchman, N. E., DeCoste, C., Castiglioni, N., McMahon, T. J., Rounsaville, B., & Mayes, L. (2010). The mothers and toddlers program, an attachment-based parenting intervention for substance using women: Post-treatment results from a randomized clinical pilot. *Attachment & Human Development, 12*(5), 483–504.

Suchman, N. E., DeCoste, C., McMahon, T. E., Rounsaville, B., & Mayes, L. (2011). The mothers and toddlers program, an attachment-based parenting intervention for substance using women: Results at 6-week follow-up in a randomized clinical pilot. *Infant Mental Health Journal, 32*(4), 427–449.

Thornberry, T. P., Henry, K. L., Smith, C. A., Ireland, T. O., Greenman, S. J., & Lee, R. D. (2013). Breaking the cycle of maltreatment: The role of safe, stable, and nurturing relationships. *Journal of Adolescent Health, 53*(4, Supplement), S25–S31.

Trickett, P. K., Aber, J. L., Carlson, V., & Cicchetti, D. (1991). The relationship of socioeconomic status to the etiology and developmental sequelae of physical child abuse. *Developmental Psychology, 27*, 148–158.

Trout, A. L., Ryan, J. B., La Vigne, S. P., & Epstein, M. H. (2003). Behavioral and emotional rating scale: Two studies of convergent validity. *Journal of Child and Family Studies, 12*, 399–410.

U.S. Department of Defense. (2011). *Demographics report: Profile of the military community*. Retrieved September 29, 2014, from http://www.militaryonesource.mil/12038/MOS/Reports/2011_demographics_Report.pdf

U.S. Department of Health & Human Services. (2009). *National health security strategy of the United States of America*. Washington, DC: Author. Retrieved September 29, 2014, from http://www.phe.gov/Preparedness/planning/authority/nhss/strategy/Pages/default.aspx.

U.S. Department of Homeland Security. (2010, February 5). *National disaster recovery framework (draft)* (FEMA-2010-0004-0001). Washington, DC: Author.

Van Ijzendoorn, M. H., Bakermans-Kranenburg, M. J., & Juffer, F. (2005). Why less is more: From the Dodo bird verdict to evidence-based interventions on sensitivity and early attachments. In

L. J. Berlin, Y. Ziv, L. Amaya-Jackson, & M. T. Greenberg (Eds.), *Enhancing early attachments: Theory, research, intervention, and policy* (pp. 297–312). New York: Guilford Press.

Wald, M. (2009). Preventing maltreatment or promoting positive development: Where should a community focus its resources? In K. Dodge & D. L. Coleman (Eds.), *Preventing child maltreatment community approaches* (pp. 182–195). New York: Guilford Press.

Walsh, F. (1998). *Strengthening family resilience.* New York: Guilford.

Werner, E., & Smith, R. (1989). *Vulnerable but invincible: A longitudinal study of resilient children and youth.* New York: Adams, Bannister, and Cox.

Wolfe, D. A. (1994). The role of intervention and treatment services in the prevention of child abuse and neglect. In G. B. Melton & F. Barry (Eds.), *Safe neighborhoods: Foundations for a new national strategy on child abuse and neglect* (pp. 224–303). New York: Guilford.

Yates, T. M., & Masten, A. S. M. (2004). Fostering the future: Resilience theory and the practice of positive psychology. In P. A. Linley & S. Joseph (Eds.), *Positive psychology in practice* (pp. 521–539). Hoboken: Wiley.

Zielinski, D. S., & Bradshaw, C. P. (2006). Ecological influences on the sequelae of child maltreatment. *Child Maltreatment, 11*(1), 49–62.

Zolotor, A. J., & Runyan, D. K. (2006). Social capital, family violence, and neglect. *Pediatrics, 117*, 1124–1131.

Tova B. Walsh is a Robert Wood Johnson Foundation Health & Society Scholar at the University of Wisconsin-Madison. In Fall 2015, she will join the faculty of the School of Social Work at University of Wisconsin-Madison. Dr. Walsh's research focuses on the role that expectant and new fathers play in the health and wellbeing of their partners and children, and the influence of parenthood on men's health. She aims to use research to develop interventions and public policy to improve the health and wellbeing of infants, young children, and their families. She has a specific interest in efforts to support and strengthen parent-child relationships in military families. Prior to entering graduate school, Dr. Walsh worked in Jamaica and the United States with home visiting services for low-income families with children ages 0–3. She received a Ph.D. in social work and psychology from the University of Michigan, and a B.A. with honors in sociology and politics from Brandeis University.

Sandra Nay McCourt is a child clinical psychologist and visiting research fellow at the Social Science Research Institute at Duke University. Dr. McCourt's research focuses on developmental processes that underlie maladjustment or resilience in response to early traumatic experiences. She aims to use applied research to facilitate the translation of social science into policies and practices that promote optimal child development and effective preventive interventions for children at risk in the areas of child maltreatment, family violence, and chronic antisocial behavior. Her current research examines the effects of state child welfare reform and state expenditures on early childhood programs on academic outcomes among children reported to child protective services. Dr. McCourt received a Ph.D. in clinical psychology from Duke University, a J.D. from the University of Michigan Law School, and a B.A. in Classical Greek and Political Science from DePauw University. She completed her clinical psychology internship and post-doctoral fellowship at the Indiana University School of Medicine.

Whitney L. Rostad is a developmental psychologist and postdoctoral research associate with the National SafeCare Training and Research Center (NSTRC) at Georgia State University in Atlanta. At NSTRC, she is currently working on several projects examining the dissemination and implementation of SafeCare—an empirically supported, home-based intervention for the prevention of child maltreatment—as well as a modified version of the program for use with fathers. She recently conducted her dissertation at the University of Montana examining the effectiveness of a DVD-guided, attachment-based parenting program with a sample of primarily low-income caregivers. In addition, Dr. Rostad has assisted and conducted multiple projects on the influence of parent-child relationships on child and adolescent development, and continues to assist on projects that aim to understand and reduce child abuse and neglect. She received a M.A. in developmental psychology from the University of Montana and a B.A. in psychology from Gonzaga University in Spokane, Washington.

Kaela Byers is a Ph.D. candidate in social welfare at the University of Kansas where her research focuses on early childhood toxic stress screening and intervention to promote child and family protective factors supporting healthy social-emotional development. Ms. Byers is currently a project manager at the Center for Children and Families at KU where she conducts research on the implementation and evaluation of evidenced-based interventions in community mental health, child welfare, and early childhood service settings. Ms. Byers' professional experience includes providing home and community-based early childhood mental health services and community mental health consultation. She received a B.S. in social welfare from the University of Kansas and a M.S.W. from the University of Maryland-Baltimore.

Kerrie Ocasio is a Ph.D. candidate in social work at Rutgers, The State University of New Jersey, and senior research associate at the Institute for Families (IFF) at the Rutgers School of Social Work. At IFF, Ms. Ocasio's most recent work includes a federal initiative to reduce the time to adoption for special needs children that are legally free for adoption, investigating child and adult long-term recovery following Hurricane Sandy, and evaluating an intervention for families with domestic violence concerns that are involved with the child protection system. In addition, Ms. Ocasio partners with New Jersey's Department of Children and Families on numerous on-going research and program improvement efforts. Her professional experience includes practice and policy experience in child maltreatment prevention and protection services. She received a B.A.S.W. from Rutgers University and an M.S.W. from Fordham University.

Part IV
Moving Forward

Chapter 10
Common Themes, Questions and Opportunities: Creating a Context for Continued Improvement

Deborah Daro, Anne Cohn Donnelly, Lee Ann Huang, and Byron J. Powell

Overview

A great deal has been learned about child maltreatment over the past 50 years. Much of this new learning, however, simply underscores how much more we need to learn. Today, child maltreatment is perceived as more complex than first described in terms of its interaction with other forms of risk and trauma; in terms of how best to design and implement strategies to address it; and in terms of how to tailor these strategies across different populations and contexts. Facing this reality should generate a certain degree of humility in all who work in this field.

Looking across the chapters in this book, several common themes surfaced regarding how the problem is currently being defined and how programs and policies are being crafted and implemented. As a group, the chapter authors underscored the importance of adopting a developmental framework in understanding the continuous, and often different, impacts of maltreatment. They called for a more inclusive definition of culture and its application in understanding the definition, roots, and consequences of maltreatment and efforts to prevent it. They spoke of the importance of recognizing that child maltreatment is often one of multiple adversities experienced by children and the parents who mistreat them. The authors recommend that an interdisciplinary, multilayered response be fostered, in which all

D. Daro (✉) • L.A. Huang
Chapin Hall at the University of Chicago, Chicago, IL, USA
e-mail: ddaro@chapinhall.org; lhuang@chapinhall.org

A.C. Donnelly
Kellogg School of Management, Northwestern University, Evanston, IL, USA
e-mail: Annecohndonnelly@gmail.com

B.J. Powell
Center for Mental Health Policy and Services Research, Department of Psychiatry,
Perelman School of Medicine, University of Pennsylvania, Philadelphia, PA, USA
e-mail: byronp@upenn.edu

© Springer International Publishing Switzerland 2015
D. Daro et al. (eds.), *Advances in Child Abuse Prevention Knowledge*,
Child Maltreatment 5, DOI 10.1007/978-3-319-16327-7_10

aspects of the social ecology are considered both a source of the problem and potential opportunity for prevention.

The purpose of this chapter is to expand on these themes and note areas in which they collectively deepen our understanding of the problem and how we assess our interventions. The chapter also discusses how these themes offer important opportunities to reconnect the field's treatment and prevention functions. Noting the need to build a more interdisciplinary and cross-sector workforce, the chapter discusses the development strategies required to build a pool of professionals deeply committed to interdisciplinary practice and capable of sustaining diverse and generative learning. The chapter concludes with a set of promising strategies for building on the lessons presented in this volume and continuing the field's long tradition of integrating research and practice.

The Nature of the Problem

All (or most) social dilemmas operate within a broader context. Rarely do they occur in isolation from other adverse events nor are they triggered by a narrow range of circumstances limited to a single ecological level. At a minimum, a child's safety and ultimate well-being is a function of her parents' capacity to meet her basic needs, the other adverse conditions she and her family have experienced or may experience, the resources available within her local community, and the normative standards that determine appropriate and inappropriate parent–child interactions. Despite this obvious integration with other familial and contextual conditions, child maltreatment has historically been viewed as a separate, stand-alone social problem requiring a unique public policy response. More recently, however, child maltreatment has been viewed as a behavior so deeply influenced by other issues (such as poverty, inequality, and violence) that sustaining progress in addressing its incidence and consequences can only occur from a more integrated platform.

The contributing authors, while recognizing the relationship between child maltreatment and these broader issues, endorse a set of policy and practice reforms that would retain child maltreatment as a unique topic of study and field of practice. Their perspective, however, is tempered by intentionality in recognizing points of interaction between child maltreatment and myriad other issues that facilitate or hinder progress in defining and confronting it. While supporting a research and policy agenda that centers on child maltreatment, the contributing authors fully understand that this type of single-issue focus will be insufficient to achieve a meaningful reduction in incidence rates. As noted by Atul Gawande, "We always hope for the easy fix: the simple one change that will erase a problem in a stroke. But few things in life work in this way. Instead, success requires making a hundred small steps go right—one after the other, no slip ups, no goofs, everyone pitching in" (Gawande 2008, p. 21). Strategies suggested by the contributing authors to create a rich, multifaceted lens through which to view the problem include embracing the perspectives of multiple disciplines in conceptualizing the problem; casting a broad, inclusive net in defining what constitutes abuse or neglect; and simultaneously seeking to both reduce risk and enhance protective factors.

Engage a Broad Array of Disciplines

The complexity of child maltreatment accentuates the importance of applying the perspectives of multiple disciplines to all aspects of the problem—from incidence and prevalence through intervention and prevention. This theme, evident in nearly every chapter, suggests that truly understanding child maltreatment requires the active participation of those operating with research and theoretical frameworks representing diverse areas of study, including (but likely not limited to): anthropology, biology, business, computer science, economics, education, engineering, family and consumer science, gender and sexuality studies, genetics, law, medicine (emergency medicine, pediatrics, psychiatry, etc.), neuroscience, philosophy (ethics), psychology, public administration, public health, social work, sociology, statistics, and systems science. (These areas are listed alphabetically to avoid assigning primacy to a single discipline.) It will also need to include experts from a variety of fields that are not necessarily discipline specific, such as scholars from the fields of implementation and prevention science (Institute of Medicine and National Research Council 2013).

The productive use of an interdisciplinary platform demands authentic, joint planning and integrated thinking. As described by Rosenfield (1992), a taxonomy of cross-disciplinary research (and practice) suggests that these relationships develop over time and move through specific stages. At the basic level, *multidisciplinary* approaches involve researchers working in parallel or sequentially from their own disciplinary-specific base to address a common problem. An example of this would be the early multidisciplinary teams established to review reported child abuse cases and fatalities. In *interdisciplinary* work, researchers work collaboratively, but retain their specific disciplinary base, as reflected in the relationships commonly found on public task forces and interdisciplinary study teams established to examine a specific program or complex social issue. In the final stage of collaborative work, *transdisciplinary* approaches, researchers "work jointly using shared conceptual framework drawing together disciplinary-specific theories, concepts, and approaches", a qualitatively different way of interaction (Rosenfield 1992, p. 1351). Rather than simply representing a combination of ideas, this new level of collaboration is capable of birthing a new identity and potentially generating innovative approaches. Indeed, Johnson, in his book *Where Good Ideas Come From: The Natural History of Innovation* (2010), notes that one of the factors that often underlies innovation is the availability of "loosely formed multidisciplinary teams that work on the edges of new ideas and by virtue of their proximity and specialization generate new ideas" (as cited in Hogwood et al. 2014, p. 154).

Addressing and untangling the complexity of child maltreatment through transdisciplinary research will not be possible without a great deal of patience, respect, trust, and institutional support from universities, funders, foundations, governmental agencies, and other stakeholders. On the academic side, it may also require recalibrating metrics for promotion and tenure so that they reflect the value of academic and community collaboration. Despite the challenges, the contributing authors are optimistic about the promise cross-discipline collaboration and partnerships present for advancing the field.

Broaden the Concept of Child Maltreatment

The specific behaviors and conditions which constitute maltreatment are far reaching and not simply limited to the way in which adults treat children. From the onset, researchers and practitioners have recognized that social conditions not only contribute to the likelihood that parents or caretakers may mistreat their own children but that conditions such as poverty, inequalities in how resources are allocated across populations and communities, community violence, and social norms around gender and race can have a direct, cumulative effect on the lives of young children and their overall well-being. While guidelines for reporting and substantiating child maltreatment have expanded over the years, the official behaviors that trigger a formal report of child abuse or neglect, or are perceived by the public as child maltreatment, remain narrowly focused on the behaviors individuals perpetrate against children.

Those examining the issue of child maltreatment, including the authors contributing to this volume, are now seeking ways to explicitly expand the discussion about which behaviors and conditions might be considered abusive and neglectful and how this broader range of issues might enhance our understanding of the problem. Moving forward, child maltreatment "perpetrators" might come to include not only individuals—most often parents, guardians or caretakers—but also the families, institutions, culture, and environment (e.g., the society) in which children are reared. This multilayered view of maltreatment reinforces the notion that while historically maltreatment has been defined as a collection of discrete actions or inactions (e.g., physical abuse at the hands of a parent), victims of maltreatment are often exposed to multiple forms of abuse and trauma at one time or over time. This layering of so many different traumas has cumulative effects on a child's well-being and life course development. The more adversity a child experiences, the stronger the effects. While not every act of commission or omission constitutes a reportable act of child abuse or neglect, all of these actions reflect society's inability to fulfill its collective responsibility to care for its children and create a context in which children are safe and nurtured. Recognizing this collective responsibility allows for a more effective and purposeful integration of the child maltreatment concept within the social fabric and opens up new prevention opportunities.

Establish a Dual Focus on Risk and Protective Factors

As highlighted in several chapters, efforts are being made at the local, state, and federal levels to improve utilization of prevention and treatment frameworks that focus on building upon individual and family strengths. Strengths commonly cited as reducing the likelihood for maltreatment and assisting parents in overcoming adversity include parental resilience, social connections, knowledge of parenting and child development, concrete support in times of need, and social and emotional competence of children. However, the field continues to depend largely on risk assessment and abatement strategies when working with or studying families. While it is not a viable option to abandon any discussion of risk, researchers, practitioners, and policymakers are making strides in better balancing their focus between risk and resilience.

Promulgating this dual perspective in the public discourse around child maltreatment not only impacts how practitioners and policymakers perceive the issue but also may alter how families perceive and respond to interventions addressing the problem. Effectively recruiting and engaging families are ongoing challenges for all voluntary interventions. Increasing the focus on strengths building as a critical goal of preventive services may improve the ability to attract, enroll, and retain potential participants. Programs that are built around building resilience and enhancing parental capacity create a more inclusive and welcoming window for families concerned about their ability to meet their child's needs but who are not comfortable defining these concerns as an indicator of a potential risk to abuse or neglect them. A protective factors or strengths-based framework creates a more inclusive intervention, one which may be more acceptable to a higher proportion of families across income, family structure, culture, and social stratification.

While those contributing to this volume acknowledge that there are factors present at the individual, family, and community level that may stand to protect against maltreatment, they also agree that more research is needed in several areas to provide practitioners with the information they need to develop or modify programs to reflect this reality. Community-level protective factors are not well understood—both in terms of how those factors influence the actions of individual families as well as how they effectively increase community or collective efficacy. When examining the transmission of violence across generations, the field needs to focus efforts on identifying which protective factors have the greatest likelihood to help individuals break the cycle of violence. Once identified, the field needs to develop programmatic and policy innovations to more explicitly nurture these conditions among current victims, to increase their resilience and help them avoid maltreating their own children. In addition, greater understanding is needed of the role culture and gender identity may play in the differential impacts of these factors and how to accommodate these differences when working with victims.

The Nature of the Response

As noted in Chap. 1, the policy and programmatic response to child maltreatment has grown exponentially over the past 50 years. Every state has a child welfare system to investigate all child maltreatment reports and to respond in an appropriate manner when maltreatment has occurred or is at high risk of occurring. Outside of the formal child welfare system, most (if not all) communities have some number of therapeutic and support services available to victims and their families as well as a range of preventive services to strengthen parental capacity, promote healthy child development, and address immediate needs. This system is not perfect and often inadequate to meet total demand; its depth and breadth, however, is increasingly robust.

While recognizing this progress, the contributing authors envision a response system that does more and does it in a more efficient and effective manner. Specifically, in several chapters the authors discuss the importance of building a strong continuum of interventions and public policies that support children and their families from birth through the child's transition to adulthood. Authors utilize a range of diverse research designs and methods to document the implementation and impacts of these interventions and create a "learning culture" in which data is used to inform program development and interagency collaboration. Underlying all of these pathways to improvement is the realization that the most effective response system will indeed be one which is diverse and one which avoids creating a hierarchy of what is "best." One of the major themes surfacing throughout these chapters is the importance of *always* considering context when determining what interventions will be used, what research methods will be employed, and how data can best inform a given policy or practice.

Develop an Integrated Response Across the Lifespan

Confronting child maltreatment has, for decades, involved the development and implementation of diverse services provided by a range of public and private agencies. As noted in Chap. 1, most recently the prevention field has placed particular emphasis on investing in early intervention services and those programs targeting newborns and their parents. Reflecting on this reality, several of the authors make a compelling case for not allowing concern with one developmental stage to minimize the importance of supporting a child's development at every stage, utilizing a developmental lens to create a comprehensive array of mutually reinforcing supports. As Isabell Sawhill and her colleagues at the Brookings Institute have demonstrated, interventions offered at multiple points during a child's development produce a level of additive value unable to be achieved through a singular offer of assistance, even when that assistance begins early in a child's development (Sawhill and Karpilow 2014). While investment in early childhood interventions makes solid programmatic and financial sense, such investments will never yield the anticipated level of returns unless high-quality clinical interventions and prevention services are offered throughout the life span, including adolescence and young adulthood. And, as cited earlier, such efforts need to target not only individuals but also the context in which these individuals live and the systems and institutions that shape these contexts.

Future public policies targeting child maltreatment will need to embrace multiple programs provided through multiple institutions. These policies will also need to build in an intentional focus on addressing the factors associated with an elevated risk of maltreatment at every stage of a child's development. Collectively, the contributing authors believe the programmatic response to maltreatment needs to be deeper, broader, and more fluid. Allocating prevention resources more equitably across all populations at risk rather than focusing so heavily on early childhood—which is certainly what has occurred in the child maltreatment prevention field—will be required to maximize impacts over time. It is becoming increasingly difficult to justify investing in the *one* thing you think is most promising. What is needed are investments in multiple strategies operating at varying levels of the social ecology.

Embrace Methodological Pluralism

A new balance is needed between effectiveness and efficacy studies when investing in program research. When promising programs are taken to scale, the limitations of relying on randomized clinical trials in determining "what works" becomes more evident. As noted in several of the chapters, improving the quality and replicability of interventions requires greater investment in research studies built around implementation science. At a minimum, improving practice will require a more detailed and nuanced documentation of how programs operate and their key levers of change, the organizational and contextual factors that facilitate or hinder successful program replication, and the "meaning" participants ascribe to the interventions they receive. Obtaining these data and effectively using them to guide practice reform and policy innovation requires the development and implementation of a new research framework. Addressing this need, Lisbeth Schorr and her colleagues have called for an expanded definition of what constitutes "useful and usable" evidence. The core operational elements of their framework, the majority of which mirror recommendations made in several chapters, include the incorporation of multiple sources of evidence, goal-oriented networks to accelerate knowledge development and dissemination, multiple evaluation methods suitable for diverse purposes, and a strong infrastructure to support continuous learning over time (Schorr and Farrow 2014).

The range of issues addressed in this book further speaks to the need for the field of child maltreatment prevention to employ a diverse set of research methods and analytic approaches. This is directly related to the need to engage various disciplines; no one method or approach to analysis will be sufficient for all situations. For example, randomized controlled trials are not always feasible, because they need both design alternatives (Brown et al. 2009) and analytic methods that can approximate the conditions of a randomized controlled trial (e.g., propensity score matching). Chapter 6 deals with this most explicitly. Other chapters also suggest the need for quantitative, qualitative, and mixed methods research approaches. Mixed methods approaches are particularly attractive. These approaches address the need to demonstrate the impact of interventions in a rigorous way. They also foster a better understanding of the processes and mechanisms by which they exert their effects and the subjective experience of relevant stakeholders who are involved in providing or receiving the intervention. Economic evaluation is another underutilized methodology that deserves greater attention. Finally, systems science has promise for capturing, explaining, and intervening in the complex pathways that lead to child maltreatment (Office of Behavioral and Social Science Research 2014).

Promote Greater Data Use and Sharing Within and Across Programs

Creating a more diversified body of evidence is one challenge. Equally important is improving the capacity of policymakers, agency managers, and practitioners to access these data in a timely and appropriate manner and to make sure that they know what to do with the data once they access it. In several chapters, authors underscore the need to create methods in which direct service providers can document what they do and how participants are responding in a seamless manner. In addition, providers must view such data collection is as an integral part of the service delivery process, not an added burden. These data can then inform the supervisory process as well as guide agency decisions regarding appropriate target populations, methods of participant engagement, dosage levels, and service duration. When data is collected as a matter of practice and the information fed back to staff in a timely manner, practice and resource decisions are well-served. Choices regarding resource allocations, modifications to an existing protocol, and opportunities for interagency planning are guided by current reality and the best available information.

Great progress has been made toward accomplishing the ideals of open access to research findings and the sharing of data. The contributing authors are optimistic that a commitment to increased data sharing will continue. With respect to interagency data sharing, a growing number of state agencies are encouraging policy innovations and methods that will allow for cross-referencing the experiences of families across various institutions as well as tracking performance over time. These "integrated data systems" are allowing state child welfare directors, for example, to better understand the long-term developmental and educational outcomes of children in foster care and to examine the characteristics of those children in care who are at highest risk for poor outcomes (Wulczyn et al. 2005). Similarly, those interested in documenting the potential savings of early intervention services are investigating ways to use administrative data to track future expenditures as well as performance (Aos et al. 2011). This ability to be more intentional and creative in using the data currently available regarding service use and expenditures has strong potential to improve the public policy debate regarding alternative strategies and, more importantly, to enhance participant outcomes (Haskins and Margolis 2014).

In addition to the more effective use of administrative data, researchers are seeking ways to share their data and build on each other's findings in a more efficient and time-sensitive manner. In the area of child maltreatment research, the federal Children's Bureau has supported the National Data Archive on Child Abuse and Neglect at Cornell University since 1988. The goal of the Data Archive is to make available to researchers and doctoral students all of the studies that have been funded by the federal government regarding this topic, as well as several other large national studies that have examined the issue. (The Data Archive can be accessed at www. ndacan.cornell.edu.) Similarly, all publications from taxpayer-funded research in the United States are required to be made freely available after one year's delay (http://blogs.nature.com/news/2013/02/us-white-house-announces-open-access-policy.html). There are also increasing numbers of open access journals available (see the website for the Directory of Open Access Journals at http://doaj.org). Data sharing may also soon be incentivized, if not required. A recent editorial in the *Journal of the American Medical Association* advocated for the value of scholars' research being evaluated on a specified list of criteria, one of which was the sharing of data and other resources as indicated by the proportion of publications that share data, materials, or protocols (Ioannidis and Khoury 2014). These and other efforts suggest that, going forward, researchers examining child maltreatment and related issues cited by the authors in this volume will have more direct access to each other's work.

Building and Sustaining a Unified Approach to Child Maltreatment

Practitioners, policymakers, researchers, and advocates need to learn from and inform each other's decisions. Those focusing on developing treatment and preventive services need to identify shared challenges and opportunities for joint learning. Reflecting on their own experiences and interests moving forward, the authors identified at least three areas where all of those contributing to the child maltreatment response can find common ground regardless of their specific target of interest: the application of neurobiological research findings in identifying new pathways for understanding and confronting child maltreatment; better designed program evaluations and implementation studies to inform the design and quality of both treatment and prevention programs; and examining the ways in which community context can be altered to better support participant engagement in services and reinforce the gains such programs are able to achieve for the families they serve.

Neurobiological Research

The application of neurobiological research offers a unique and robust opportunity to identify both the consequences of abuse as well as the possible interventions to pursue in remediating or preventing these consequences. As this line of research refines and clarifies how behavior and context influences early brain development, program planners and policy advocates are developing a clearer understanding of how exposure to ongoing stress, economic deprivation, and violence can alter a child's cognitive and neurological development. The use of physiological measures to assess outcomes (e.g., saliva cortisol to measure neuroendocrine levels) provide new, more consistent ways to assess constructs, such as emotional dysregulation, that cannot be directly observed but can now be inferred by measuring neuroendocrine levels. Such information can inform both the treatment and prevention planning process by documenting the impacts of maltreatment and other trauma on child well-being and more effectively monitoring the impact interventions have on these constructs. While capturing only one aspect of trauma, this line of research offers a common source of new knowledge equally useful to those focusing on new treatment interventions and those seeking ways to design more effective prevention services.

Neurobiological research also furthers our understanding of the developmental challenges facing children who are born into families affected by intergenerational maltreatment. These children face not only the adverse consequences resulting from direct environmental stress, such as maternal drug use, mental illness, or intimate partner violence, but also may be born primed to respond to stress much differently as a result of their genetic makeup. As with an increased risk for cancer, diabetes, and heart disease, it is now hypothesized that trauma, including trauma resulting from abuse or chronic neglect, can be passed down generation to generation through genetic patterns. While far from a fully understood process, this line of research will most certainly influence the next generation of researchers and provide a rich context for joint discussions at both ends of the intervention continuum.

Implementation Research

Just like other fields, such as health, behavioral health, and social services, the field of child maltreatment prevention has been hampered by the slow translation of research into practice; effective prevention and treatment programs have been developed but they are seldom implemented widely or with a high degree of fidelity (see Chaps. 7 and 8). Implementation research is fundamentally about bridging the gap from research to practice by developing and testing strategies to change the behavior of individuals, families, teams, organizations, and systems. Implementation research also enables greater understanding of the contextual factors that influence those behaviors (Eccles and Mittman 2006). Further, it is increasingly recognized as a necessary element for improving the response to child maltreatment (Institute of Medicine and National Research Council 2013; Paulsell et al. 2014).

Implementation science has the potential to serve as a strong, generative platform to promote a shared purpose across all stages of the child maltreatment research and service continuum. First, implementation research can bridge multiple phases of research. While we sometimes think of the progression from efficacy studies to effectiveness studies to dissemination and implementation studies as linear, all of these stages of work inform one another in an iterative fashion (Institute of Medicine 2009). At the early stages of intervention development, there is utility in "designing for dissemination" by taking into account the characteristics of interventions that may render them easier to implement in the real world (Brownson et al. 2013; Klesges et al. 2005). Similarly, learning about how these interventions are actually implemented and adapted in community settings (see Chap. 8) will inform future efforts to develop and test any intervention regardless of its focus in efficacy and effectiveness trials.

Second, the field of implementation science does not belong to a single discipline, so it has the advantage of facilitating the type of interdisciplinary and transdisciplinary research needed to advance the field as discussed earlier. There are also ample opportunities to apply the lessons learned about the implementation of complex interventions in health, behavioral health, and other settings that may or may not focus specifically on child maltreatment.

Finally, implementation research inherently requires partners (Chambers and Azrin 2013; Kirchner et al. 2014); thus, it demands that a wide range of stakeholders be brought to the table to address the challenges of child maltreatment prevention. The traditional siloed approach to research will not suffice. The contributing authors believe that the work of researchers and program developers are enhanced when they partner with children and families, community organizations, treatment providers, and other key stakeholders to develop effective and culturally informed prevention and treatment programs.

Community Context Research

Understanding the role context plays in determining both the potential and feasibility of evidence-based interventions and public policy to succeed is increasingly salient to those now entering the field. Although the development of model programs and interventions grounded in a solid theory of change is of high importance, as discussed in Chap. 6, the chapter authors are keenly aware of the influence context and culture will have in how potential participants view these models and how these models adapt to diverse settings. Understanding these processes are of equal importance and interest to practitioners and researchers formulating both treatment and prevention services. The fundamental question of what can be accomplished through interventions targeting individuals in the absence of adjustments to community context is equally important across all interventions. All interventions, even those highly specified, will need to make some adjustments and adaptations in going to scale. Given the complexity in the causal factors contributing to the likelihood of maltreatment and the diversity of needs presented by families who have either experienced maltreatment or are trying to avoid it, any intervention's long-term success is inherently dependent upon how context supports or contradicts its mission. Rather than addressing these issues on their own, the next generation of program developers and those who evaluate these models will need to work in partnership—sharing ideas, formulating a common message, and advocating for similar changes in the institutional response to the problem and in the normative context in which parents care for their children.

Building and Sustaining New Leadership

Throughout this book, the authors have highlighted their interest in working more intentionally across disciplines, subject areas, funding streams, and agencies. Despite these good intentions, experience suggests that collaborative problem solving and true transdisciplinary inquiry will not happen in the absence of intentional and sustained efforts—it is simply easier to continue doing things the way they have always been done. Fortunately, the next generation of leaders, as represented by the chapter authors, appears willing to take on the challenge of change and are defining their work and research questions in ways conducive to a more collaborative and integrative planning process. The structure and implementation of the Doris Duke Fellowship, and efforts underway in many academic institutions across the country, suggest at least three strategies will be important in supporting the next generation of researchers:

- **Nurturing transdisciplinary practice**: In the coming decade, the child maltreatment field will require "renaissance researchers" or individuals who are comfortable working in diverse settings as well as across diverse disciplines. The Doris Duke Fellowship fosters this type of scholar through a variety of strategies, including organizing the fellows into small groups that are intentionally multidisciplinary yet loosely focused on a particular line of research (e.g., early childhood, adolescents, child welfare, parenting, etc.). Fellows are required to complete a collaborative project within that group, increasing their exposure to actually working jointly with colleagues from other disciplines. These joint projects, along with the development of this manuscript, have required the fellows to accommodate diverse perspectives as they grappled with how to frame and prioritize an integrated response to a common problem.
- **Introducing young scholars to the policy world**: As public policy adopts a more intentional focus on using research to guide decisions and determine the allocation of programmatic resources, researchers face increasing pressure to insure that their research questions and findings are in line with the questions of high interest to those making these decisions. To this end, the Doris Duke Fellowship explicitly emphasizes the link between research and public policy, both in its selection methods and mentoring structure. As part of the application process, all candidates are required to address the practice and policy implications of their dissertation. Candidates also are required to identify a policy or practice mentor who is committed to working with them and participating in fellowship activities should they be selected. These mentors are typically senior-level professionals in nonprofit organizations, state or federal agencies, or university-based policy centers. The policy mentor's role is to assist the fellow in understanding the policy challenges facing their agency or service delivery process and the way in which data is integrated (or not) into their decision making process. Expectations for the policy mentor during the fellowship period include engaging in regular communication with the fellow, establishing goals for the relationship, providing feedback on the dissertation to sharpen its policy or practice focus, assisting the fellow

in improving her ability to communicate research findings to a nonacademic audience, and facilitating networking with colleagues.

- **Enriching the pipeline**: Traditionally, a doctoral student works directly—and often in isolation—with a faculty member at his university. The student may or (more likely) may not have substantive exposure to other researchers within his department; only rarely is a doctoral student substantively engaged in working with researchers in other contexts or from other disciplines. Yet experts continue to call for scholars to be willing and able to work jointly with scholars from other disciplines, utilizing different funding streams and targeting their findings to diverse audiences in order to maximize their learning (Walker et al. 2007). The Doris Duke Fellowship is built upon the idea that in order to become leaders in the child abuse and neglect prevention field, it is imperative that students have meaningful interactions with others from different disciplines who represent different professional perspectives (i.e., policymaker, practitioner, program developer, funder). Opportunities for these types of substantive interactions are built into the fellowship through small group collaborative projects, mentorship from individuals engaged directly in creating policy or implementing programs, and multiple opportunities to learn from experts and other students.

In the end, the primary lesson from all of this work may lie less in the merits of a specific strategy and more in the need to create *multiple opportunities* for emerging scholars to interact with those in other disciplines and to commit to working jointly on projects that involve coauthorship. Such opportunities can be created through a specific fellowship program or embedded within organized research centers that draw together different academic departments from within a specific institution or between a university and local or state agencies. Professional associations that focus on a substantive area of study rather than a single discipline also offer opportunities for cross-discipline learning and joint relationships between research and practice. Such associations often have specific strategies for engaging students and early career professionals. Some examples include the Society for Prevention Research's Early Career Preventionists Network (ECPN) and the American Professional Society on the Abuse of Children's Prevention Committee and Early Career Sub-Committee. Where these opportunities exist is far less important than ensuring that emerging scholars have multiple opportunities to "look over the fence" and learn from other disciplines and theoretical frameworks.

Conclusion

The authors who contributed the central content of this book challenge all concerned with child maltreatment to think anew about the problem and the public policy response. They have articulated a set of issues, big and small, that will influence their work and the direction of the field. These authors collectively recognize the complexities of child maltreatment as a societal and a human problem; it is not a singular phenomenon but rather multiple, often overlapping ones. Within this context they acknowledge that there is no "silver bullet" for addressing the issue and that building and sustaining an effective response requires a thoughtful and nuanced approach. No research portfolio, no matter how inclusive or sophisticated, will produce a singular and lasting resolution to the problem. Each study adds to the knowledge base and while some insights are robust and enduring most have a limited shelf life, or must share "the shelf" with hundreds of other possible solutions. That said, each finding or promising intervention offers an important building block for advancing our thinking and stimulating innovation, particularly when considered in tandem with other results.

Drawing on the lessons learned and recommendations articulated by the chapter authors, several operational pillars emerge as being important to this group of leaders as they think about their future work. The most salient of these features include:

- **Implementation science**: Examine programs not simply from the perspective of outcomes but also with an eye toward more fully understanding the implementation process and the factors that contribute to successful replication.
- **Data integration**: Find ways to share information on program participants across institutions and across the life span for purposes of better understanding who is being reached and who is most successfully served. Equally important is using administrative data to identify promising pathways for prevention—better understanding how families come to require remedial services can offer critical insights into how to find them before such assistance is needed.
- **Continuous quality improvement**: Raise the performance bar and set the expectation that researchers and practitioners alike have a responsibility to find ways to do better, even when they believe they are doing a great job.
- **Family and participant voice**: Listen to those you intend to help and incorporate their thoughts and perspectives into planning and implementation.
- **Policy integration**: Do not implement policy reforms alone when it can be done in partnership with others. This principle applies to work across agencies as well as across sectors (public, private, and nonprofit).

Making progress in understanding and resolving social dilemmas requires a balance of generating innovative ideas and rediscovering the potential of old ideas when applied to a new context. The next generation of scholars is well-positioned to lead the field in ways their predecessors could not have imagined. This fact alone suggests great promise for the field and great hope for the well-being of all children.

References

Aos, S., Lee, S., Drake, E., Pennucci, A., Klima, T., Miller, M., et al. (2011). *Return on investment: Evidence-based options to improve statewide outcomes. (Document No. 11-07-1201)*. Olympia: Washington State Institute of Public Policy.

Brown, C. H., Have, T. R. T., Jo, B., Dagne, G., Wyman, P. A., Muthen, B., & Gibbons, R. D. (2009). Adaptive designs for randomized trials in public health. *Annual Review of Public Health, 30*, 1–25.

Brownson, R. C., Jacobs, J. A., Tabak, R. G., Hoehner, C. M., & Stamatakis, K. A. (2013). Designing for dissemination among public health researchers: Findings from a national survey in the United States. *American Journal of Public Health, 103*(9), 1693–1699. doi:10.2105/AJPH.2012.301165.

Chambers, D. A., & Azrin, S. T. (2013). Partnership: A fundamental component of dissemination and implementation research. *Psychiatric Services, 64*(16), 509–511. doi:10.1176/appi.ps.201300032.

Eccles, M. P., & Mittman, B. S. (2006). Welcome to implementation science. *Implementation Science, 1*(1), 1–3. doi:10.1186/1748-5908-1-1.

Gawande, A. (2008). *Better: A surgeon's notes on performance.* New York: Picador.

Haskins, R., & Margolis, G. (2014). *Show me the evidence: Obama's fight for rigor and results in social policy.* Washington, DC: Brookings Institution Center on Children and Families.

Hogwood, K. E., Olin, S. S., Horwitz, S., McKay, M., Gleek, A., Gleacher, A., … Hogan, M. (2014). Scaling up evidence-based practices for children and families in New York state: Toward evidence-based policies on implementation for state mental health systems. *Journal of Clinical Child & Adolescent Psychology, 43*(2), 145–157. doi: 10.1080/15374416.2013.869749

Institute of Medicine. (2009). *Preventing mental, emotional, and behavioral disorders among young people: Progress and possibilities.* Washington, DC: National Academies Press.

Institute of Medicine & National Research Council. (2013). *New directions in child abuse and neglect research.* Washington, DC: The National Academies Press.

Ioannidis, J. P. A., & Khoury, M. J. (2014). Assessing value in biomedical research: The PQRST of appraisal and reward. *JAMA.* doi:10.1001/jama.2014.6932.

Johnson, S. (2010). *Where good ideas come from: The natural history of innovation.* New York: Penguin.

Kirchner, J. E., Kearney, L. K., Ritchie, M. J., Dollar, K. M., Swensen, A. B., & Schohn, M. (2014). Lessons learned through a national partnership between clinical leaders and researchers. *Psychiatric Services.* doi:10.1176/appi.ps.201400054.

Klesges, L. M., Estabrooks, P. A., Dzewaltowski, D. A., Bull, S. S., & Glasgow, R. E. (2005). Beginning with the application in mind: Designing and planning health behavior change interventions to enhance dissemination. *Annals of Behavioral Medicine, 29*, 66–75.

Office of Behavioral and Social Science Research. (2014). *Systems science.* National Institutes of Health, Office of Behavioral and Social Sciences Research. http://obssr.od.nih.gov/scientific_areas/methodology/systems_science/

Paulsell, D., Del Grosso, P., & Supplee, L. (2014). Supporting replication and scale-up of evidence-based home visiting programs: Assessing the implementation knowledge base. *American Journal of Public Health, 104*(9), 1624–1632. doi:10.2105/AJPH.2014.301962.

Rosenfield, P. L. (1992). The potential of transdisciplinary research for sustaining and extending linkages between the health and social sciences. *Social Science & Medicine, 35*(11), 1343–1357.

Sawhill, I. V., & Karpilow, Q. (2014). *How much could we improve children's life chances by intervening early and often? CCF Brief #54 (July).* Washington, DC: Brookings Institution Center on Children and Families.

Schorr, L., & Farrow, F. (2014). *An evidence framework to improve results.* Background paper presented at the 2014 Harold Richman Public Policy Symposium: The Future of Evidence. November. Washington, DC: The Center for the Study of Social Policy.

Walker, G. E., Golde, C. M., Jones, L., Bueschel, A. C., & Hutchings, P. (2007). *The formation of scholars: Rethinking doctoral education for the twenty-first century.* New York: The Carnegie Foundation for the Advancement of Teaching.

Wulczyn, F., Barth, R., Yuan, Y., Harden, B., & Landsverk, J. (2005). *Beyond common sense: Child welfare, child well-being, and the evidence for policy reform.* Piscataway: Transaction.

Deborah Daro is a senior research fellow at Chapin Hall at the University of Chicago. Dr. Daro's current research and written work focuses on developing effective early intervention systems to support all new parents and examining the impacts of reforms that embed individualized, targeted home-based interventions within universal efforts to alter normative standards and enhance community context. Reflecting her strong commitment to developing leadership in the area of child maltreatment prevention, she designed and directs the *Doris Duke Fellowships for the Promotion of Child Well-Being*. Dr. Daro has served as president of the American Professional Society on the Abuse of Children and as treasurer and Executive Council member of the International Society for the Prevention of Child Abuse and Neglect. Dr. Daro holds a Ph.D. in Social Welfare and a master's degree in City and Regional Planning from the University of California at Berkeley.

Anne Cohn Donnelly is a child abuse prevention researcher and lecturer at the Kellogg School of Management, Northwestern University. She is the founding director of the school's Board Fellows Program. Dr. Donnelly conducted the first national evaluation of child abuse treatment programs. Dr. Donnelly served for 17 years as the head of Prevent Child Abuse America where she launched the Healthy Families America Initiative. Prior to this, she served as a White House Fellow and a Congressional Science Fellow. Dr. Donnelly received a B.A. degree from the University of Michigan, an M.A. from Tufts University and both the M.P.H. and D.P.H. degrees in health administration and planning from the University of California (Berkeley) School of Public Health. She is a Fellow of the American Association for the Advancement of Science.

Lee Ann Huang is a researcher at Chapin Hall at the University of Chicago. Ms. Huang has a strong commitment to supporting all families and children through effective programs. Her work focuses primarily on evaluating child maltreatment prevention initiatives that serve the parents of young children. Ms. Huang manages the *Doris Duke Fellowship for the Promotion of Child Well-Being*, and initiative of the Doris Duke Charitable Foundation that identifies and develops new leaders in the prevention field. She is evaluating a doula/home visiting program for young parents in Chicago, as well as managing Chapin Hall's work on the MIECHV Technical Assistance Coordinating Center. Ms. Huang has a Master of Public Policy degree from the University of Chicago and a bachelor's degree in social work from Texas Christian University.

Byron J. Powell is a postdoctoral researcher at the Center for Mental Health Policy and Services Research, Department of Psychiatry, Perelman School of Medicine, University of Pennsylvania. Dr. Powell's research focuses on efforts to improve the quality of mental health and social services that are provided in community settings. Specifically, he is working to develop a better understanding of the types of strategies that can be used to implement effective services, and the organizational and systemic factors that can facilitate or impede implementation and quality improvement. Dr. Powell received a B.A. in psychology from Taylor University, an AM in social work from the University of Chicago, and a Ph.D. in social work from Washington University in St. Louis where he was a National Institute of Mental Health Pre-Doctoral Fellow (T32MH19960). The Doris Duke Charitable Foundation, Fahs-Beck Fund for Research and Experimentation, and National Institute of Mental Health (F31MH098478) have supported his research.

Index

© Springer International Publishing Switzerland 2015
D. Daro et al. (eds.), *Advances in Child Abuse Prevention Knowledge*,
Child Maltreatment 5, DOI 10.1007/978-3-319-16327-7

CPSIA information can be obtained at www.ICGtesting.com
Printed in the USA
BVOW05*1413050116

431850BV00005B/5/P